The Anti-ageing Beauty Bible

The Anti-ageing Beauty Bible

Josephine Fairley & Sarah Stacey

Illustrations by David Downton

Kyle Books

Contents

It's this simple:

there has never been a better time to age. Every year, billions are poured into research into the creams, the vitamins, the age-spot-zapping lasers (and even magic tummy-flattening pants!), and the light-reflecting make-up innovations which can help us look great for our age, whatever our age

There are fabulous role models out there, too, to give us all hope. Women we know as friends. Women we see in magazines, or on screen, from Helen Mirren (who wouldn't want to look that good in a bikini at any age?), Julianne Moore, Cate Blanchett, Susan Sarandon, Oprah Winfrey, Isabella Rossellini and Sophia Loren. (Even, God bless her, Joan Collins, who just keeps pushing back the threshold for what's considered 'old': first forty, then fifty, sixty, and now – who knows where it'll end…?) We know plenty of women who once would have been written off as 'middle-aged' at forty, who are back-packing, dating, even clubbing (a dance-step too far, for us, but why on earth not…?) up to their eighties.

If you're reading this book, we know one thing: you want to stay looking and feeling your absolute best, for as long as possible. (Without, necessarily, going under the knife or having invasive treatments. Although in *The Anti-Ageing Beauty Bible* we've some advice on that, too – even if personally we'd never help nature along quite so drastically for ourselves.)

The real challenge for so many women is that as the years go by, our confidence wobbles. We can lose our way. We don't look the way we always did, but we haven't worked out how to embrace this new phase. One key thing we've observed as we look around: women can start to 'fade away'. Complexions get paler. Hair colour, ditto. And if we're not careful, we start dressing to match, to reflect the fact we feel a bit low-key, a bit less va-va-voom – in muted shades that eventually make us look like a ghost of our former, younger, more attractive-feeling selves.

But it doesn't have to be like that!!!!! Women really don't have to do a vanishing act. We know, because we've talked to the experts – from globally renowned hair colour wizards to A-list nutritionists, facial massage gurus to experts who know how to keep our brains sharp, too. (Because it's all very well knowing which concealer's going to blitz your under-eye circles, but it really helps if you can remember where you put your make-up bag…! Not to mention the car keys, your glasses, etc.) And if you're bothered by the effects of gravity, we've talked to people who can help everything become that bit more 'pert' again – from faces to thighs, even foot arches!

Crucially, we've tapped into the wisdom of

You're *never* too old to become *younger*

make-up professionals who understand mature faces, because they're facing the challenge of lines and wrinkles or 'sun spots' themselves, every day when they look in the mirror. Because make-up – applied well – can be your quickest way to drop a decade in little more than a flash. In fact, our advice to women who write to us for advice because they're contemplating a facelift is simple: get a makeover first. It is truly, truly, truly miraculous what the right foundation (with primer first), concealer, lipstick and brow pencil can achieve.

But which concealer, which moisturising lipstick, which age-defying foundation? (Not to mention which are the best anti-ageing eye creams, or shine-restoring hair masks, or body firming creams…?) As beauty editors, that's what we're asked all the time, and the signature of our best-selling Beauty Bible series of books has been pointing you in the direction of the products which really, truly perform.

We've now had over 4,200 real women testing products – all aged from 35 to well into their sixties – who've put container-loads of anti-ageing products through their paces over a period of three months or more. There are super-whizz-bang, high-tech options, and all-natural choices (and our 'daisy rating' – see box right – helps you identify those).

There are dozens of new entries for this edition, but what our testers' incredibly consistent comments and scores (out of ten) confirm yet again is what we've known for a while: that there truly are many, many products out there which can help you look younger. Not as young as your 19-year-old daughter (let alone granddaughter), or the intern in your office. But radiant. Glowing. Not someone fading into the distance, but who's enjoying your life, looking and feeling the best you possibly can.

This book is exceedingly close to our own hearts – having a joint age of 119, as we sat down to put manicured digits to Apple keyboard. But yes, we do constantly get compliments about 'looking good for our age'. Which, frankly, are the compliments that any woman *d'un certain âge* wants to hear.

Through the pages of this book – organised as an A to Z of everything that our friends and readers have told us bothers them about ageing – we are about to help you feel your best. Look your best. And be your best, too. Life is no dress rehearsal and we only get one chance to enjoy this one.

The truth is that when your daily 'self-care' ritual is sorted – from the right skincare to the perfect make-up to haircare to at least a little bit of exercise – then you can do the things you still long to do, explore the passions you yearn to pursue, be the woman you'd really like to be.

Trust us: age really can be a thing of the past. With love,

Jo – Sarah x

www.beautybible.com Don't forget: you can follow us on Twitter: @Beauty_Bible!

10 important things you need to know about make-up

While perusing 24,000 forms (yes, it nearly killed us) from the ten-women tester panels who trialled literally thousands of products for this latest Beauty Bible (which we believe is the definitive guide to ageing gorgeously), we realised there were some key myths and misconceptions about make-up. And also some key secrets that everyone simply needs to know – because make-up isn't cheap, and you want to get the very best value out of the cosmetics you buy.

So (with apologies to those of you who basically have a degree in make-up and know this stuff already), here goes.

A primer goes over moisturiser, under foundation. Used on their own, primers aren't moisturising enough. And if you're not sure why you need this extra step in your make-up regime, turn to page 89 to find out how primers will help you create the most flawless canvas ever for your foundation – and make it last longer.

Apply eyeshadow and other eye make-up before your base, though. That way, if it 'sheds', it's easy to clean up and won't spoil your foundation.

For eyeshadow, it also helps to own a 'blending brush'. This is quite simply the best way to make sure all the edges of your shadow are seamless. Jemma Kidd recommends dipping the blender brush in a little translucent powder and buffing over eyes to soften. ('The idea is to "sheer down" the colour, not remove it,' she advises.) All brush ranges feature a 'blender' brush, and if you can't identify it – well, that's what sales consultants are for.

The time to apply light-reflecting concealer (or a brightener) is before foundation. If applying under eyes, use the brush/wand to trace a triangle down from the corners of the eye to meet in the middle of the under-eye zone, and then blend with brush or ring finger. On eyelids, start in the inner corner by your nose.

Apply flaw-correcting concealers over foundation. Once you've evened out your skintone, you may not need so much.

Dry, dull-looking skin makes you look much older than you are. Youthful skin isn't powdery and one-dimensional; it's radiant. So we swear by this tip from Laura Mercier to achieve that, fast: 'Use the tiniest bit of a light moisturiser patted around the outer eyes and along the top lip over your make-up. It makes skin look fresh, not dry, and it's a great de-ager as it stops make-up settling into any fine lines.' (You can do this during the day to refresh make-up, too.)

You really don't have to live with dry, cracked lips. But lip balm is only half the answer. Lips respond beautifully to buffing: press a wet flannel on to your lips, then use it to gently rub away flakes and roughness. And then slather on your balm or lip treatment (we've lots of good ones on page 137). Your lip pencil will glide on more smoothly, too: even the creamiest of these can be drying.

There's a quick way to deal with eye-make-up smudges. Don't ask us why make-up seems to flake and speck more now we're older – but it often does seem to, and during a busy day you don't have time to start again. MAC Cleansing Tips are infused with make-up remover, so very handy – but better still, roll a Q-tip in a very little bit of foundation, then roll it back and forth over the eye zone. It removes smudges – but doesn't leave skin 'naked'.

Remember: self-tanner will always look patchy unless you exfoliate and moisturise first. It really is that simple, and not buffing and hydrating skin is the number one reason why we get negative comments from our testers about some fake tans. (OK, this isn't strictly make-up. But we have lots of testers who need to understand this!)

And whatever else you do, get a regular makeover. It's easy to treat make-up like a trusty recipe – finding something that works and clinging to it long after it's stopped doing what it once did for you – so we recommend regular makeovers. These are free (or at the very least, redeemable against purchase). There is no better way to discover what make-up can do to counterbalance the fact that skin has become thinner, thirstier and more transparent, or its tone has altered and faded. A good in-store make-up pro – we particularly recommend the make-up artists at Laura Mercier, Bobbi Brown, Trish McEvoy and on the By Terry counter in Space NK branches – can also help show you tricks to deal with lips that are thinning, eyes that are drooping and a chin or nose that is becoming 'longer'. As the ads say, Just. Do. It. (Please!)

Cosmetics:
your top 10 products

Before you consider a facelift, buy these Make-up Musts

We have four words to say when friends and readers tell us they're considering 'having work done', or even Botox. 'Have a make-up makeover.' Make-up really can work miracles. And showcased here are the ten make-up essentials that we know can melt away the years – blurring lines, delivering radiance and making skin look dewily fresher, smoother and younger. We feel strongly that cosmetic surgery (and even cosmeto-dermatology) should be a last resort. Trust us: by ensuring that your make-up kit features these ten categories of cosmetics, you really can drop a decade – with the wave of a magic (concealer) wand.

1 **A make-up primer.** With silicones (to smooth the skin) and light-reflective pigments (to 'blur' the appearance of fine lines), a make-up primer also helps solve the problem of make-up that 'disappears' into thin air, which can be a particular problem for drier, mature complexions. (For specific recommendations, see page 89.)

2 **A 'line-smoother'.** Real magic, these. Again, they feature silicones and sometimes even nylon particles, and can be applied as required to deep grooves and finer lines. (Personally, we favour the type with a teensy nozzle, for targeted application.) They simply 'sit' on the skin's surface, and can be patted into the skin to create a truly velvety surface. Lines? Now you see them. And now, with these, you don't. (Our testers' favourites are on page 95.)

3 **An anti-ageing foundation.** Many foundations now have age-defying properties. These can work in several ways: through the addition of skin-caring ingredients, plus moisturisers to ensure skin looks 'plumper'. This new generation of 'anti-ageing' foundations also harnesses the power of 'optical pigments'. (Want to know which ones are worth investing in? Turn to page 90 for our testers' experiences.)

4 A light-reflective concealer. We probably get more anxious queries addressed to www.beautybible.com about dark circles than any other beauty woe. As well as effective lifestyle tips (on page 54), we bring you the low-down on the wand-style concealers which go a long way to disguising the darkest circles, and can lessen the appearance of deep grooves and lines. (For Beauty Bible award-winning concealers, go to page 91.)

5 Cream blusher. Lots of reasons to love this. First, the texture 'melts' into skin, so doesn't look dusty (which is always a risk, as we age). That makes it fairly goof-proof, too. But another reason cream blush should nudge the powder option out of your kit once you hit 35 plus is that it adds another layer of moisturising protection against the elements. (Which versions did our testers rate? Look at page 23.)

6 Lip pencil. Does double-duty, at this phase in life: it not only defines lips (the contours of which can become blurrier with the years), but it helps prevent lipstick from 'travelling' into feathered lines. (For the best, see page 135.)

7 Lip gloss. Recent research showed that the plumpness of lips is a way that we (subconsciously) gauge an individual's age. Lip gloss is the fast-track to a juicier pout: a smoosh on the lower lip makes them look instantly fuller. (But because not all lip glosses are created equal, you'll want to read our panellists' opinions, on page 134.)

8 A bone-coloured cream eyeshadow. You can shade your eyes with a rainbow of colours, but our prescription is always to use a neutral eyeshadow as a base, first. Why? Because it evens out the skintone of the eyelids, which tends to darken and redden as we age, while at the same time creating a velvety-smooth, even base for shadow – whether that's another cream version (turn to page 70 for our testers' favourites), or powder.

9 Brow colour. Because 'not fade away' should be your beauty mantra, at this time in your life – and because defined, groomed brows help give your face much-needed structure. (The most outstanding brow pencils on the market are listed on page 64.)

10 Waterproof mascara. A boon, as we age, because waterproof mascara stays put through hot flushes and survives watery eyes. It's a fact: eyes get touchier and well up more as the years roll by. (It's hard to find a good version – one which neither gives you panda eyes by teatime, nor requires industrial-strength remover – so our testers tried them all on your behalf. See page 73 for those that 'wowed'.)

LOVE
the BODY
you're in
...and it will
LOVE YOU
right back

Be more active
(your body will love you for it)

A simple programme of daily exercises will help tone your body – and make you feel happier, too. So counteract the force of gravity by following our 10 easy steps to a firmer, fitter, more confident you…

As the T-shirt slogan goes, 'Gravity sucks'. Because after 35 (if not before), bodies start to head south. At the same time, our bodies get stiffer and less flexible. Some people embark on a major blitz to counteract this – the gym, jogging, Pilates, whatever. But the best strategy to start with is simply to become more active, all the time – then you can add your favourite exercise, as we suggest below. Being more active boosts the rate at which the body burns calories. It firms you up and (done properly) stretches you out. And it also produces feel-good hormones called endorphins so that your mood, as well as your body, feels less saggy.

So if you're standing disconsolately in front of a long mirror in your undies and wondering what on earth you can do to shape up and/or slim down, take heart. Embarking on a simple daily programme of little shifts will really make a difference to your body (and at the same time, to how you feel about showing it – on the beach, to a new lover, or in that Little Black Dress that used to fit but doesn't now). Best of all, you can start in your very own bed. (Although probably better alone, in this instance…)

1 **When you wake up,** lie straight and flat in your bed, take a few slow, deep breaths (in through your nose and very slowly out through your mouth), then lift your arms above your head and point your toes, feeling the stretch right through your body on both sides. Stretch your whole body, then each side, and finish with your whole body again.

2 **While the kettle boils,** tense your buttock muscles ten times for ten seconds each time. The more you practise this, the firmer your bottom will become, so practise whenever you're standing: waiting at the bus stop, stirring a pan, queueing to pay in a shop, etc.

3 **While you brush your teeth** for the recommended three minutes morning and evening, squat down with your back against the wall or door. (It feels weird, but it's a great stretch.)

4 **When you're watching TV,** hide the remote control and when you get up to change channels, do ten squats to tone your upper thighs. As you squat down, with your back straight, push your weight down through your heels so the front of your thighs work harder.

5 **Tone up your arms and bingo wings** by pushing light weights above your head: do ten pushes at a time, as many times a day as you can. No weights? Use cans of baked beans. (We love baked beans – to eat! – especially with a slurp of olive oil and grated Parmesan.)

6 Lose five pounds by improving your posture…

• Stand up straight, as if the crown of your head is suspended from a thread in the ceiling/sky.

• Let your shoulders sink down and back: feel as if your shoulder blades are meeting at the back.

• Do a few shoulder rolls both ways while you are sitting at your desk or on the train.

• Walk like a cat (think model on catwalk…), hips swinging forward with your big toe leading.

7 Walk briskly everywhere you can, swinging your arms (put belongings in a back pack – the kind that fastens across your front is easiest if you carry a lot). Look for hills and climb stairs rather than using the lift. Get in the habit of striding out for at least 15 minutes in the evenings to help you relax. You should aim for 10,000 steps a day – easy to calculate if you have a pedometer.

8 Every time you get up from a chair, consciously pull your belly button in towards your spine to work your tummy muscles. If you are picking up things from the floor, bend sideways while pulling in your tummy to help smooth your love handles.

9 Finally, do exercise you enjoy. Whether it's walking or swimming, dancing or yoga, riding or fencing, if you look forward to it you are far more likely to stick with it and get a feel-good double whammy. Aim for at least 30 minutes, five days a week.

10 Make all of this a habit. It takes 16 to 21 times of repeating an activity for it to become a habit – so in less than a month, all this can become second nature. And by then you should look very luscious in that Little Black Dress.

First, find your MIRACLE

Since the first edition of this book appeared, we've had another 1,800 women trialling anti-ageing products for us: 4,200 testers in all, who've put hundreds and hundreds of 'dream creams' through their paces. But with some even higher-scoring contenders in this edition, this serves to further confirm what we've known for years: that there really are creams and serums that magic the years from your face. The challenge is: how on earth do you find out which ones…? Well, there's no need for (expensive) trial and error – because our testers have done the research for you.

The diligence of our trials means that we get support for what we do from the whole beauty industry, who happily supply products for our trials – from high street/supermarket anti-agers right through to the priciest creams on the market. Our ten-women tester panels were under strict instructions: use the treatment on one side of your face, observe and note any immediate improvements, then after two weeks, and finally, at the end of the tube or jar. (NB: many of our testers started out cynical – and were converted.)

OK, so no cream is going to make you look 17 again, waving a wand to magic away every line and wrinkle. But the scores here are high. So: there really ARE products which, as well as softening and smoothing your complexion, can help plump out deeper lines, make smaller ones disappear, firm skin tissue – and turbo-charge the glow. (For more 'miracles' – in the form of specific night treatments – please see page 156, while miracle serums are on page 172.)

Now, just before you dive in… While, as we've said, we tested all price ranges for this book, the simple truth is that all the top scoring ones are pretty pricey – even after this latest extensive round of testing. But on page19 you will find a rundown of more moderately-priced creams (£20-and-under) that we tried for our previous book *Beauty Bible Beauty Steals* (which also comes as an iPhone App, see Directory).

Something for every age-defying beauty, we think…

Anti-ageing miracle creams: *our award winners*

REVIEWS

Temple Spa Skin Truffle Total Face Rejuvenation

 9.31/10

A truly stupendous score: the highest we've ever had for an all-round, all-singing-and-dancing miracle cream, in 17 years of Beauty Bible testing. (Not that Sarah's surprised: she's long been a Skin Truffle-ette.) Diamond powder, gold and silk clearly do illuminate the skin from first application, testers report; other key ingredients include black truffles, grapeseed champagne, purifying strawberries and lush cocoa butter, in a cashmere-soft formulation.

Comments: 'Oh, this is a wonderful cream: I'm so in love with it you can look out for the announcement in *The Times*! Skintone is brighter and all my nasty lines – even the deeper ones – appear to have lessened' • 'face looks younger and not a needle in sight' • 'skin looks glowy and dewy, forehead grooves smaller – and husband says I look great' • 'the best anti-ageing moisturiser I've ever used – fantastic miracle product; skin looks like I have a luminising primer on, even when not wearing make-up' • 'gives a definite glow to the skin with improvements in brightness, softness, crêpiness, fine lines' • 'noticed a difference in texture, smoothness and brightness within days' • 'gives an "instant lift" to skin' • 'my husband and my mum both said I looked really healthy – fine lines were rendered invisible and I really loved the radiance: a "lit-from-within" effect'.

Pevonia Timeless Repair Cream �

 9.06/10

Best known through its widespread spa distribution, Pevonia's age-proofing award-winner also features luxe ingredients like caviar, pearl and something called 'Escutox', alongside green olive squalene, brightening lemon peel oil, chamomile – and an SPF8 (not enough for protection in all but the dingiest months, we'd counsel). It's got a pretty fragrance – a touch of honeysuckle, we'd say, to further enhance application pleasure.

Comments: 'My face literally felt as if it was drinking it in: after application, one half of my face felt supple and soft and looked rested' • 'a Holy grail find' • 'after two days, let alone two weeks, I was in love with this product my skin's brighter, softer, smoother and it has helped with fine lines and skin tone' • 'didn't want to see the bottom of the pot! I love this and hope if I hint strongly enough my husband/sons might be generous enough to buy me some more' • 'love this: have never used anything before with such a dramatic effect on my skin – after six weeks my face was starting to look lop-sided – seems to be acting like a facelift on the side I'm using it on' • 'fabulously soft skin, much better under chin' • 'bigger wrinkles in particular were reduced; I have some large grooves which seemed to improve' • 'skin firmer and plumper, even forehead grooves less prominent – and big thumbs-up from my husband!'

L'Occitane Immortelle Divine Cream ✿

 8.98/10

This truly 'divine' high-scoring award-winner has gone on – justifiably – to become a global anti-ageing bestseller and a new anti-ageing 'classic' since the first edition of this book. (Jo's a massive convert, too). It's helped put L'Occitane firmly on the map as a serious skincare brand, with its fabulously aromatic formulation (featuring lavish quantities of Corsican Immortelle, 'the flower that never dies'), together with myrtle and other key anti-agers. Enriched with 34 per cent plant oils, Divine Cream is formulated to boost cell regeneration and 'increase cellular vitality', which translates to enhanced radiance.

Comments: 'Love the texture and smell, it took a little while to sink in but it was worth the wait; skin instantly looked brighter and much smoother and plumped; after two weeks, fine lines around mouth much less noticeable and skin much more supple,

AT A GLANCE

Temple Spa Skin Truffle Total Face Rejuvenation

Pevonia Timeless Repair Cream

L'Occitane Immortelle Divine Cream

Decléor Excellence de l'Âge Sublime Regenerating Cream

Dermalogica Power Rich Cream

Melvita Naturalift Anti-Ageing Cream

This Works No Wrinkles Extreme Moisturiser

Elemis Cellular Recovery Skin Bliss Capsules

If you know you have sensitive skin and you want to try a powerful anti-ageing treatment, go carefully. Start by using the product two or three times a week, and build up from there. Alternatively, do a 'patch test' (using the crook of your elbow or the skin just behind the ear), and check for any redness/irritation/flakiness 24 hours later. If that happens, you may be one of the people who simply can't tolerate some ingredients – and if you do suffer a reaction, it is always worth taking the product back to the counter (although the beauty industry will probably have hit-men trained on us for suggesting this). Sometimes a sympathetic sales consultant feels empowered to give you a refund, confident that you'll be back again in future. (Which you certainly won't be, if they don't.)

and the improvements continued: my husband said my skin was looking nice and for him to notice is quite remarkable' • 'my skin hasn't looked so good for a long time, so much brighter I look as if I've had a good night's sleep; crêpiness, fine lines, grooves all reduced – a fantastic product and I got lots of positive comments' • 'lovely thick product with fabulous smell, absorbed very well and skin felt so hydrated and really supple; definitely boosts the skin; but do give it five or ten minutes before applying make-up' • 'complexion was more plump, less drawn, less sagging, with really nice bright glow, eyes glowed too and normally ruddy complexion reduced'.

Decléor Excellence de l'Âge Sublime Regenerating Cream

 A day cream (Decléor like their customers to use oils at night), this meltingly-smooth cream-textured cream works to enhance firmness, smoothness, hydration, and to even out skintone. As you'd expect from an aromatherapy brand, fragrance is an important part of the pleasure factor, although this is powdery/creamy (with notes of sandalwood, amber and peach) rather than 'botanically-scented'.

Comments: 'I was dubious as this cream looked too rich and thick for my oily combination skin but it is amazing, after five weeks skin looks luminous, almost glass-like, firmer, smoother and springy to the touch – rejuvenated' • 'fine lines reduced, deeper grooves too, and crêpiness? There is none! This cream really makes me look better and younger, lots of people have commented' • 'immediate discernable improvements, skin felt softer, less dry, fine lines plumped out and after two weeks, skin looks more youthful, fine lines less visible, skin around eyes and lips less dry and crêpey, overall more radiant and fresh-looking – works wonders on an ageing face' • 'skin looks brighter and love the texture and scent'.

Dermalogica Power Rich Cream

 This is Dermalogica's state-of-the-art anti-ageing cream. It claims to use a trio of 'pharmaceutical-strength' ingredients, and comes in the format of a 35-day supply of (five) sealed metal tubes, complete with a key (think glamorous sardine tin!), to squeeze out every last skin-regenerating, vitamin-and-antioxidant-powered molecule.

Comments: 'The first night I applied this I woke up

and thought the spa fairies had been at work all night: my skin glowed, had a wonderful aliveness and look of youth and vitality; after two weeks complexion was great despite the harsh weather outside and heating inside – wonderful plump, smooth skin; youth in a tube (the only downside was the rather sweet smell)' • 'wow! What a product, the holy grail of creams, delivered all it promised and more; massive difference between the tested and not tested side: smaller wrinkles faded, pores so much smaller, skintone so much brighter, I LOVE it' • 'skin was much more radiant; after a few days that went, people have commented on how smooth and radiant my skin looks: I would use it every few months as a treatment' • 'the grooves down the sides of my mouth look as if I have been using a filler, they're so plumped up and smoothed out, absolutely fabulous product'.

Melvita Naturalift Anti-Ageing Cream
✿ ✿ ✿

 Melvita is a big name in France, now spreading its reach overseas (it's part of the L'Occitane empire). This Ecocert-certified creation blends oligopeptides from hibiscus seed to protect collagen and elastin, argan (for an instant firming action), revitalising chestnut and New Zealand mamaku (derived from a fern), plus potent antioxidants. Subtle but nice scent from rose and geranium.

Comments: 'A friend noticed that my skin looked firmer and my face slimmer; I had seen my skin get brighter and clearer in tone, with less noticeable fine lines: am very happy with this' • 'my fine lines have improved and that's great, a real visible effect, I enjoyed using the cream because it's very light and yet moisturises very well, also smells delicious and you don't need to use much' • 'as well as skin being brighter, pores finer and less noticeable, and fine lines slightly reduced, this definitely lessened my hyperpigmentation brown patches: I would buy it' • 'fine lines and wrinkles plumped out with continued use, and skin soft; did like the lightweight texture and the lovely lemon smell' • 'absolutely wonderful. After finishing the jar, I noted 50 per cent improvement in brightness, 100 per cent in softness and also crêpiness and about 75 per cent reduction in fine lines, plus the two large wrinkles above my eyebrows have reduced in length and depth. I can't believe it! My friends and family have certainly noticed a difference and paid me compliments on looking younger'.

This Works No Wrinkles Extreme Moisturiser

Hurrah for our beauty editor friend Kathy Phillips's contender – the hero product in her recent chunkily/chicly-packaged anti-ageing skincare collection. Intensely hydrating, this lush cream is packed with moringa oil and UK-sourced crambe oil, amino acids and time-released retinol (vitamin A), to brighten skin, while plumping with lots of hyaluronic acid (a magic ingredient, in our book…)

Comments: 'Skin felt softer, with a brightness which has been maintained, with fine lines less noticeable' • 'I've had comments saying my skin is looking nice!' • 'skin illuminated and feels "looked-after"' • 'no dry patches any more – this really is a miracle cream as fine wrinkles seem to have disappeared; skin looks so much brighter and "cared-for"' • 'skin plumper and fresh-looking' • 'loved the creamy smooth texture, the slightly lemony smell and how it soaked into my skin' • 'I wish I'd heard of this before and introduced it into my regime years ago; lots of people have commented I look better/younger' • 'I've already recommended this to friends'.

Elemis Cellular Recovery Skin Bliss Capsules

This winner – featuring a programme of single-dose capsules containing facial oils which you open and apply – proves to us that our system works. Elemis actually submitted this twice (an admin error, we think). We sent the product to two different sets of women, six months apart. And the average of their scores was absolutely identical: 8.5/10, from both groups! Use one pink capsule (rose-smelling) in the morning, one green (lavender fragrant) capsule at night, ideally using a facial massage to apply the oil.

Comments: 'Silky, oily texture sank in almost instantly and made skin softer and smoother; after two weeks, I could see a big difference; handy that you can take just the right number if you go away but make sure they're well-wrapped so they don't puncture and leak' • 'beautiful product with gorgeous smell' • 'definite improvement in softness and brightness, due to the product and the massage, seemed oily to start with but it wasn't; great product overall, lovely smell and I actually looked forward to using them; because of the consistency you are more likely to massage your skin which can only help' • 'this is a really clever product, gives radiance and less crêpiness, fine lines less noticeable as well as smoothness and softness'.

Beauty Steals

As we explained on page 16, these 'miracle' products did incredibly well in our book *Beauty Bible Beauty Steals*, which is also available as an App for your iPhone (see DIRECTORY). So if you're having a budget-watching time, they're really worth considering.

Neal's Yard Remedies Frankincense Nourishing Cream

Beauty Bible has trialled this natural product over several years and it has always scored spectacularly with some testers (a few found it too heavy). The rich botanical cream has very high levels of frankincense essential oil, which was used in mummification – so no wonder it's so good at preserving skin. The blend includes oils of wheatgerm, almond and myrrh – renowned for their regenerating and moisturising properties. It can be used under make-up or at night.

Comments: 'I thought it would be too rich for my oily skin but it was miraculous! Skin looked so much younger and plumper and seemed to reduce breakouts: I've never seen such initial dramatic effects which were maintained' • 'the immediate feeling of plumpness has been replaced by a smooth uplift and youthful tightness' • 'I always felt my skin looked colourless and grey until I tested this product'.

Soap & Glory Make Yourself Youthful Rejuvenating Face Serum

A triumph for the amazing Ms Marcia Kilgore with this light, sinks-in-fast serum. It is probably all oily skins need (under fifty), but can be layered under something richer if you're dry-complexioned or post-menopausal. It contains a collagen-stimulating tetrapeptide, a 'superactive stimulating organic oxygenating complex', ginseng, shea butter, sweet orange peel essential oil (which gives the lightest of fragrances) and a 'moisture-trapping complex'.

Comments: 'Glided on the skin wonderfully and sank in quickly; after two weeks a marked improvement to skintone and softness, fine lines slightly less evident, skin had a lovely bright glow' • 'significant improvement in radiance in first 24 hours, skin on neck and chest looked smoother, fine lines a little softer' • 'skin looks younger because more glowing and well hydrated'.

Nivea Visage DNAge Cell Renewal Night Cream

Slightly further down the ranking, iconic brand Nivea's contender targets women from 40–55, seeking to boost firmness and elasticity. Key ingredients are creatine (an amino acid) and folic acid, which work to guard skin cells' DNA against damage.

Comments: 'After two weeks, fine lines smoother and wrinkles not as deep, skin healthier and plumper, very noticeable between the side I used it on and the other' • 'absorbed very quickly with no residue' • 'skin looked lovely and clear and definitely brighter and smoother, as if I'd had a good night's sleep which unfortunately I hadn't' • 'nose to mouth groove greatly improved' • 'definite improvement in brightness – really loved the rich, creamy texture'.

Plump up your cheeks!

If you're looking pale and wan and your cheeks (like the rest of you) are beginning to head south, you can create a brighter, more uplifting appearance in next to no time…

Every woman with a thinnish face knows that when you're tired or under par, you're liable to look a lot less than radiant – peaky, sad and, at worst, like Lady Macbeth's rather haggard first cousin (as Sarah knows all too well…). As the years go by, the upsides of a slender form mean your cheeks tend to drift downwards with the rest of your body. But there are immediate ways to give your cheeks (and thus your whole face) a lift – plus some mid- to long-term strategies which we promise can transform you.

For instant lift, apply a 'pop' of blush to your cheeks (see overleaf for more). And marvel at the mirror…!

Pinch your cheeks. No blusher? Gently pat and pinch your cheeks for a few seconds until they glow rosy pink. Better still, if you have five or ten minutes, do some star-jumps.

Pop on some earrings.
Sparkly, shiny or lovely fat pearls, in colours that flatter your skintone – and never, ever dangly. If you can, find ones that wing their way upwards taking your face with them. (Sarah's favourite pair are rather Art Nouveau-ish wings in blue, green and amber-y faceted glass.)

Sweep your hair up. Brush your hair back and up, clip it on top, pop in pretty combs, roll into a pleat… Anything to take the eye of the beholder upwards.

Try milk! Drinking it, that is – which is a suggestion given to us by Beverly Hills make-up artist Valerie Sarnelle. One of her starry clients (there's a galaxy flashing in and out of her elegant salon) – a *femme d'un certain âge* with divinely plumptious cheeks above her slender form – told Valerie they were due not to cosmetic fillers but milk! We suggest organic full-fat milk from grass-fed moos because it should have more conjugated linoleic acid (CLA), which may help your facial muscles. (Cheeks are the 'meatiest' part of your face, and increasing muscle mass will make them look fuller.) Milk will definitely give you magnesium – great for your mind as it's a natural tranquilliser, and helps with teeth, bones, muscles and sleep, among lots of other things. (We love magnesium!)

Apply skincare products upwards. Whenever you apply skin cream, oil or lotion, always stroke upwards from your chin to your cheekbones, then out to your temples. Facial therapist Suzie Mitchell suggests: 'Put a little facial oil or cream in one palm and rub your hands together, then smooth over the face, neck and bosom. Rather than fingertips, use the big muscle in the cushion at the base of your thumb, always working upwards. Start by fanning out over and round your neck, then work round and up your jaw and cheekbones to the temples, then across and up your forehead to your hairline. Repeat, covering the whole face for five to ten minutes. The oil or cream will be absorbed, skin velvety, and your face look rosy and "lifted".'

Pop some supplements. Consider supplementing with omega-3 essential fatty acids, hyaluronic acid (HA) plus Sun Chlorella. The first two keep skin cells

For *instant* lift, apply a 'pop' of *BLUSH* to your cheeks, and *MARVEL* at the mirror!

NB: we recommend
doing these exercises
in private…!

1 Put a finger in your
mouth, close your lips
round it and suck on
your finger for five to
ten seconds, as hard as
you can while sucking
in your cheeks. It's
like a child making a
fish face. Release, and
repeat 15 more times.
This will help strengthen
your cheek muscles and
enhance the circulation
and oxygen flow to
your face, so your
cheeks look more pink
and full. It also helps
prevent lip lines.

2 Tone your cheeks
by placing your
fingertips on top of
your cheekbones. Now
inhale and tilt your chin
down towards your
collarbone; exhale
and push the skin and
muscle fibres of the
cheekbones upwards.
Then open and close
your mouth five to
ten times, feeling the
muscles tightening as
you do so. Do this three
times a day or as often
as you can.

3 Place your index
finger and middle finger
on each cheek and then
slowly rub in a circular
motion. This will
stimulate the muscles,
which will thicken
them up and cause
them to look fuller.
(It also makes your
cheeks rosy!)

at optimum lipid (fat) and hydration levels, and
we also suggest Sun Chlorella A, a Japanese
brand, to keep your gut happy; it really does
show on your face, due to the two pairs of
stomach meridians which run down the face –
one pair down the sides to the chin, one pair
from under the eyes to the chin. If your tum's
upset, your face gets longer and more gaunt;
keep your gut in good shape and you won't
believe the difference! Sarah's skin plumped
and peachified almost incredibly when she
started taking Sun Chlorella, which she
anticipates taking for life. (Also see the
Supergreens Facelift Diet, page 176.)

Sign up for a course of facial acupuncture.
And have regular maintenance sessions (see
page 155).

TIP

**Supermodel Carmen dell'Orefice
recommends doing any inverted
(upside down) yoga pose, such as
Downward-facing Dog, to bring
colour to your face. If you don't
practise yoga, simply plant your
feet a hip-width apart then try
touching your toes. Hang there for
a few seconds as the blood pours
to your head.**

**Keep regular appointments with the
dentist.** Teeth and gums need to be in
optimal shape to support your facial
bone structure.

And if slimming down rather than plumping
up your face is your problem, see our section
on facial contouring, on page 44.

Blush becomingly

A subtle hint of pink blusher applied to the cheeks will bring a youthful glow to your complexion (and we mean subtle – you certainly want to avoid an alarming doll- or clown-like appearance). And it's uplifting too. Here's how to make it work for you…

Choose a transparent rose blusher. 'By mid life you are naturally losing that youthful "rosiness",' explains Terry de Gunzburg, 'and you want to recreate that. That doesn't mean turning into a babydoll, but finishing with a hint of blush: a nude rose or a transparent rose, even a pinkish coral, high on the cheeks. Even if you have "couperose" [rosacea/redness], it's very important, but in that case use a beige-y rose. Blusher gives an instant "lifting" effect.'

If you prefer powder blushers, try Chanel Joues Contraste in No 15 Orchid Rose. We're mostly cream blusher girls but less dry skins may be fine with powder. This looks really muddy in the compact but in fact it's a whisper-light soft rose that Mary Greenwell uses on everyone on the planet, with (as we now realise) good reason.

Use the right brushes. Of course cream blushers can be applied with fingers, but we find the best way to apply cream blusher (and to get longer-lasting results) is with a foundation brush; just 'feather' it into the skin with the lightest touch. Jo uses the flip side of her regular foundation brush, but if you do the same, you need to be religious about washing your brushes once a week or the blusher shade starts to 'pinkify' the foundation (to be avoided at all costs). For a powder blusher, apply an angled blusher brush with the short side on top, laid against your

TIP

Cream (or gel) blusher tends to fade on your cheeks, so 'set' it with a touch of translucent powder, and remember to take it with you for touch-ups.

cheekbone, to wrap the colour around without overloading it. Try them out in store to find one with a handle that suits your grip – personally we don't like too-short handles, but they might suit you.

Remember: nobody blushes brown. Because many women with high colour are scared that pink blusher will draw attention to that, they're tempted to use bronzer instead of blusher, so that it won't pick up the redness. Don't go there. Instead, use foundation to tone down that redness and then – as above – a very soft pinky shade on the top.

And never forget that less really is more. You need a whisper of colour not warpaint.

Cream blushers: *our award winners*

We trialled many new launches for this edition of the book (making almost 40, in all), requesting suits-all-skintone shades – usually a mid-rose tone. The challenge we set our testers: identify the brands which deliver a healthy flush that looks subtly, naturally glow-y – but crucially, stays put too.

REVIEWS

Bobbi Brown Pot Rouge for Lip and Cheeks

9/10

Sometimes this happens. Bobbi Brown resubmitted their existing winning product for this updated book – and it scored even higher marks, rising to the top of the blusher charts! Use this as a cheek tint – as our testers do – but it also does double-duty on lips, too. (Bobbi's memory of her grandmother using lipstick on her cheeks inspired this product.) It's creamy but sheer – with a matt finish – and comes in a pot (as the name suggests), with a twist-off top. Nine shades; our lot got Pale Pink this time. Here are testers' thoughts, this time round.

Comments: 'Loved this: can be adapted to suit the effect you desire and stays put all day' • 'naturally glowing, long-lasting – didn't need reapplying all day' • 'first time I've used a cream blush – love it, and the fact you can use it on lips too' • 'so easy to apply with fingers – very smooth, no dragging, with a colour that appears natural and bright' • 'gives a fantastic glow – like the healthy cheeks I used to have 30 years ago'.

Clinique Blushwear Cream Stick

8.28/10

Silky and oil-free, this water-resistant formula is specifically created to deliver long-wear results. It's non-drying (thanks to plant sterols and lecithin in the creamy blend), and comes in just four versatile shades which are designed to be universally flattering. It swivels up for direct application to cheeks – but ideally, we advise using a brush for blending.

Comments: 'Top marks; very easy to apply stick straight on to skin then blend with fingertips, looked natural, glowing' • 'am buying more and for

AT A GLANCE

Bobbi Brown Pot Rouge for Lips and Cheeks

Clinique Blushwear Cream Stick

Elizabeth Arden Ceramide Cream Blush

Jemma Kidd Blushwear Crème Cheek Colour

♡ WE LOVE...

In Jo's kit you'll find two new favourites: Liz Earle Colour Healthy Glow Cream Blush in Nude (an ultra-slim compact which now goes everywhere with her for on-the-go 'face-revival'), and Chantecaille's equally silky-soft Cheek Crème, in 'Shy' (!) Sarah loves Jemma Kidd Blush Wear Crème Cheek Colour in apricot-y Paw Paw – looks bright orange until you blend it, then abracadabra, it's a natural glow. See right for testers' raves, too.

my friends!' • 'colour looks vivid at first but mellows and lasts for hours' • 'worked well over liquid foundation, but not over mineral powder' • 'great product; much more dewy and healthy looking than powder blush; applied in the morning and still had a glow by evening' • 'don't usually wear blusher as end up looking like Coco the Clown, but was very happy with this'.

Elizabeth Arden Ceramide Cream Blush

7.67/10

We normally request brands to send products in just one shade, for our trials, but Elizabeth Arden sent a selection of Honey, Nectar and Plum blushers – and testers found them all pleasingly natural-looking. Skin-caring ceramides are a key ingredient for this brand, here helping to deliver a silky, dewy finish – and this is also enriched with vitamins A, C and E, in a mirrored brushed gold-effect compact.

Comments: 'Very natural glow without that harsh blusher line you sometimes see' • 'I'm a new mum who's had about two hours' sleep for the past 10 weeks and this blush perked up my skin beautifully' • 'I now use this every day and have binned the powder blush!' • 'made my cheeks look like I've been out in the fresh air: a soft, natural glow' • 'useful mirror' • 'colour and finish long-lasting even on hot days' • 'a good product to perk you up whenever you're looking tired'.

Jemma Kidd Blushwear Crème Cheek Colour

7.5/10

Smiles from Sarah: this mirrored compact happens to be her fave blusher (and it's always reassuring when testers fall for our own favourites!). This is designed to be long-wear (the only downside of cream blushers is they sometimes need re-applying during the day), and it too features antioxidant vits A, C and E. Testers were sent soft rose Pomegranate – and loved it.

Comments: 'Am a complete cream blush convert after using this; even my mum commented on how youthful I looked and asked if I'd had Botox!!!' • 'the best blush I've ever used: I train for up to three hours a day including cardio, and it lasted without any bother' • 'received compliments from people suggesting I had a "glow" about me' • 'felt and looked very natural on skin' • 'I have sallowish skin and this has given me a new look of life!'.

'When you're *younger*, you want to be PERFECT, but *later* you learn that perfect isn't really that INTERESTING'

Susan Sarandon

Body: how to look better naked (*truly*)

We have a sneaking admiration for nudists of mature years, who throw caution (and just about everything else) to the wind, and go naked. (And even play badminton or volleyball *au naturel*.) Are we about to do the same? Not for all the tea in Fortnum's…

Bodies, like our faces, show signs of gravity and sun damage. And often they're more neglected than our faces: swathed in layers of clothing for much of the year puts crêpey skin, bingo wings and even saggy knees out of sight – and off our beautycare radar. Even when it's roastingly hot, we see many women hiding under kaftans and sarongs feeling self-conscious about a body that's less than Elle Macpherson-esque.

But the naked truth is that nobody is ever going to judge you as harshly as you judge yourself. Just think of that little mental dialogue when you shop for a swimsuit: 'Omigod, look at my backside.' Contrast that to the thoughts running through a man's head when he catches sight of you naked: 'Whoo-hoooo!'

However, there are ways for every woman to feel a bit more 'Whoo-hoooo' about her own body. Overleaf, you can read about creams to slather on which, according to our testers, really can help body skin be more resilient, more velvety, more bare-able (and stroke-able, too). But there's a lot more that you can do to look better naked – which in turn, makes you feel better in your clothes. We just love that French phrase: '*être bien dans sa peau*' – literally 'to be good in your skin' – meaning 'to be content with yourself', which we think is definitely worth aspiring to. So, here are some suggestions that we're confident will make you feel that bit more comfortable in your own skin…

Stand up straight. Good posture not only makes you look an inch or two taller, but magically takes an inch or two off your mid-section, by un-sagging it. We've explained this on page 15, but it's so vital that here it is again! Imagine lifting your rib-cage as if there was a string going up from your breastbone to the ceiling. At the same time, gently pull your shoulder blades back and down. It's pretty easy to remember to do this every time you catch sight of yourself in a mirror, but you want to make more of a habit of it than that. For enhancing posture permanently, nothing beats Pilates (though yoga and the Alexander Technique come pretty close), through which you become much more aware of how you're standing, sitting and moving. And strengthening the core muscles in the tummy (the aim of Pilates) and the obliques creates an invisible 'corset' around the body, flattening your abs with absolutely no need for Playtex or Spanx.

Soften your water... and you'll soften your skin. Hard water is really drying, leaving skin looking and feeling papery. If you aren't sure whether your water is hard or soft, try the soap test: if your soap lathers extremely well and is hard to rinse away, it's soft. If it lathers only moderately and leaves skin rapidly squeaky-clean upon rinsing – or if there's a chalky residue on your shower door or curtain – then it's hard. You can actually buy a gizmo which fits into your shower to help remove the minerals, softening the water you use for washing your body. (See DIRECTORY, or simply Google 'shower water filter'.) The lower-tech alternative for dealing with the effects of hard water is to keep baths and showers short – under five minutes, if possible. Use a mild soap and use it only in areas of skin folds – underarms, neck, feet and, er, 'bits'.

Quit smoking... We can give you a gazillion reasons why you'll be better off not smoking, but in this case it's because the swirl of smoke around your body has an ageing effect on skin, bombarding it with free radicals – which break down collagen and elastin. There's some suggestion that smokers have a more negative body image, and the more a woman smokes, the worse she feels about herself.

...and get moving. On the other hand, the act of exercising actually makes you feel better about your body (never mind the physical improvements), according to a study from the University of Florida.

Get rid of 'goosebumps'. Shy to take that summer cardie off because of your bumpy upper arms? Blitz with a twice-weekly scrub. If that doesn't beat the problem, you may have an inherited skin condition called keratosis pilaris (KP), for which a consultant dermatologist recommends using a product called Dermol 500, with Vaseline Intensive Care Lotion to remoisturise afterwards. In fact, we recommend body-scrubbing to everyone as a preparation for any anti-ageing body lotion/butter/oil: a top-to-toe rub-down with a sugar- or salt-and-oil-based scrub, followed by moisturiser, is an instant skin makeover.

Tackle dry shins. Skin over the shins is particularly prone to dryness and can even develop cracks that look like a dry river-bed. Also, observes beauty therapist extraordinaire Nichola Joss, 'We're generally unaware how much waxing and shaving can dry out the skin.' There's another good reason for keeping shin skin supple: later in life, this is where leg ulcers can develop – hard to shift and unpleasant to live with. Prevention is very definitely better than cure, here. We cannot recommend too highly that you try This Works Skin Deep Dry Leg Oil, which we love because it's absolutely miraculous for easing the itchiness and

TIP

If you're heading for a 'red carpet'-type event, you might want to consider this advice from Kylie Minogue: 'My real skin tip is that I use all-over body make-up, which makes a real difference because you get this even, lovely finish everywhere. When you hit forty, you need a little more help.' Recommended products are Per-fékt Body Perfection Gel, a gel-mousse that slides on to give a natural build-upable coverage and smooth airbrushed glow, and Prtty Peaushun Skin Tight Body Lotion, a natural product with light-reflecting particles devised by Hollywood make-up artist Bethany Karlyn, which helps even out skin tone and enhance muscle tone. MAC does a range of body make-up, including Face and Body Foundation, which is water resistant and available in a wide range of colours.

tautness of dry shins. You could also follow Nichola's advice: 'Use a body oil first because it penetrates deeper into the skin, then double up with cream on top to hold the moisture in.'

Apply a self-tanner. According to all the beauty pros we know, the very fastest way to look slimmer is with a body self-tanner, which helps create the illusion of a slimmer body (a little like the way darker clothes do). Self-tanner can also help conceal the dimpling and puckering from cellulite. If you're self-tan-phobic, we recommend one of the gradual options which can be massaged into the skin in circular movements, just as if you were applying a body lotion: favourites with Beauty Bible testers include St Tropez Gradual Tan Everyday Body, Nivea Sunkissed Skin, Palmer's Cocoa Butter Formula Natural Bronze and Hawaiian Tropic Gradual Bronze Moisturiser.

Use camouflage. If you're self-conscious about red veins on your feet and legs, you have three options: make-up, sclerotherapy or lasers (see page 203). Sclerotherapy (generally using local injections of saline) has been tried-and-tested over the years and it's a fraction of the price of lasering (for questions to ask before venturing into either of these procedures, see page 46). But for occasional pin-baring, Nichola Joss recommends concealing veins (or other blemishes) with Laura Mercier Secret Camouflage concealer, which works as well on legs as it does on faces: she advises applying with fingers as the warmth helps the make-up 'meld' into skin for a seamless finish. It's pretty budge-proof, too. (And see also our suggestion above about self-tanner: flaws of all kinds are infinitely less visible when the rest of the leg is 'sun-kissed'.)

Gloss up. Polish off your body make-over with a spritz of 'dry' (ie, non-greasy) body oil on shoulders and bosom (we love Soap & Glory Easy Glistening Dry Oil Body Gloss), and a slick of varnish on toes and hands.

Anti-ageing body treatments: *our award winners*

The women we know are finally waking up to the fact that, yes, skincare should extend below the neck-line. In fact, right down to your toes. Firming, smoothing and moisturising ingredients can deliver rapid results, improving dull, papery, flaky (and even saggy) body skin – and with it dramatically boosting body confidence

AT A GLANCE

Decléor Aroma Sculpt Divine Rejuvenating Cream

This Works Skin Deep Dry Leg Oil

Pevonia Botanica Ligne Tropicale De-Aging Body Balm

Elemis Pro-Collagen Body Cream

Natio Wellness Body Lotion

Guerlain Super Aqua-Body Body Serum

Balance Me Super Toning Body Oil

We tested several dozen more entries for this paperback, dispatching creams, butters and oils which made a big difference to the resilience, smoothness and touch-me-softness of arms, legs, bums and tums. (Though if it's cellulite you want to blitz, see page 38.) So which texture – lotion, oil, cream, serum – and fragrance (or not) should you go for? We suggest choosing whatever you'll enjoy most – because as our testers found, that's what inspires regular use. And goodness, how they enjoyed these!

REVIEWS

Decléor Aroma Sculpt Divine Rejuvenating Cream

 A really outstanding score from the well-known aromatherapy-powered brand, with a scrumptious cream featuring a cocktail of essential oils (rose, chamomile, lemongrass, lemon, grapefruit, frankincense, myrrh), plus shiitake mushroom extract, tamanu and macadamia oils. Pearlescent particles deliver a lovely instant radiance, while the cream is designed to have a draining, firming and even a 'lifting' effect, making it ideal (so Decléor promise) for use after weight loss, as well as for general anti-ageing. **Comments:** 'I would give this 12/10 if I could; it's a smooth, silky cream that's firm enough to take a scoop and rub it in; I used to be a bit slapdash but the improvement is so noticeable that I apply every morning: I can now go out bare-legged!' • 'skin no

longer flaky, tone has improved, and I got a compliment on how smooth my legs are' • 'fabulous fragrance, my skin feels so much fresher and softer, and looks almost shimmering; compliments from my other half were a nice side effect' • 'I have to confess that I only did the trial on one side of my body for two days: the instant difference in skintone – especially on my legs – made me switch to using it all over'.

This Works Skin Deep Dry Leg Oil

 Shins start out with few oil glands, but as we age they can become super-dry and paper-thin. And there's a health issue there: poor circulation and a fragile skin barrier can increase the chances of 'leg ulcers' in later years: painful, hard to budge and depressing. This blends over a dozen rich plant oils – including jojoba, macadamia, evening primrose, plus rose oil, tuberose and sandalwood (hence the heavenly smell) – to nourish skin deeply. Not just thirsty shins, but all over… **Comments:** 'I've always had rough, dry patches on knees and elbows but they're much smoother now, with an overall healthy glow that makes me feel happier to wear clothes that expose more skin' • 'lizard legs now non-flakey and look younger' • 'delicious aromatherapy smell' • 'skin appears totally revitalised and it's perfect to use on your whole body, not just the legs' • 'although it's an oil, it doesn't seem to get everywhere (as other oils do)' • 'such a gorgeous smell I kept putting some on hands, to smell them!'.

Pevonia Botanica Ligne Tropicale De-Aging Body Balm

Gosh, this is luscious: a really rich, creamy product (designed, ideally, to be used following the scrub which features on page 30). 'Micro-emulsified' shea butter delivers its truly voluptuous texture, alongside pomegranate and acknowledged anti-ageing tropical botanicals, plus 'tegospheres with Retinol'. Hey, we're beauty editors, and we don't even know what those are – but the bottom line is that it truly seduced testers with its feel and exotic, tangy fragrance.

Comments: 'A dream: light, smooth, creamy; my upper arms benefited most – they're less bumpy and more toned' • '10/10: overall skintone better' • 'amazing smell: quite sharp, tangy and pineapple-y!' • 'used to suffer dry, flaky skin on lower legs/shins, and dry arms that appear finely wrinkled when pinched: the treated side seems to "bounce back" more quickly and looks firmer and plumped-up' • 'so luxurious, and smells divine' • 'improvement in skintone after a couple of days, noticeable to others'.

Elemis Pro-Collagen Body Cream

This Pro-Collagen range is now a beauty 'classic', having consistently scored well in our books – and this new addition also performed outstandingly well in our most recent trials. The silky cream stars a trio of oils – babassu, castanha and bilberry seed oil, plus laminaria brown seaweed and marine algae padina pavonica. Look closely and you'll see subtle radiant particles, though the cream's key action is 'firming': Elemis aim for what they call a 'body stocking effect on the skin, using 'micro-lattice' technology.

Comments: 'Skin looked more toned, supple; it smoothed out dryness and wrinkles, and looked younger' • 'a genius product: I was sceptical but skin is butter-smooth, very soft and looks younger due to benefits of light gleam – wish it came in giant 500ml tub!' • 'skin feels great: moisturised, plumped, glowing and years younger – a revelation' • 'beautiful fragrance lingers all day'.

Natio Wellness Body Lotion ❀

Not quite a 'steal', but a reasonably-priced product from an Aussie brand with a natural focus (Natio is that country's fastest-growing beauty brand, though they've actually been producing cosmetics for 75 years). A non-greasy formula, rich in aloe vera and

vitamin E plus potent antioxidant pomegranate.

Comments: 'Very effective body moisturiser, skin is much softer, silkier, smoother and has healthy glow; and yes, younger-looking – smoothed it into recent surgery scars and they are less visible' • 'skin feels velvety, absorbed quickly so no worries about using before you get dressed and fantastic smell' • 'liked everything about this: and the benefits are lasting with regular use' • 'skin a lot less dry and plumper, very easy to smooth in, and instant results – skin lovely and silky-smooth'.

Guerlain Super Aqua-Body Body Serum

This serum is a bit of a legend in body-care circles, a super-luxurious 'soft touch' treatment that gives long-lasting hydration, boosting skin's resistance to environmental stresses and ageing, and revitalising with cell-renewing Desert Rose Flower Complex. Soft-focus powders deliver an instantly even-toned, luminous finish.

Comments: 'Lovely to use if you had a special function coming up, after a week skin felt very smooth, well-hydrated and silky, drier areas disappeared' • 'skin appears more youthful, radiant and healthy after using this for a few weeks, I feel my skin has had a real treat! It's soft, smooth and supple, has a healthy sheen and feels as if it has more elasticity' • 'loved this product, smell was divine, and skin condition has improved significantly, now very smooth, toned and even. Gorgeous!'.

Balance Me Super Toning Body Oil ❄ ❄

You could try this as a cellulite treatment: it's designed to have a firming action on wobbly bits. It earned a place in the new line-up for its super-conditioning blend of macadamia, jojoba, sweet almond oil and wheatgerm. Deliciously fragrant with juniper, lavender, bergamot and lavender, this was the first product Brit brand Balance Me created – for themselves! – and many happy women already thank them for sharing it with the world.

Comments: 'Skin on décolletage smoother, less dry and nicely perfumed' • 'amazing transformation: dry skin on shins and elbows became smooth and soft' • 'I have a monthly sports massage and the masseur was so impressed she's now using it on her clients' • 'fewer wrinkles and plumper, more hydrated skin' • 'skin instantly firmer, smoother and less dimpled at the top of my legs; elbows and heels softer than they've ever been' • 'body skin definitely more youthful'.

♡ WE LOVE...

One thing you should never be without as the years fly by is a good body cream. Our motto is more is better, and slathering is fantastic! Sarah likes a really rich butter on the very dry bits (such as organic Neal's Yard Remedies Rose Body Cream) and has never found anything better for the rest than another natural (though not organic) product, Seven Wonders Miracle Lotion. Meanwhile, Jo's a bit of a body creamaholic, with a distinctly over-crowded bedside table that features ultra-rich and nourishing Liz Earle Superskin Body, Aromatherapy Associates Enrich Body Serum (she's noticed a very definite 'firming' action) and Trilogy Aromatic Body Treatment Oil. She slathers them on (sometimes layering them) just before bedtime, so they sink in overnight. (We prefer more natural body treatments over high-tech creations and feel that botanicals have excellent skin-smoothing properties while doing a perfectly good job of keeping 'wobbliness' at bay.)

Body scrubs: *our award winners*

When you want fast body improvements, we say: reach for a scrub. These are pretty darned miraculous for transforming dry and rough skin in about 30 seconds flat. (Especially when the exfoliating particles are suspended in an oil base that delivers a softening, sensual 'slick' on the surface, to nourish as it sinks right in.) What's more, if you then choose to layer another body oil, lotion or cream on to body-scrubbed skin, the ingredients will work their cell-plumping magic more effectively because you've buffed away the dead surface cells first

AT A GLANCE

Ila Beyond Organic Body Scrub for Energising and Detoxifying

Soap & Glory The Breakfast Scrub

Pevonia Tropicale De-Aging Saltmousse

REN Moroccan Rose Otto Sugar Body Polish

Liz Earle Naturally Active Skincare Energising Body Scrub

Balance Me Skin Brightening Exfoliating Body Polish

So: our Beauty Bible recruits trialled several dozen body scrubs, plus many more for this paperback edition – and these were their super-smoothing favourites, with some truly stellar scores. Several also earn at least two daisies for naturalness. (See page 7 for more about our daisy rating.)

REVIEWS

Ila Beyond Organic Body Scrub for Energising and Detoxifying

 Ila's the Sanskrit word for 'earth', and this all-British luxury spa brand – founded by an aromatherapist who set out to fuse holistic wellbeing with beautiful skin – prides itself on being all-natural, too. Hand-blended in the Cotswolds, the scrub's based on Himalayan mineral salts to detoxify and restore energy, with a sense-awakening essential-oil blend of organic rose geranium and juniper. Congrats to Ila for a truly outstanding score (very few products ever exceed an average of 9/10 from our testers).
Comments: '10/10! The skin on my legs looked dull and tight, overall my skin lacked lustre; after using this it shone, smelt fragrant, was smooth and very moisturised – and didn't need any body lotion; after a few uses skintone visibly improved' • 'I looked like a pork sausage before it's been cooked! But instantly my skin really glowed,

with a lovely sheen, and after using twice a week it looks more toned and less pasty' • 'gorgeous smell of rose geranium' • 'luxurious packaging and nice-sized pot, slightly drier than other oil-based scrubs, with nice grainy bits of salt which dissolved in water, now have silky soft thighs and arms'.

Soap & Glory The Breakfast Scrub

 Another off-the-wall name – and another serious performance from Marcia Kilgore's so-affordable brand. Thick, luscious and almost gloopy as an uncooked banana muffin (and with something of the same scent!), this serves up skin-calming oats, alongside luscious shea butter, honey and almonds – and all sprinkled generously with maple sugar.
Comments: 'I have the skin of a reptile but now it feels a lot smoother; little white spots on upper arms appear less obvious and some have gone completely' • 'not only did it smell absolutely heavenly, it was extremely effective and after just one use I noticed how soft my skin was – may actually persuade me to exfoliate more!' • 'didn't feel I needed moisturiser afterwards and smells amazing: buttery/maple syrup fragrance' • 'loved this product – self-tan went on much more smoothly' • 'I was absolutely amazed how after just one use, my skin felt so different – like a baby's; I just kept running my hands up and down my legs in disbelief; my beauty therapist asked what I'd done

as patchy bits of rough skin had completely disappeared'.

Pevonia Tropicale De-Aging Saltmousse

9.27/10

Question: what's a 'Saltmousse'? Answer: a salt scrub with a slightly mousse-y texture (and in this case, a quite scary tangerine colour!). Pevonia's award-winner features sea salt harvested from the Brittany coast, in France, blended with minerals, vitamins and enzymes. The 'Tropicale' refers to the use of papaya and pineapple enzymes (which have an exfoliating action in their own right), and it has an 'exotic fruit sorbet' aroma, as a result.

Comments: 'Gorgeous and fruity and I wanted to eat it' • 'it smelt gloriously dreamy – very fruity and fresh' • 'it was like a breath of sunshine to the skin' • 'this has converted me to the benefits of body scrub: skin feels soft and moisturised and elbows much smoother' • 'skin looks as if it has come alive again! It was like a breath of sunshine to skin that had been covered by winter clothes' • 'when I showered it washed away easily, unlike other scrubs' • 'can see improvement in rough, dry knees and elbows' • 'you get addicted to this product – an even bigger tub would be great!'.

REN Moroccan Rose Otto Sugar Body Polish

9.27/10

Oh, we love it when this happens… Yes, this product has featured previously in *The Green Beauty Bible* – but we sent it out to ten different testers specifically for this book, who awarded the scrub virtually the same impressively high score as when previously trialled. With Paraguayan cane sugar, skin-conditioning olive and almond oils, kola nut and tea extracts – and the heady fragrance of rosa Damascena oil (you lot really are suckers for rose scents), we're elevating this to the Beauty Bible Hall of Fame.

Comments: '10/10! Not really messy, easy to rub in, beautiful rose smell, good texture like soft sugar, washed off quickly leaving nice soft film on body; lovely to use in bath – rose-scented water – or shower. Very luxurious lovely product, and softer skin!' • 'left skin very smooth and moisturised, no need for body cream on my very dry skin; bumpy skin on upper arms has gone after a month of using regularly' • 'like a spa treatment! Skin more even in tone now, I loved this – the best scrub ever!' • 'moisturising lasts for days, skin silky and much softer and clearer, particularly around my thighs and buttocks, and bumpy arms reduced – fabulous'.

Liz Earle Naturally Active Skincare Energising Body Scrub

8.87/10

What universally seduced testers with this product was the rev-you-up, sense-awakening smell (a combination of sweet orange, grapefruit, geranium, peppermint, eucalyptus, pine, rosemary, patchouli and petitgrain). With a more liquid texture than other scrubs in this category, this could almost qualify as a skin-buffing body wash.

Comments: 'Very impressed: skin felt smoother, no need for body lotion' • 'I like the eucalyptus scent, as it makes me feel clean; the texture's not too abrasive and I like the way it feels like a body wash as well as a scrub' • 'it's like a spa treatment and using it leaves the whole bathroom smelling like your own spa – very relaxing!' • 'skin looked brighter after first use; lumps and bumps also improved over time' • 'application very pleasant: easy to rub into skin, helped by a slight foaming action' • 'kept the flaky patches at bay on my legs and I saw an improvement in the amount of ingrowing hairs I had; the top of my arms looked less bumpy and I have fewer flaky patches there too' • 'left skin feeling really "alive" and fresh due to the menthol and peppermint' • 'definitely uplifting and made me feel nice and "tingly"' • 'has just the right amount of exfoliation and feels great on the skin; will definitely buy again'.

Balance Me Skin Brightening Exfoliating Body Polish

8.67/10

One for the mornings, we'd say, with its zingy, wake-you-up spearminty scent. A blend of natural salt, coconut and sweet almond oils, it buffs and moisturises in one – in common with most of these winning scrubs.

Comments: 'Top marks! Skin on my legs was dry and quite flaky – lizard-like – texture is perfect, and skin felt fabulous, moisturised and smooth with no stickiness or irritation. The best exfoliating polish I have ever used, didn't need a body cream after' • 'stubborn rough patches on knees and feet from kneeling to bathe my toddler are definitely smoother and more moisturised; rinsed away well, leaving no gritty bits; would be great to use before waxing – I shave and found I had fewer ingrown hairs than usual' • 'lovely minty smell, perfect texture; skin felt gorgeous after, really soft and smooth – as good as my expensive brands – a great product'.

♡ WE LOVE…

Well, first of all we'll tell you what we personally don't love: those body scrubs based on crushed nuts and seeds, which drift to the bottom of the bathwater and make you feel like you're sitting in a tub of grit. (Not such an issue if you shower, but we're mermaids.) REN Moroccan Rose Otto Sugar Body Polish (which scored so well with our testers), ESPA Detoxifying Salt Scrub and Les Soins aux Fleurs de Bach Body Scrub (with its amazingly effective 'Anti-Stress' fragrance) all have a place on Jo's bath-side, while Sarah's shower features Essential Care Organic Coconut Candy Scrub (literally good enough to eat), Wild Organics Marshmallow Butter Sugar Scrub, and – a double-duty skin whammy – Yes to Carrots Pampering Hand & Nail Spa, which works all over!

We must, still must, improve our busts...

And we CAN! Starting now, with the right bra – because choosing the right 'underneath' (as fashion guru Amanda Platt calls your bra), is as crucial to looking great as what you put on top

When you can't rely on youthful perkiness, you need a better bra to give you uplift. Undies have become increasingly important in our lives. To put it plainly, at this stage in life you need a bra that's not only pretty but does its job impeccably (and don't forget equally well-fitting knickers). We'd always urge you, if possible, to go to an expert: the difference it can make is staggering. And it's not just a question of looking good: your bra can affect your health.

Think of your bra as a suspension bridge.
You may never have linked your bosom and engineering, but according to chiropractor Tim Hutchful, it really is like a suspension bridge! 'You need a well-engineered bra so your shoulders don't end up doing all the work. Bras that don't fit affect the shoulders and chest and usually cause pain as you get older.' Poorly-fitting bras can lead to all sorts of physical problems, including head-, neck-, shoulder-, and/or back-aches (back pain is common among large-breasted women). Too tight a bra can even restrict your breathing.

Most importantly, wear the right size.
Amazingly, about 80 per cent of women are wearing the wrong-size brassiere. In one study, most women with shoulder pain found it lifted completely when they removed their bra. (Though the researchers didn't try kitting them out in the right-size bra to see what happened then...) Add to this the fact that our bosoms lose firmness with age and you can see why it's vital to confront the bra issue if you want your *poitrine* to look alluring and feel comfy. Be aware too that, however carefully you handwash them (and never tumble dry), bras lose their oomph as they get older, so depending on how often they're worn you should replace them every six months. (If necessary please shuffle your budget – it's really worth it.)

Become a savvier bra-shopper. There are more types of bra than we've had hot dinners (well, nearly) but whether you choose wired (or not), padded or plain, demi-cup or full, black lace, crimson satin or classic white cotton, there is basic advice that's common to all styles. Plus, for energetic exercisers, you can now find a range of sports bras that is specially designed to keep your bosom stable rather than bouncing with every movement (think of the way a ponytail bobs up and down as you run, play tennis, even do yoga). So...

● First and most importantly, says June Kenton,

BRAS AFTER BREAST SURGERY

June Kenton of Rigby & Peller, who has had a mastectomy herself, is passionate about the concerns of women who've had this surgery. 'Getting a prosthesis and bra after mastectomy is often treated in the same way as getting a pair of crutches, but it should be about fashion, not a medical appliance,' she says. The key is to find a bra which fits the other breast perfectly before choosing a prosthesis. 'Get bras to fit your "good" side then fit the prosthesis so it matches,' she advises. (Find more advice at www.rigbyandpeller. com, and other specialist mastectomy lingerie suppliers.)

owner of Rigby & Peller (the legendary lingerie emporium in London), 'Be really grown-up and have a proper expert fitting. Try on lots. Move around, sit down, stand up, lift your arms – make the bra work for you. Then choose the style which performs best.'

● The two crucial measurements are cup size and band size (the bit at the bottom) – so make sure the fitter measures those each time. The perfect position for your breasts is midway between your shoulder and your elbow. The most common problem is wearing a bra too small in the cup and too big in the band at the back. Most women wear their bra bands too high (see next point), so their measurements are wrong. Often the key is to get a deeper cup and a smaller band. This usually eliminates the dreaded 'back sausages' too.

● The band should sit evenly around the chest, ie, the back shouldn't be higher or lower than the front. It shouldn't ride up but stay parallel to the floor.

● Breasts should be supported primarily by the band around the rib-cage, not the straps.

● Breasts shouldn't bulge over the top or sides of the cup, even with a low-cut style such as a balconette.

● The nipple should be in the centre of the cup.

● The cup should fit smoothly, and not wrinkle, be loose, or cut in at the top so you get a bulge (called 'double-cupping' in the trade).

● The centre piece of the bra should lie flat against the chest.

● If it's underwired, the wires should go under the bust contour and follow it snugly – not cut in or rub.

● Straps should not dig in or slip off the shoulder. Choose straps that are comfortable and make you feel supported. Generally that means wider straps – but they don't need to look bulky.

● A well-fitting bra shouldn't leave marks on your skin – and that means the straps too.

BOOST YOUR BUST... AND BANISH BINGO WINGS!

There are very simple actions that will help firm your bosom – and arms too. Fitness trainer Andy Wadsworth suggests the following for bust uplift, followed by a couple for debagging the dreaded bingo wings! But most important of all for the bustline, he says, is your posture: stand tall, keep your shoulders down and wide, lift your chest. Don't round your shoulders or slouch.

1 **Palm push:** standing or sitting, extend your arms in front of you at chest height, elbows bent as if you are hugging a tree (or a person...). Now push your palms together with force. Hold for ten seconds. Repeat ten times. Do this as often as you can. Watchpoint: keep your shoulders relaxed, pushing your shoulder blades down and together.

2 **Floor press-up:** do full press-ups on the floor if you are strong (and used to this type of exertion); if not, keep your knees to feet (you're on tiptoes) on the floor and press-up the rest of your body. Once you can do 20 knee press-ups, try doing a full press-up. Aim to build up to three sets of ten press-ups.

3 **Wall press-away:** stand facing a wall, then extend your arms at chest height a bit wider than a shoulder-width apart, so your hands touch the wall. Bend your arms and let your body fall towards the wall, then push away by straightening your arms. Aim for three x ten repetitions.

4 **Chest press:** lie on the floor (or bench or fitness ball), with a weight in each hand (either a 2kg weight or a full bottle of water). Raise your arms up in the air above your chest. Aim for three x ten repetitions.

5 **Butterfly:** standing with feet a hip-width apart and with a weight (as above for Chest press exercise) in each hand, start with hands at about 45 degrees to the floor; then lift the weights up in an arc to meet in front of your chest. Aim for three x ten repetitions.

FOR BINGO WINGS...

6 **Tricep dip:** sitting on a chair or the edge of the bath, with your feet under your knees a hip-width apart, grasp the sides of the chair or bath while you lift your bottom from the seat and let it drop down and forward; keep your elbows behind you rather than out to the side. Straighten your arms to come up. Move down and up without pausing for three sets of ten, building up to 20.

7 **Overhead triceps press:** put your hands behind your neck with a weight in each (as in exercise 4), then push them up above your head in a straight line. Go up and down smoothly without pausing for three x ten repetitions.

PS Any activity that uses your arm and chest muscles will help tone and firm: Jo swims and does yoga, Sarah brushes big horses, mucks out stables – and finds that scrubbing the bath with both arms is an amazing workout for arms and tummy!

Bust treatments: our award winners

You've found the perfect-fitting bra to give maximum support – now lavish your bust with treats that not only leave the skin feeling soft and smooth but, amazingly, claim to make your breasts feel firmer and more pert… So you can reveal your décolletage with confidence

AT A GLANCE

Lulu's Time Bomb Trouble Shooter Neck, Jaw and Chest Cream

Liz Earle Superskin Bust & Neck Treatment

Caudalie Firming Concentrate

Liz Earle Superskin Moisturiser

Motherhood, gravity, going bra-less when you were a carefree twentysomething – they all take their toll on the bust area. Add to that the effects of gravity over the decades and none of us is as pert as we once were – although good underwear, fitted properly, can be nothing less than a miracle-worker (see page 32 for more). Frenchwomen swear by the perkifying effects of cold water (once upon a time, Clarins even made a device that blitzed boobs with icy water – and rather effective it was, too), but nowadays there are more treatments than ever which allege that they'll firm and uplift breasts, not simply leave the skin soft and silky. (Any body lotion would achieve velvetiness in the boob zone, frankly.) So do these targeted bust treatments achieve the near-impossible and deliver real uplift? To find out, we've now dispatched well over two dozen products to testers, and are showcasing two new entries here. NB: they were instructed to use the product for four weeks on one breast alone and note any difference.

REVIEWS

Lulu's Time Bomb Trouble Shooter Neck, Jaw and Chest Cream

7.94/10 Having already put on a pretty stupendous performance in the so-challenging neck category, Lulu (yes, that Lulu) and her team submitted this for our 'boob treatment' trials, and it slipped straight into the top slot. (NB: all this team also noted neck/décolletage improvements, too). Ingredients include vitamin E, pea extract, sunflower and shea butter extract; it has a fabulous, waft-you-to-Provence lavender scent, which

encourages diligent application – and that's half the battle, with bust treatments. Like every product, these are only effective with regular use.

Comments: 'Prior to use I felt my bust skin was starting to develop a crêpey look but this not only made me feel as if I was receiving a luxury salon treatment, seeing results serves to confirm these impressions' • 'skin on my bust is now soft, smooth and supple – and also good for droopy jaw-line and crêpiness' • 'smells lovely – like lavender-y baby powder, but nicer' • 'loved this – it's done what it says it will, improving both my bust and neck/jaw area, which are more toned and soft to the touch' • 'surprised by its effectiveness and will buy again' • 'from bust to neck, skin looks fresher and more youthful, with improved texture and tone'.

Liz Earle Superskin Bust & Neck Treatment

7.57/10 This smoothing serum is a personal favourite of Jo's (see We Love…), and we're not surprised that it also did very well in our trials. Lightweight and cooling, it sinks in fast and is packed with the botanical ingredients you'd expect from the 'naturally active' brand: omega-3 and omega-6 essential fatty acids, antioxidants, quince and green tea extracts, white lupin, plus an ingredient extracted from Kigelia africana (aka the 'sausage tree'!), sourced from a community-based sustainable forestry project in Malawi. Some testers applied it to their necks too, and loved the double whammy.

Comments: 'Skin felt moisturised, softer and firmer; natural herby smell soon went, and skin dried very quickly, not sticky at all' • 'felt like I'd had a mini bust-lift, skin looked luminous and softer; results were excellent though I wasn't fond of the brownish colour' • 'definite improvement in décolletage area, although not in that small area between my breasts; had lost elasticity due to pregnancy and age, and definitely has improved a little; love the smell' • 'bust and neck much softer and less crêpey, and fine lines less noticeable' • 'I am cursed with a very large chest and there was never a chance it was going to make a huge difference, but it improved my skin, felt gorgeous and smelt divine!'.

Caudalie Firming Concentrate

7.5/10 As with all Caudalie products (which are inspired by the owners' family vineyard in Bordeaux), this 100 per cent natural lightweight oil features vine-derived ingredients – here, grapeseed oil. They recommend it's used not just on the bosom, but to firm the arms and stomach, and what we love about it is the delicious blend of aromatherapeutic oils: sweet mint, peppermint, douglas fir and lemon.

Comments: 'Skin felt soft, moisturised and also more firm and toned, immediately; liked the light, natural fragrance a lot. After two weeks, bust more toned and felt firmer – and it definitely improved the crêpey skin on the underside of my upper arms (put it there too)!' • 'really liked the fresh citrussy smell, skin was softer and smooth, and I really got into the routine of application – no miracle cure for pert boobs but maybe a bit firmer' • 'improved texture and firmness of décolletage, skin looked smoother and more evenly toned' • 'my partner didn't know I used this, and spontaneously commented on the lift

and appearance of my breasts – was absolutely amazed it worked, though not sure who'd want their breasts to smell of chewing gum…' • '10/10: skin felt immediately firmer and softer, and I adore the minty fresh smell; bust feels firmer and more lifted and stretch marks less visible. Have bought some more supplies. I feel more confident and can't live without it'.

Liz Earle Superskin Moisturiser

7.44/10 They know a thing or two about customers' habits at Liz Earle – and inspired by that feedback loop, the Isle of Wight team put this rich, fragrance-free moisturiser – something we've always considered for faces – forward for our bust category. And what do you know? Several Beauty Bible panellists awarded it an excellent score – so Liz Earle now have two winners in this section, here with a luscious product based on cranberry seed/rosehip/borage oils, plus pomegranate extract and vitamin E. The one caveat: it did perform better in the 'smoothness' than the 'pertness' stakes.

Comments: 'I was lucky enough to be given Liz's "official" bust treatment shortly before starting this trial so thought I'd compare them – after four weeks, the Superskin side was noticeably softer, smoother and preferred by my partner!' • 'a joy to use whether for face or bust, leaving breasts beautifully smooth and well-moisturised' • 'area looked more even and felt more moisturised with this lovely, subtly-scented cream'.

♡ WE LOVE…

We don't really 'do' bust treatments. But Jo does slather Liz Earle Superskin Bust & Neck Treatment on her décolletage, for suppleness. (At Jo's suggestion they renamed this as '& Neck' because it's so great for that – see page 153 for more.)

Give **cellulite** the brush-off

Tone those thighs and de-dimple that derrière. (Because there's a lot you can do to smooth out cellulite)

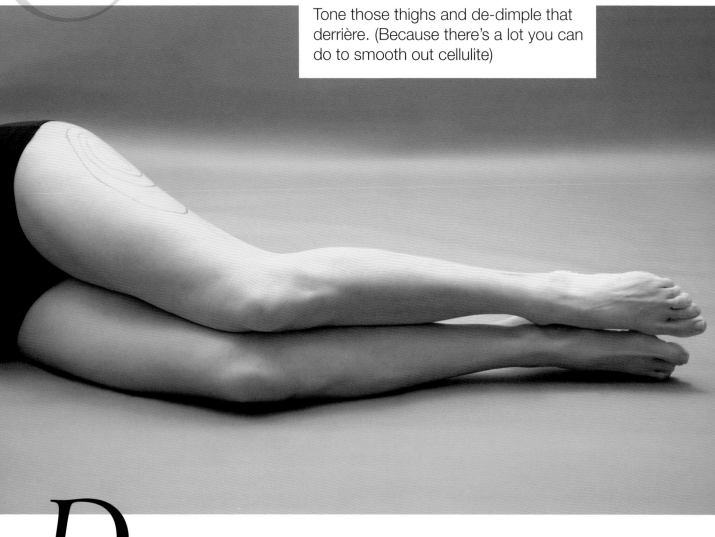

Dimples may be appealing on babies (and handsome men), but on your thighs and backside? Not so charming. So the bottom line on cellulite – hallelujah – is that there's much that can be done to improve it (and thus, in turn, your body confidence). You may never conquer the problem completely – but a combination of nutrition, body-brushing, exercise and localised massage can make a visible difference...

Scrub off the dead skin cells. As well as dry-skin body-brushing (see right), do use a scrub on your backside, thighs and hips, because any cellulite product you apply to the area is going to penetrate better if it doesn't have to make it through dead skin cells. Targeted body exfoliation also brings about incredibly rapid improvements in skin texture: in our experience it can take less than a week of daily blitzing to combat 'goosebumps' in the cellulite zone and thereby transform skin smoothness.

Body-brush the bumps bye-bye. The skin is a vital (and often overlooked) organ of elimination and nothing is better at stimulating localised circulation than daily brushing. It wakes up a sluggish lymphatic system – and many women have told us it works astonishingly well to improve digestion and aches and pains as side benefits.

First, find your brush: most diligent body-brushers choose a brush with a strap that slips over your hand, and has a removable long handle to get at your back, etc. (Sarah finds her favourite Origins Raffe brush which has a short-ish handle reaches everywhere.) The brush shouldn't be scratchy: if it makes little white scratch marks when you brush the back of your hand with it, it's too hard.

We recommend total body-brushing rather than targeted brushing of the affected area, because you get the all-over lymph drainage and circulation-boosting benefits – here's the how-to:

● Body-brush dry skin, not damp or wet, and never areas that are bruised or irritated, or your breasts.
● Begin by standing in a comfortable position. Place one foot on a higher surface, such as the edge of the bath or a bed.
● Start by brushing the soles of the feet from toes to heel. Move on to the top of the foot and then upwards, with smooth, long strokes – always in the direction of the heart.
● Give extra attention to the skin between the knees and the waist, going over the cellulite area several times. Don't ignore the lymph nodes in the groin. Upwards, upwards, upwards.
● Next, move on to the top half of the body: palms of hands, backs of hands, sweeping towards the armpits (plenty more lymph glands there). Now do your shoulders and back – you'll probably need your long-handle brush here.
● Continue the sweeping movements on the front of your torso, going a little more lightly as the skin can be very sensitive here. (But miss out your breasts and nipples.)
● Brushing should be firm and vigorous, but shouldn't hurt. A rosy glow is fine; red or irritated skin isn't.
● Three to five minutes is ideal. Realistically, two minutes is OK. But the key is: do it daily, and if you can only manage even one solitary minute every morning, that's infinitely better than a once-a-week longer blitz.

Give your fat a mini-massage. Dermatologist Dr Elizabeth Tanzi explains: 'Fat doesn't have a lot of blood flow, so kneading the skin helps increase circulation – and in turn, lessens the appearance of lumps.' Massage with your knuckles, moving up the fronts of your thighs, across your rear and then up the back of your thighs. (If this requires a little contortionism, so be it.) Alternatively, book regular massages with a deep tissue masseur

or practitioner of manual lymphatic drainage (MLD): these can help both to improve circulation and to drain away any excess fluid, which can exacerbate the appearance of cellulite.

Take exercise! As usual, more is better…it works. And you might want to try FitFlops, the footwear range with the inbuilt gym in the sole, for its proven leg-toning benefits.

Eat more veggies and high-fibre foods. They'll help in the war on dimples (and benefit your whole body): loads of veggies and salads (green leaves, onions and garlic); fruit (especially deep reds and purples – so make the most of berries and dark grapes); some wholegrains (brown rice, oats, and anything sprouted); olive oil and herbs. Also go for good-quality protein: oily fish and shellfish, eggs, poultry, tofu and natural live yoghurt. When you're out and about, choose a freshly-squeezed veggie juice or berry smoothie over tea and coffee, and take snack-packs of seeds and nuts (especially Brazil nuts and almonds). Basically, let 'fresh' be your watchword.

And it's about what you don't eat, too. Avoid processed and preserved foods, sugar, refined salt, 'fungal' foods (which means mushrooms, vinegar, blue cheese). Some people find that giving up gluten helps, too, and we also suggest you avoid caffeine and alcohol as much as is realistic. (NB: we do appreciate you're not a nun.)

Take goji. Dermatologist Dr Howard Murad (who's written an entire book on the subject) calls goji 'the cellulite assassinator' (it comes as berries and also juice). We've long espoused an inside-out as well as an outside-in approach to cellulite, and pharmacist Shabir Daya has put together a Cellulite Busting Kit (see DIRECTORY), incorporating the latest guidelines to help minimise the look of cellulite. This includes a food state multi-nutrient, vitamin B50, omega-3 essential fatty acids, glucosamine sulphate and goji berry juice.

And give yourself a break. We know women get incredibly angst-y about cellulite, but we would encourage you to relax a bit about the problem. Cellulite is never as apparent to others as it seems to our own so-critical selves (we've never yet met a man who even quite knew what cellulite was, let alone complained about it on a woman) – and other people see the 'big picture' (your sense of humour/great cooking skills/ your laugh). And if all else fails – well, that's why sarongs were invented.

> FAT doesn't have a lot of blood flow, so *kneading* the skin helps INCREASE circulation

Cellulite treatments: *our award winners*

It's a fact that even if you've been mercifully dimple-free until mid-life, the breakdown of collagen and elastin which leads to lines and wrinkles in the face can become all-too-apparent on the hips, derrière and (especially) thighs – in the form of cellulite. Certainly, diet plays a role, as does exercise, and we always advise body-brushing which is our own secret weapon. And now there's an abundance of cellulite-blitzing products. Do they really work? Our research with younger readers showed that yes, some definitely do. But we wanted to know – can they rise to the challenge of a more mature body? Almost three dozen cellulite products later – each dispatched to ten testers who 'fessed up to *peau d'orange* – here's the bottom line. Look out for three new entries

REVIEWS

Thalgo Crème Thalgomince

8.28/10 Thalassotherapy spa brand Thalgo actually prescribe this for massage twice daily, so that key ingredients – horse chestnut, caffeine complex, plus a plant extract they call 'Adipo-reset' (!) – are able to get to work round-the-clock. It's rich and creamy, enveloping skin 'like a slimming patch', Thalgo tell us, and though it's designed to complement two specific salon cellulite treatments Thalgo offer, our testers trialled it as a stand-alone product, observing impressive results. Several gave it nine or ten marks out of ten.
Comments: 'Lovely light but rich cream, which sunk in immediately; I used it on one leg which was instantly smoother and softer, and after six weeks cellulite definitely less noticeable, orange peel almost gone, firmer, and smoother than it has been for years; lost half an inch around my thigh – loved it' • 'very luxurious product with wonderful aroma, really feel good and my cellulite was a little improved' • 'after six weeks, skin looks and feels smoother and firmer – really loved using this treatment' • 'cellulite markedly reduced, thighs much less uneven and lumpy; when you pinch the skin, the orange-peel effect is much less obvious, plus thighs look and feel much firmer and tighter: expensive but I will be buying more – I love this and recommend it unreservedly' • 'silvery stretch marks and orange peel were much improved'.

Decléor Aromessence Slim Effect Localised Contouring Gel-Cream

7.33/10 It's an inescapable fact that cellulite products only work with diligent use – and the so-fresh aromatic fragrance of this alone, is to us a reason to get to work with it daily (or twice daily) on trouble zones. Scrumptious gel/cream texture, too, featuring essential oils known for their 'draining' action: sweet marjoram, elemi, grapefruit. There are actually three cellulite-fixers in the Slim Effect range which can be used in synergy

– or individually, as our testers did. (See WE LOVE, though, because Jo's a big fan of the other two products.)

Comments: 'Legs feel smoother at the rear; can see how using this could become effective' • 'this works a bit like a "beauty flash balm" does for the face; liked it as a super treat for my arms, legs, bottom and tummy – and my skin smelled really lovely' • 'liked the smell and the gel-like texture which goes on well and spreads easily, leaving skin feeling toned after use' • 'my cellulite looks much better after using this product over six weeks – I've lost a centimetre at the top of my thighs and they appear smoother' • 'a lovely, luxurious product to use – the non-sticky texture makes it easy to apply in the morning without needing to wait to get dressed' • 'smells wonderful – my skin has truly never looked so good'.

The Organic Pharmacy Resculpting Body Gel
❋ ❋

7.31
10

This glides on as a cooling gel, but since it features chilli in the ingredients (as well as green coffee), there's then a definite 'warming' (they call it 'thermogenic') action after application, helping to boost circulation. With high levels of organic ingredients this is the most natural of our high-scorers – and you might like to know that Organic Pharmacy also recommend it for use on wobbly tummies (men's, too…!) Testers were particularly impressed with its effect on the 'tone' of skin, after regular use.

Comments: 'Have lost an inch – which is fantastic for me – off each thigh; cellulite is improved, texture smoother and skintone firmer' • 'an exciting, vibrant product with a lovely citrus scent' • 'I've never used cellulite products as I was never convinced there'd be any improvement, but the texture of my skin has so improved I'll continue with this' • 'skin looks smoother and cellulite not as pronounced' • 'lovely gel which smoothed in easily with no dragging' • 'definitely made my skin smoother and the cellulite bumps appeared "softer"' • 'skin is smoother, softer and tighter'.

Mary Kay TimeWise Body Targeted Action Toning Lotion

7.22
10

A 'double shot' of caffeine in this one, plus (so we're told) pumpkin – and testers loved the invigorating fragrance of this lightweight formulation. Though we trialled this in

Jo was cellulite-free until she hit 50. Then, she observes: 'I suddenly understood what all those "resort wear" sarongs were created for…' She regularly uses a cellulite brush discovered in Germany with copper bristles, and is now devoted to the Decléor Aromessence Slim Effect Draining Contouring Serum and Baume Slim Effect Draining Massage Balm: 'Both the balm and the oil are divine, and 100 per cent natural.' Sarah's dimples are relatively shallow – possibly due to riding and walking for miles every weekend – but she scrubs thighs regularly, applies body lotion most nights and skin-brushes as often as she remembers.

TIP

Double up your daily application of product morning and night. You may get through more, but the active ingredients will have twice the opportunity to tighten and drain. If you just apply once, do it before bedtime: loose night clothes are less likely to rub the product off again than tight daytime clothing.

the cellulite category, it can multi-task as an all-over de-ager: there are ingredients to reduce the appearance of age spots, as well as minimising crêpey skin, alongside a general firming action.

Comments: 'Skin definitely smoother and more taut, less dimply: I loved the fact I actually lost an inch-and-a-half off each leg without actually having to do anything' • 'wish I'd used this on both legs (rather than use the whole tube on one leg, for comparison) – because the results were very impressive' • 'also used on décolleté area – wow! Softness, smoothness, eye-appealing…!' • 'subtle fruity smell; no dragging at all – works into skin evenly and smoothly, leaving it smooth and hydrated' • 'didn't notice any cellulite changes, but great for smoothing skin, which gets better with continued use'.

Turbo-charge your cleansing regime

We are the Queens of Clean – always have been – but we know many, many women who are so bored by cleansing they skimp (and even occasionally skip) this important part of the anti-ageing ritual. You can spend hundreds of pounds on an anti-ageing cream (if you really must…) but it's money down the drain if you aren't cleansing properly

T he reason is simple: unless you've got rid of the daily build-up of dead skin cells, your anti-ager is just going to sit there. Doing not very much at all. Quite expensively…

Cleansing in this specific way – as espoused originally by Eve Lom and then Liz Earle and now many, many happy and fresh-faced followers – is, in our experience, the most effective way to swoosh away the day and 'prep' skin for everything that comes next.

Step 1 Massage your cleanser into dry skin – balm, lotion, cream, whatever your preference. (Ideally at this stage in life you will have progressed from foaming cleansers, which in general are too drying for mature complexions. And if you're still using soap and water? Stop. Right. Now.)

Step 2 When we say massage, we mean massage. Ideally, use a pressure-point massage, making firm, small circular movements starting at chin-level and working up the cheeks to the eye zone, then shifting along the jaw-bone towards the ears (a distance of around 1.5cm), mid-cheek, cheekbones. And then the same on your forehead. Sweep your fingers more gently around the eyes in a circular but outwards direction. But – important BUT – if you can't be bothered to follow that precise prescription, just general firm massage of your face using circular movements will work wonders for melting make-up, improving circulation and decongesting the skin. You can do this for as long as you like. We recently talked to a Frenchwoman who explained that in France, it's not unusual to spend ten minutes on cleansing. We award ourselves Brownie points if we manage two, but really, the longer you knead your face with your fingertips the more it will reward you for it.

Step 3 Take a hot, wet cloth – a muslin cloth, or a flannel (Sarah prefers that). Press on to the face to remove the first load of cleanser and debris. Rinse under hot water (warm-to-hot water if you are prone to broken veins), then be a bit more vigorous as you swipe away more of the cleanser. (NB: never rub at areas where you have those aforementioned vein problems.) Repeat, until you feel you've swooshed away all remaining cleanser.

Step 4 Rinse the cloth again and wrap a corner of the flannel or cleansing cloth over the tip of your index finger. Rub at areas where skin and make-up build up – particularly in the crease around the nose, the cleft of the chin, and the sides of your face. If you do this, you may never need to use a specific exfoliator. (We rarely do.)

Step 5 As a final step, try swishing the flannel/cloth in cool water and press it on your face. (Jo does this while imagining the day and all its stresses are trickling away down the plug-hole. It isn't compulsory, but she finds it a relaxing technique…)

And overleaf, see the run-down of specifically anti-ageing cleansers. But we say: they'll all work best if you use this technique.

Cleansers: *our award winners*

A good cleanser is in itself a wonderful weapon against ageing. Unless you get the gunk off your face at night thoroughly, you're wasting your money on age-defying moisturisers and serums – because they simply sit on cellular debris and the day's make-up, with no chance of performing miracles. Now, though, there's a new category of cleansers which claim, in themselves, to offer anti-ageing benefits

AT A GLANCE

Elemis Pro-Radiance Cream Cleanser

Dr Brandt Lineless Foaming Cleanser

Balance Me Cleanse and Smooth Face Balm

Rodial Glamtox Cleanser

MV Organic Skincare Gentle Cream Cleanser

Pure Lochside Organic Orange Cleansing Oil

We've been a bit cynical about that, frankly: a cleanser is meant to be swiped or sluiced away, so how can it do anything more than cleanse and maybe brighten…? This book, however, gave us the opportunity to put several dozen 'anti-ageing' cleansers through their paces, to find out whether you really can cleanse the years away. These scores (and new entries) suggest the answer is a resounding 'yes'.

REVIEWS

Elemis Pro-Radiance Cream Cleanser

 Elemis suggest massaging this richly-nourishing, antioxidant-powered cleanser directly into skin, or – if you like a lather – to mix with warm water first. Active 'anti-ageing' ingredients include moringa seed peptides, 'super berry' açai and burdock, while shea butter moisturises, in addition to melting make-up. (Yes, even eye make-up.) It comes with a cotton facial mitt, to be used with warm water for optimum cleansing.

Comments: 'I really love this product – I thought my face was clean when I first used it but when I removed this cleanser with the cloth provided, I was shocked at the make-up that had remained on my face; it also left my skin moisturised' • 'a fabulous cleanser, thick but easily spread, removed all traces of make-up, even eyes and a waterproof lip stain' • 'this cleans effectively, doesn't dry skin, and leaves it looking brighter' • 'I looked forward to the ritual of using it, and skin felt so soft and velvety after that it makes you feel uplifted and good about yourself'.

Dr Brandt Lineless Foaming Cleanser

 We know – because you're always asking for recommendations – that many of you don't feel properly clean without a bit of foam from your cleanser. A real beauty innovation – from Dr Fredric Brandt, one of the US's leading skin cosmeto-dermatologists – this has a 'self-foaming action', yet doesn't strip skin of moisture. Botanical elements include circulation-boosting tangerine leaf oil, apple fruit extract (for firmness), green and white tea (antioxidants), plus grapeseed extract to protect collagen and elastin.

Comments: '10+! Loved its deep-cleansing properties – all my life I've been troubled with clogged pores, but now my skin has never been clearer; I just wouldn't want to be without it, left skin feeling fabulous, superclean and very soft' • 'easy to use, smooth, creamy consistency, skin has benefited' • 'loved the balm-like texture and pump action' • 'liked fresh smell, skin was improved – looked fresher and possibly firmer'.

Balance Me Cleanse and Smooth Face Balm ❀ ❀

8.88/10 One key action of an anti-ageing cleanser is to brighten skin – which Balance Me's does beautifully by buffing away flat, dead surface skin cells with the teensiest, gentlest particles of complexion-friendly oatmeal. The oil base blends antioxidant-rich Arctic cloudberry, shea and cocoa butter, rosehip, camellia, virgin coconut and kukui nut oils, deliciously fragrant with essential oils from Roman chamomile, lemon and red mandarin – all designed to be swiped away after 30 seconds of 'polishing', with a muslin cloth.

Comments: 'SPECIAL! The scent is lush, it leaves skin soft and glowing and himself (who notices nothing) told me he liked my perfume, even though it was just the cleanser!' • 'fantastic product: lovely to use, cleanses quickly, gently but thoroughly and leaves skin feeling soft, plumped and moisturised' • 'noticed blackheads disappearing from my nose with each use' • 'my skin's never been as good as this in my whole life: I love the feeling I'm "feeding" my skin with this' • 'would recommend to anyone with a dry, parched skin like mine'.

Rodial Glamtox Cleanser

8.75/10 This luxe cleanser, formerly known as the A-List Cleanser (as in the 'red carpet of facial cleansing'…), contains skin-lightening amino acids to target pigmentation and uneven skintone. We're told it has many celebrity fans – but we're more interested in these real-life comments from our somewhat more down-to-earth, un-famous testers.

Comments: 'Pleasure to use this smooth creamy gel balm, with gorgeous smell, removed all traces of make-up including waterproof mascara, the loveliest cleanser I have ever used!' • 'lovely silky, non-sticky texture like honey, left my skin feeling soft and moisturised, even and smooth – but price might make it sit in the "treat" category' • 'felt warm on skin, when washed off skin felt very fresh and clean, not at all dry' • 'removed all traces of make-up, no need for toner' • 'seemed to help the spots I get on my chin at certain times of the month; they disappeared and didn't come back'.

MV Organic Skincare Gentle Cream Cleanser ❀ ❀

8.57/10 Although this pump-action cleanser doesn't specifically promise anti-ageing benefits, our testers were so impressed by the radiance-boosting results it delivered, we felt we should include it. MV Organic Skincare is an Aussie brand formulated with many certified organic ingredients (although the final product isn't independently certified). One of our fellow beauty editors has raved: 'It's no exaggeration to say that the longer you use this range, the less make-up you'll have to wear.' It's suggested you remove the creamy, make-up-dissolving aromatic formula with a hot compress to decongest skin.

Comments: 'So loved this product: rich, not greasy, not runny, just lovely! Removed all make-up and skin felt great' • 'worked really well, smelt lovely, easy to use, great!' • 'nice and rich for my dry skin' • 'love the rose and chamomile smell, fantastic cleanser which calmed and soothed my skin and left no tightness, everything an all-in-one cleanser should be' • 'perfect texture once hands are damp – if dry it's too hard to spread'.

Pure Lochside Organic Orange Cleansing Oil

8.55/10 Cleansing oils are suddenly taking off in a big way (and we're not just talking about make-up…). This existing favourite with testers for *The Green Beauty Bible* was resubmitted for the new edition of this book, earning praise from mature testers, who in particular raved about the lovely soft orange/mandarin scent and skin-nourishing action. It's packed with omegas 6 and 9, antioxidant vitamin E – and is swiped away with a muslin cloth.

Comments: 'A lovely product which lasted a long while – and I'm truly hooked on the most wonderful scent' • 'made cleansing my skin a treat' • 'very versatile: as well as cleansing effectively morning and night I've used it as a facial oil' • 'skin felt beautiful afterwards – you could even give your skin a breather and skip cream' • 'I thought it might be a palaver to massage into skin and emulsify with water, but I love this more than my longstanding fave cleanser' • 'left it on for a deep cleanse and moisturise during a long bath and skin felt superbly soft and plump afterwards!'.

Learn to contour and sculpt your face

Over the years faces lose definition, with saggier and more padded cheekbones and jawlines. Here, make-up expert Mary Greenwell shares the secrets to creating a more sculpted, slimmer look

A little extra weight as we age can be flattering to the face. There's an old saying: 'After a certain age, you have to choose between your face and your a**e', and it's true. A little fat on the face plumps out the lines from within (as you'll know if you've seen, say, a fiftysomething friend lose a lot of weight – and watched what happens to the depth of her wrinkles).

However, the flipside is that as faces fill out they lose definition. Cheekbones and jawlines get more padded, pouchier and saggier. Even beauties like Grace Kelly and Catherine Deneuve look heavier-jawed, with less gloriously-winged cheekbones. Here, international make-up pro Mary Greenwell – who's made up many a gorgeous older face in her three-decade career – gives us the secret of 'contouring', for a slimmer-looking, more sculpted face. (And it's not the conventional wisdom.)

Always even out your skintone with primer and foundation first. Contouring on to bare skin, even if moisturised, could look dingy. Prepping properly gives the best effect plus staying power.

Use a fawn-y eyeshadow or a mineral powder. The traditional wisdom is that you should use bronzer for contouring but both Mary Greenwell and Terry Barber, director of make-up artistry at MAC (whose products Mary recommends for contouring) say, simply, don't! 'Look at the colour of the shadow under your chin,' says Mary. 'It's fawn. To mimic that, you need something with no red in it, and zero sparkle or shimmer.' Terry recommends

MAC's new-generation powder called Mineralize Skinfinish Natural, in a shade a couple of notches deeper than your skintone. It's 'satiny matt to give a moisturised finish', and will add definition without creating dull 'theatre' shadows. Terry advises a two-step approach: 'Add a hint of bright, fresh rose or apricot quite high on your cheekbones, then sweep the deeper colour in from your temples, under the lower half of your cheekbones.'

Use a blusher brush to apply the shadow (an angled one is good). 'Think "shade" here. Sweep the brush across the eyeshadow and tap the handle on a hard surface to remove any excess. To refine the jawline, sweep the brush along the underside of the jaw from edge to edge,' says Mary.

Don't forget right underneath the jaw. 'If you look at someone's chin and jaw, you'll notice that a real shadow goes all the way back to the angle at which the underneath of the chin meets the neck. So should the contouring. Apply lightly, and then add more until the jaw is more defined.'

Give yourself cheekbones, too. 'The principle is the same for under your cheekbones as under your jaw: same product, same brush. Start at the hairline by your ears, and sweep the shadow under the cheekbone. For a truly natural effect, you can apply a whisper of blusher (or blusher and bronzer) to your cheeks, as you normally would, on top of the contour powder.'

Spend an evening practising at home in front of the mirror. Ideally, use a 'triptych' mirror or angle a couple of mirrors so that you can see yourself from the side. If you long for a slimmer-looking face, contouring is an art worth mastering.

> If you *long* for a slimmer-looking face, *contouring* is an *art* worth mastering

Before you sign up for cosmetic fillers, read this!

If you're considering filler injections, laser treatment, a peel, Botox or even a facelift, it's essential to get as much information as you can first. Cosmetic surgery expert Wendy Lewis tells you all the questions you need to ask to help you get the best possible result

Whenever we want the lowdown on cosmetic procedures and clinical treatments, we turn to Wendy Lewis – aka The Knife Coach, who runs the truly independent Global Aesthetics Consultancy in the UK, Europe and America (as well as writing books, which we list at the back of this one). There is nothing Wendy doesn't know about who's the best, what's new – and the questions that every single woman should ask, not just before undergoing major surgery, but even having what may seem like a minor procedure such as Botox.

As Wendy says, there are – amazingly – people who sign up for fillers, Botox, lasers, peels and even full-blown facelifts without giving the issue much more thought than if they were shopping for a new face cream.

We can't tell you whether you should have a filler injection, or whether you really need a facelift. We believe this is very much a matter of personal choice (though ours is not to). But it is vital to know the right questions to ask before you take the plunge – to optimise your chances of a successful treatment and a good outcome.

Get real. Although some of the most popular procedures are non-surgical, none of them are non-medical. They should be performed in a clinical environment under good lighting and under the direction of a qualified and medically-trained professional. For example, wrinkle-relaxing and filling injections should only be done by a medical aesthetics practitioner, which in the UK includes doctors, nurses and dentists.

Have an initial consultation. Make an appointment with one or preferably two healthcare practitioners. Insist on having adequate time with the individual who will actually be carrying out the procedure – not an assistant or sales person. Your relationship with the person who will be doing your treatment is most important, and he/she is not interchangeable.

Ask serious questions (see box right).

Ask for detailed printed information on every procedure you are considering. Every doctor should have his own materials, pre- and post-treatment instructions, or at least brochures from companies whose products he/she is using, and there should be more consumer information on the websites of all of these brands. However, be aware that no honest or responsible practitioner can guarantee a specific result – we are all individuals and everyone responds differently.

Ask to see photographs of other patients. You should be able to look at real photos of clients who have undergone the procedure/ technique carried out by this specific practitioner. This is most important: there have been instances where one doctor may be showing patients another doctor's results, or labelling the filler company's 'before-and-after' photos as his own work. The caveat: be aware that you can expect to see only photos of the best-case scenario and judge from there – no one will show their worst results. It is impossible to predict the

TIP

Before treatment, Wendy recommends:

● Avoid aspirin products (Nurofen, ibuprofen), blood thinners or vitamin E for one to two weeks before treatment to prevent increased bleeding and bruising.
● Don't have a treatment on an empty stomach – you may get dizzy or faint.
● Ice packs before and after can help with pain and swelling.
● Bring concealer with you to cover up bruises or needle marks.

exact result that you may get from a procedure, but photographs offer a good guideline for what is reasonable to expect.

Check out the practitioner's qualifications, experience and training. Find out what professional organisations he/she is a member of and visit their websites for confirmation if needed. Check online to see if the practitioner has had any legal cases brought against them, and what the outcome was.

Tap into your intuition. How do you get along with the person who is going to be wielding the needle? You should feel you can trust him/her with your face and/or body. If you don't get a good vibe, move on. There are many practitioners and clinics to choose from.

Have a good look round. Is the clinic clean and orderly? Does he/she employ professional assistants and nurses? Ask to see inside the room where the procedure will take place, and satisfy yourself that it's the proper clinical setting necessary for a medical treatment. Also look at the other patients in the waiting room – do you like the way they look? And do you like how the staff and even the doctor look? If not, run a mile!

See DIRECTORY for organisations where you can research your practitioner and/or clinic.

WENDY'S VITAL QUESTIONS TO ASK

- What is the medical name of the treatment the practitioner is recommending?
- How long has it been on the market?
- How long has the practitioner been using it?
- What is the name of the manufacturer and where are they located?
- What clinical studies have been done?
- What is the source of the filler material – is it natural, animal or synthetic?
- What are the possible side effects?
- Could I be allergic to it?
- What does a reaction look like and how long does it last?
- What can be done if I have a reaction?
- How many treatments will I need and how often will I need to come back?
- How much will each treatment cost?
- If I don't like it, what can be done?
- Can I still have other treatments (fillers, wrinkle relaxers, lasers, peels) later?
- Is this the best laser technology/filler/injection to accomplish my goals?
- What are the alternatives?
- Does it have a CE mark (ie, comply with European Health and Safety legislation)?
- Is it approved by the US Food and Drug Administration (FDA) and UK Medicines and Healthcare products Regulatory Agency (MHRA)?
- Is it licensed for cosmetic use?

'I NEVER want to lie about my age. The actresses I *admire* are all women who have not fought growing older, but EMBRACED it – like Sophia Loren or Audrey Hepburn'

Penélope Cruz

Keep your eyes on the prize

For eyes, read 'angst'. They can be top of many a woman's list of beauty woes, as the years roll by. Think: puffy bags. Think: dark circles. Think: 'laugh lines' (that's the nice way to describe them). And then there's the challenge of applying eye make-up when a) skin's just not as smooth as it was, and b) you can barely see what you're doing anyway…

But leaving vanity aside (temporarily!), what should be absolutely paramount is eye health. Beauty may be in the eye of the beholder, but the bottom line is that we all want to go on beholding everything. So before we give you a rundown of products over the next few pages which will help with the beauty challenges, and share some fabulous make-up tips, here's how to optimise eye health – and help prevent eye-lines at the same time.

Don't frown! Forgive us for stating the obvious but how do you think frown lines get there…? Exactly. But looking after your eyes isn't just about a smooth forehead: taking very good care of eye health in general is absolutely vital as we get older. So…

Wear big sunglasses. Choose glasses which are UVA/B protective. And slap on a broad-brimmed sunhat, not just for the sake of your skin and hair but also, very importantly, for your eyes. Just look at the way people screw up their eyes and face in bright sunlight… Even in not-so-bright conditions, wind is a damage-doer too – and sunglasses provide great protection from dust, specks of dirt and the eye-drying effect of a mistral. Remember, they're also instant glam!

Take reading glasses everywhere and *wear* them. Sarah recently looked at a photo of herself trying to decipher a Christmas cracker joke and nearly choked as she saw the two deep lines scored down her forehead. Motto: must take specs – in chic case, possibly hanging round neck – with you at all times. (Jo keeps a pair in every room of the house, which is also very much appreciated by presbyopic friends.) If you are caught out and about without them, get someone to read to you – the menu, the programme, whatever. (One super-elegant friend takes a lorgnette out and about…!)

Have regular eye tests. The right specs help you read, work at a computer screen, drive safely and prevent frown lines and headaches. Testing can also pick up any other conditions such as glaucoma, which damages the optic nerve and may cause blindness if untreated. Every two years is a minimum when you're over forty, and every year if you have glaucoma in the family. NB: women over sixty in the UK can claim free eye tests and will usually get a discount on spectacles. (Remember to get at least one pair of prescription sunglasses, too.)

Attend to dry eyes. OK, it's age again! Like our skin, eyes get drier as we get older, especially if you work at a screen and/or in an office with aircon. If your eyes are itchy, sore, red, stick together on waking and, more seriously, you have any blurred vision, consult your family doctor or talk to your optician. Hopefully, it will just be a case of applying drops once or twice a day. (Sarah swears by Viscotears, a thin gel/ointment you can apply any time – but beware it can blur your sight for a few moments.)

Invest in a good, strong reading light. According to consultant ophthalmologist Professor Charles Clark, 'This can improve vision enormously, slow the deterioration of sight – and reduce

frowning!' Obviously, this isn't just for reading but for any close-up fine work, such as tapestry (which Sarah does – very slowly – in the dark winter evenings; Jo knits!). We like the range of lamps from www.seriousreaders.com, which have options for everything.

Consider a supplement. The 'Age-Related Eye Disease Study', sponsored by the US National Eye Institute, reported that two nutrients – called lutein and zeaxanthin, which are both found in healthy retinas – may help your vision and protect your eyes from the age-related condition called macular degeneration. A product called Brite Eyes Formula by LifeTime Vitamins is based on bilberry and eyebright, which contain these nutrients, plus a range of other helpful ingredients. Fish oil, which contains omega-3 essential fatty acid, may also help vision. But you should still eat lots of green, red and orange vegetables and fruit (full of lutein and zeaxanthin) plus at least two portions of oily fish weekly, if you're not vegetarian.

*A*nti-ageing eye creams: *our award winners*

Because eyes are so expressive – conveying joy, or sadness, or anger – the skin around them wrinkles faster than anywhere else on the face. The skin beneath the eyes also contains less collagen and elastin than the rest of the face. And as a triple whammy, this fragile skin is fine as eggshell – only one quarter as thick as that on the soles of your feet. (Precisely because it's so thin, moisture evaporates very easily)

But – hallelujah – we do know, from years of trials on real women, that there are plenty of products out there to make a difference to those expression lines. As of now, we've dispatched over 150 different creams to panellists for this book, requesting them to try them on one eye only. There were some truly spectacular performances – and three new award winners here.

AT A GLANCE

Clarisonic Opal Sonic Infusion System

Elizabeth Arden Prevage Eye Advanced Anti-Aging Serum

Barefoot Botanicals Rosa Fina Intensive Eye Serum

Murad Intensive Wrinkle Reducer for Eyes

Guerlain Orchidée Impériale Exceptional Complete Care Eye and Lip Cream

REVIEWS

Clarisonic Opal Sonic Infusion System

 8.88/10 We've always known that Clarisonic (despite the hefty price tag) had many devotees, but we've never put ten of them through their paces with our testers till this updated book. Testers used this smaller eye gadget with the accompanying Anti-Aging Sea Serum (with Canadian willow herb, oat kernel extract and Kigelia Africana fruit extract), but you can use it with your own eye cream, if preferred. Hugely impressive as a de-puffer for eye bags in addition to tackling lines. (See also INSTANT FACE REVIVERS, page 212, for other dramatic results.)

Comments: 'Skin under eyes looks really bright and fresh as if I'd had a great night's sleep when I hadn't' • 'after about three weeks my wrinkles are a lot less severe and early in the day, at least, one seems to have disappeared; have also used it around my mouth and nose and lines have faded there, too' • 'love the serum, which is like thick silk' • 'one of the best products I've used: skin instantly smooth and eyes less puffy, and my lines are definitely blurred' • 'feels like a little workout for your eyes, which appear brighter without any sleep – and lines definitely faded'.

Elizabeth Arden Prevage Eye Advanced Anti-Aging Serum

 8.6/10 From Arden's highest-tech range, this delivers high levels of idebenone, one of the most powerful antioxidants, alongside peptides, a green tea blend and an advanced moisture complex, designed to target puffiness and dark circles as well as lines. In general, because serums sink in faster, you can apply this type of eye treatment to lids in addition to the whole eye zone: they don't 'travel', and so avoid irritation.

Comments: 'After a few days I could see the difference and my "crow" lines seemed softer; I was also amazed by how well it worked on my puffy eyes and I had to start using it on both, as there was a noticeable difference' • 'fine lines, wrinkles, and certainly had an effect on fine lines which looked smoother because skin plumper; had a positive effect on puffiness and seemed to calm skin around eye socket; dark circles did diminish slightly' • 'really light, silky product; lines much, much fainter after six weeks; wrinkles less deep, skin much smoother; really loved it!' • 'people commented I look "fresh"'.

Murad Intensive Wrinkle Reducer for Eyes

 8.43/10 Dr Howard Murad's was one of the pioneering dermatologist brands in the skincare world, founded in 1989, and this features a breakthrough ingredient derived from the superfruit durian, alongside powerful antioxidants including goji berry, plus anti-inflammatories and moisture-boosting hydrators.

Comments: '10/10: fabulously hydrating, improved wrinkles, lines, puffiness, dark circles and crêpiness, made eyes look brighter and seemed to "lift" the area; my partner said the "test" eye looked better' • 'fine lines improved, deep lines less deep and defined, eye area looks younger, eyes much, much brighter and tired bags almost gone. I can see a real difference in the left eye. One of the best products I have used in a long time!' • 'finer lines definitely improved and skin more elastic and smoother, wrinkles less prominent, crêpiness of eyelids improved and disappeared after four weeks, puffiness definitely down, dark circles not gone completely but am hopeful. Several people said I look well'.

Guerlain Orchidée Impériale Exceptional Complete Care Eye and Lip Cream

 8.36/10 The ultra-luxe Orchidée creams have been a massive hit with *Anti-Ageing Beauty Bible* testers, who this time around highly rated Guerlain's 'double-duty' cream (it can be used on lips, too.) The range's key ingredient is a 'Molecular Extract' from four carefully-selected orchids (and of course, it comes as glamorously-packaged as you'd expect).

Comments: 'Crêpiness definitely reduced by this little darling; improved the whole general look of eye area and I got a couple of "you're looking well" comments' • 'plumped up wrinkles and works well around lips, helping to fill in lines' • 'absolutely love this and can't wait for the trial period to be over so I can use it on both eyes; beautifully hydrating without a hint of heaviness – love it, love it, love it!' • 'eyes definitely look brighter' • 'a lot of people have said I look different – "sort of radiant!"'.

dark circles, crêpiness all reduced and it seemed to "lift" the area' • 'lines reduced; I was pleasantly surprised – I've used lots of eye creams and this is the best so far' • 'skin around the eye zone a lot smoother' • 'eye make-up went on really well afterwards, including foundation and brow pencil – a real winner' • 'I know it's not cheap, but worth it: I'll definitely be buying this'.

Barefoot Botanicals Rosa Fina Intensive Eye Serum

8.49/10 This high-scoring, high-potency serum-style treatment product – despite featuring argan and rosa mosqueta (rosehip seed) oils – sinks in fast, according to delighted testers. Other key botanicals in this all-natural winner include frankincense, antioxidant vitamins A, C and E plus vitamin B5. The bonus: witch hazel promises instantly firming benefits.

Comments: 'Divine smell, I liked this product very much; I did notice a difference in crêpiness which in turn seemed to make eyes brighter. Would definitely buy' • 'the best eye cream I've tried so far; pleasant to use, didn't give me spots and lumps, fantastically hydrating, and made the skin look a little brighter and more radiant' • 'could apply make-up straight after; skin looked much more hydrated around eyes

&Lighten those dark circles

Fact: we get more anxious questions about under-eye circles to www.beautybible.com than almost any other subject (except eye bags and crow's feet). In a survey by Clinique of 13,000 users, about 53 per cent cited dark circles and puffiness as their number one concern. So here's how to make shadows, well, a shadow of their former selves

Conceal, conceal, conceal. Overleaf, you'll see the top light-reflective concealers, in our testers' considered opinions. If there's a shade choice, pick a yellow-based concealer if your dark circles have a purple or blue cast; go with a peachy colour if they are browner in tone. Meanwhile, women with darker skintones may find that light-reflective concealers just don't work for them – so you'll want to know that Guerlain Precious Light and the legendary YSL Touche Eclat come in darker shade options. And Bobbi Brown actually created her Corrector concealer specifically for dark circles, with the darkest shade being Very Deep Bisque.

Try Traditional Chinese Medicine. In TCM (as it's known in the holistic realm), dark circles can be linked to an imbalance in kidney energy – which can be helped by acupuncture. With TCM, as with all complementary therapies, seek out someone who is qualified and registered (see DIRECTORY for more details).

Drink plenty of water. For some women, dark circles can be a sign of dehydration. Another good reason to sip those eight glasses a day.

Consider using a cream targeted at 'sun spots'. For some women, dark circles can be linked to hyperpigmentation (see box opposite), in which case it may be worth trying one of the age-spot-lightening creams which performed best in our trials (see page 190). Don't apply so close to the eye that there's a risk of the product 'travelling' into the eye itself, as these can contain potent ingredients that might sting.

Try a D-I-Y Ayurvedic eye mask. Ayurvedic beauty expert Monisha Bharadwaj swears by a recipe for tackling dark circles handed down by her family. 'Crush five mint leaves in a little water with a pestle and mortar. Strain the juice and add to one teaspoon of almond oil and half a teaspoon of honey. Stir until completely mixed and apply a tiny amount under the eyes before going to bed.' Works wonders, she swears.

Clear your nasal passages. As nasal congestion is a common cause (see box right), clearing the respiratory tract may help. If it could be an allergy, try a supplement such as Aller-DMG, and also a barrier product (balm, cream or spray) in your nose which helps to prevent allergens being inhaled. A steam 'head bath' (also brilliant for your complexion) clears nasal passages a treat: fill a bowl with very hot water, add a few drops of essential oil such as eucalyptus, peppermint, rosemary, cover your head with a towel and steam gently for five minutes.

Try an antihistamine. If you think your underlying problem could be an allergy to an airborne substance (as in hayfever, or an allergy to something in a fragrance or cosmetic), an antihistamine could be a simple solution.

Eat dark-circle-busting foods. Certain antioxidant-rich foods may help to strengthen capillaries: edible eye TLC comes in the form of blueberries, cranberries, bilberries, blackcurrants, onions, peas and beans, as well as green and black tea.

Follow the dark circles blog! Believe it or not, there is an entire community on the net, written by dark-circle sufferers and focusing on women's experiences with many of the creams and non-surgical treatments on the market targeting this beauty challenge – www.mydarkcirclesblog.com is pretty commercial (and US-based), but it will at least reassure you that you are far from alone.

WHAT CAUSES DARK CIRCLES?

There are multiple causes for dark circles (medically called periorbital hyperchromia), according to medical research.

Genes They can be genetic, affecting any skin colour and type, but Asian and Afro-Caribbean races and southern Italians are particularly prone to them.

Hyperpigmentation The browner type of dark circles, rather than the bluish-hued type, could be the results of post-inflammatory hyperpigmentation due to sun damage or hormonal fluctuations, notes dermatologist Dr Nicholas Perricone.

Older, thinner skin As we age, we become more prone to permanent dark circles – simply because, as skin thins, the blood vessels in the under-eye zone show up more. Airborne allergens cause blood to pool in the vessels under the skin, worsening the appearance of any dilated blood vessels.

Nasal congestion Famously, they're linked with lack of sleep, but consider this insight from beauty guru Liz Earle: 'The most common cause of dark circles is nasal congestion. When your nose is bunged up, veins that usually drain from your eyes into your nose become dilated and darker.' Ask yourself if you tend to get them with hayfever during the summer, or ongoing colds in the winter. Equally something in your beauty regime could be the culprit (we have often found the finger pointed at a new mascara or eye cream, which may also cause puffiness).

Stress Dr Perricone also blames stress: 'When your body is in fight or flight mode, your brain, like every other organ, leaches every single molecule of oxygen it can from the blood, so a darker, more deoxygenated blood flows through your veins. This dark blood is most visible in the transparent skin under our eyes, and is what causes the appearance of these discoloured veins.' (The skin under the eyes is the thinnest on the body.)

Drugs Some drugs, including the contraceptive pill and HRT, can darken the eye area by dilating blood vessels.

Smoking Women who smoke – which affects micro-circulation long before it leads to heart and lung problems – can be prone to dark circles, too.

'I choose *NOT* to hang on to this **ideal** of looking 20 years old but **understand** that I have a wealth of EXPERIENCE to share. I make the *best* of what I have, but I don't long for who I *used* to be' Elle Macpherson

Concealers for dark circles: *our award winners*

At our age, a woman needs a (small) wardrobe of concealers. Here, you'll find the best candidates for disguising dark circles under eyes, which also work well on pigmentation

AT A GLANCE

YSL Touche Eclat

Lancôme Teint Miracle Perfecting Concealer Pen

Guerlain Precious Light Rejuvenating Illuminator

La Prairie Light Fantastic Cellular Concealing Treatment

TIP

Don't only apply light-reflecting concealer under the eye: a couple of dots at the inner corners of your eye, near your tear ducts and on the bridge of the nose, instantly makes eyes look fresher.

Three out of our top four are light-reflecting so they also blur lines – stroke them in grooves and wrinkles too, to see the effect of the 'optical pigments'. Light-reflective concealers can also be used to highlight the brow bone, or accentuate a pout, when stroked along the top lip; they can do double-duty as an eyeshadow base, too. Of the many, many choices now out there, our testers help you by narrowing it down to these top picks, including a new entry. (And for concealers to hide those other flaws, such as veins and redness/scars, turn to page 91. For products to help puffiness, see page 60.)

REVIEWS

YSL Touche Eclat

We make no apologies for the fact that this classic concealer has appeared in previous books – because we sent it out to be trialled all over again for *The Anti-Ageing Beauty Bible*, and Touche Eclat (aka Radiant Touch) romped home in first place with a fah-bu-lous score, just as it did before… Created by Terry de Gunzburg (who now has her own By Terry range) in 1992, it was the first of its type. And its legions of fans still think that this pump-action, pen-style concealer – with its built-in brush and light-reflective, line-blurring formula – is unrivalled. Our testers were assigned No 1 (Luminous Radiance), which has slightly peachy-pink hints. (NB: great news for women with darker skins: as of fairly recently, Touche Eclat is now available in a much wider range of shades. Hallelujah.) A Hall of Fame

product, if ever there was one.

Comments: 'Perfect for dark circles – the best product in my opinion! Didn't cover completely but blended them in and made them less noticeable' • 'looked very natural; I always carry one in my make-up bag' • be careful not to overdo or it can look too pale' • 'blended in well over a moisturiser or cream foundation but not as good over a mineral base; great cover-up job on thread veins round my nose and sun spots under eyes; ideal quick fix before morning school run' • '10+++ for this brilliant camouflage for dark circles, also great for lines on my forehead' • 'my magic wand – I thought it was all hype, but how wrong I was! It's easy to use, gives an amazing effect – so many comments about how well I look!!!'.

Lancôme Teint Miracle Perfecting Concealer Pen

This light-reflecting silver wand-style concealer comes in four shades (our testers had the lightest, 01), and is very lightweight in texture. Though designed to be used with Lancôme Teint Miracle Foundation, our testers trialled this alongside/over/under their regular base, with great results.

Comments: 'Looked more awake on mornings when I was tired and hadn't slept much' • 'blends easily and gives decent coverage without caking – I sometimes use it now when I'm not wearing any other make-up as it looks so natural' • 'I never bothered with concealers in the past, considering them a waste of money – but I love this and don't think I'm going to be able to live without it when finished' • 'this product fools people into thinking

Radiance Pigments and Precious Rejuvenating Complex. Which means that… Precious Light claims to offer skincare benefits as well as the instant cosmetic boost. Myrrh – known for its invigorating and rejuvenating powers – is a key ingredient. In three shades – our testers had the lightest, 01.

Comments: 'Fantastic at covering up quite dark circles under eyes, also small scars; a pigmentation mark on my forehead became invisible' • 'very easy to apply, blended well; brightened up dark circles, small scars looked less obvious; good coverage' • 'a must for your make-up bag' • 'very clever at reflecting light away from my face – great product' • 'very effective on my very pale skin; when I get tired it looks so obvious and this created a good complexion' • 'smooth consistency and didn't cake when built up thinly; made eyes look younger, also covered freckles and hyperpigmentation' • 'I used a lot on my dark circles but it didn't cake or crack, despite an evening of laughter and smiling'.

La Prairie Light Fantastic Cellular Concealing Treatment

8.11/10 The winning contender from this Swiss luxury skincare brand also promises longer-term benefits, as well as a quick dark-shadow-fix, with ingredients such as horse chestnut (to target dark circles), soothing Roman chamomile and arnica, plus papaya extract to target wrinkles, and LP's signature Exclusive Cellular Complex. It comes with the luxurious price-tag you'd expect of a La Prairie creation, but a refill (it's available in three shades) comes with the cylindrical silver-coloured container. It did divide testers, some of whom really rated it – while others were less impressed.

Comments: 'Very easy to dab in, covered and improved dark circles, worked well on small brown age spot by eye; certainly improved look of eyes without looking too made-up' • 'lightened and brightened eye area immediately, but would have preferred something more nourishing like my usual Touche Eclat' • 'not a miracle worker but I looked fresher and well-rested, can use under or over foundation to give a natural-looking foundation' • 'I like the luminosity it brings to the eye area, as if I've had a jolly good night's sleep'.

you've had eight hours of sleep!' • 'disguised dark circles and definitely gave a more luminous look' • 'definitely lives up to its promise of providing radiance' • 'looked very natural after being applied and patted into the skin' • 'pleased to find this didn't cake at all, even after wearing it all day'.

Guerlain Precious Light Rejuvenating Illuminator

8.4/10 Like Touche Eclat, this comes in a sexy gold wand, with a brush at the tip to sweep on a formula enriched with Gold

♡ WE LOVE…

To erase any hint of dark circles, Jo still turns to pen-style Clinique Airbrush Concealer in 04 Neutral Fair, which she also uses as an eyeshadow base. (It's a toss-up between Clinique's version and Dior Skinflash, which is more obviously light-reflective, and – she finds – better after dark.) Sarah gives thanks daily for Trish McEvoy's Correct and Brighten twist pen for shadows and darkness; it wouldn't cover very dark circles but is fab for brightening the eye area; swipe under eyes and over inside half of lids.

Unpack those eye bags

Maybe you get them just sometimes. (We all do.) Maybe they're the bane of your life. (As for many of our readers.) The simple truth is: none of us likes excess under-eye baggage and, as we age, skin loses elasticity, so the eye area can be more prone to swelling. Here are the best fixes we know…

Sleep with an extra pillow. If you can get in the habit of sleeping on your back (not everyone can – and remember it is the sleep position most linked with s-n-o-r-i-n-g), then this extra elevation can help to prevent fluid from building up in the eye area overnight. (Most puffy-prone women find the problem's worst before lunch – good reason never to be photographed until the afternoon…)

Check out eye products containing caffeine. In our experience (and anecdotally that of our testers), some products containing caffeine as an ingredient can be especially helpful for smoothing away puffiness.

Or give your eyes a drink of tea. Since caffeine has proven useful for banishing dark circles, a low-tech solution is two tea bags (black, caffeinated, rich in natural tannins), kept in the freezer rather than the fridge and placed on the eyes to constrict blood vessels and drain fluid.

Try a roller-ball. It makes perfect sense to us that something which has a physical action can literally smooth away puffiness – and sure enough, metal roller-balls can prove amazingly effective. You literally roll them around the puffy area in a circular/outward motion, to disperse fluid. As a low-tech version, real silver/silver-plated teaspoons kept in the fridge can be used to 'tap' away fluid. Jo uses a little silver-tipped applicator – like a baby drum baton – that she got with a Crème de la Mer eye product, for the same task: 'miraculous', is her verdict. It's an expensive way to get your hands on one of the most brilliant eye de-puffers of all time… so failing that, go the teaspoon route.

Have a chilled, gel-filled mask on standby in the fridge. There are quite a few on the market, although we prefer the type that don't have eye-holes, as they offer more even pressure (and cooling action) on the whole eye area. (The Body Shop's Aqua Eye Mask is excellent, or see DIRECTORY for other sources.) Lie prone, place mask on eyes for 10–15 minutes and let the cool gel work its soothing magic.

Eliminate your eye cream itself from the list of culprits. Sometimes a product which is designed to deal with lines and wrinkles can very annoyingly trigger puffiness. If you think there's any chance at all that your puffy eyes are product-related, stop using the potential culprit for five days and note any difference. If it's the cream, you'll know because you'll see an improvement. If it's not, your puffiness will be unchanged. Be aware that eye gels are less likely to 'travel' into the eyes themselves than creams; only gels or serums can be applied on the lids themselves, as there's a risk with any oil-based product of getting into the eye – and puffiness, as well as redness, is your body's sign of rebellion.

Reduce salt intake and drink less alcohol. Oh, we're a couple of killjoys, but if you're serious about this, cut down on salt and alcoholic drinks, both of which are notoriously linked with fluid retention. Ditto any foods containing MSG; you can ask in

WHAT CAUSES PUFFINESS?

As with dark circles, there's a long list of potential culprits and it can help to try to 'unpick' your personal trigger/s, so that you can take the lifestyle steps needed to minimise the problem. First (darn it): heredity – your genes may simply incorporate the DNA that leads to thicker fat pads under the eyes, in which case there may not be much you can do to tackle the problem. There is surgery available for fat-removal under the eyes, but if performed too early in life (or if too much fat is removed), this can lead to a really hollow look later on (not a good look). Second is water retention – which is linked with diet, sleeping habits, alcohol and even hormonal roller-coastering. Third, allergies can be responsible if you're allergic to pollen, pesticides, latex, certain foods, including grains and additives including MSG, cosmetics or fragrance. These can all trigger puffiness. And even the most smooth-eyed among us can get all pouchy with a cold.

Chinese restaurants for this ingredient to be left out, but it features in a lot of ingredient lists on processed foods, often by different names such as glutamic acid, vegetable protein extract, hydrolysed vegetable protein/HVP, sodium caseinate or even yeast extract. The safest way to avoid it is always to eat fresh, unprocessed foods. Foods which have a diuretic (water-banishing) effect include celery, cucumber, watermelon, radishes and parsley.

Do plenty of cardiovascular exercise. It revs up your circulation, which helps to eliminate excess water through sweating. In our experience, everything just 'flows' better when we've exercised – and a brisk 30-minute walk can work wonders for unpacking that eye baggage. A workout followed by a sauna or steam bath can flush out puffies almost miraculously.

Make like Linda Evangelista. Readers of our earlier books may be familiar with this trick, but it sure as hell is worth repeating: stroke an ice cube over the skin, working in an outwards direction. If you're prone to broken veins, wrap it in clingfilm first. Jo watched Ms Evangelista do this on a photoshoot and it was right up there with the miracle of the loaves and the fishes in terms of transformations. (Sarah has been known to order a bowl of ice simply to stroke round her super-sensitive, prone-to-puffies eyes.)

Treats for tired & puffy eyes: *our award winners*

There are two issues that we get more emails about to www.beautybible.com than almost anything else. First, dark circles (which we help you to conceal on page 56). Second, under-eye puffiness. Even if you've never had tired-looking eyes in your youth, the mid-years can be a time of excess eye baggage and shadows. Since bright, sparkling eyes make you look instantly rejuvenated, we're delighted to bring you the updated results of this trial – which proves that there are effective treatments to tackle these Big Beauty Challenges. Yes, in the blink of an eye…

AT A GLANCE

Estée Lauder Stress Relief Eye Mask

Repêchage Cell Renewal Eye Rescue Pads

Lavera Faces My Age Cooling Eye Roll-on

Clarins Skin-Smoothing Eye Mask

TIP

'I keep a bottle of witch hazel lotion in the fridge for when I wake up a bit puffy around the eyes. Soak two cotton pads in it, place them on your eyes and lie down for a few minutes. It really takes away the tiredness.' – Mary Greenwell

REVIEWS

Estée Lauder Stress Relief Eye Mask

 8/10 These see-thru gauze pads come in sachets (two pads per single-use sachet), to be pressed on to the under-eye zone while you relax for ten minutes and allow ingredients such as vitamin A palmitate, hyaluronic acid (for a moisture boost), aloe vera, cucumber, allantoin and bisabolol to soothe, hydrate and reduce redness.

Comments: 'A bit of a hero product this: puffy eyes from a cold visibly reduced, and my life-long dark circles much improved; also I am a big investor in eye creams and concealers and both work much better if I have used the mask before; when eyes are tired, tight and sore, the effects are very soothing, cooling and moisturising' • 'my sensitive eyes look brighter, fresher and more hydrated, made me awake again after a very hard day – brilliant when you want to go out after a long day' • 'love the cooling sensation, and made the dehydrated skin around my eyes look more plumped and moisturised – does what it says and is worth the money'.

Repêchage Cell Renewal Eye Rescue Pads

 7.98/10 These are pads, too (from a Manhattan spa brand): circular cotton versions, infused with moisturising seaweed elements and no less than four types of antioxidant tea to reduce puffiness and tone the area. Again, ten minutes should do the trick.

Comments: 'Eyes felt clear and bright and skin smooth and moisturised; the packaging for these pads says these are a vacation for the eyes and it really is the case' • 'because I felt so refreshed I needed less concealer around my eyes, and didn't pile on so much make-up; would absolutely buy' • 'really liked these pads which I kept in the fridge for extra de-puffing; using them in the morning after a late night was bliss!' • 'reduced puffiness and eyes did look brighter and renewed – very relaxing and great for a little pamper session'.

Lavera Faces My Age Cooling Eye Roll-on ❁ ❁

 7.98/10 For wannabe-natural beauties out there, a NaTrue-certified formulation which glides on to skin via a metal roller-ball (which delivers a lovely instantly-cooling sensation). Soothing botanicals include white tea to boost micro-circulation, vitamins, minerals, aloe vera and salicylic acid, a red and brown algae extract plus nurturing karanja oil (known to help prevent formation of new pigmentation marks), and beachberry to target existing age spots.

Comments: 'Putting this on after a long day was wonderful, very refreshing; my husband loved it too – and you can't get higher praise than that; fantastically – and surprisingly – reviving' • 'lovely cooling effect that reduced puffiness and eyes were

ANTI-AGEING
AWARD
WINNERS
BEAUTY BIBLE

♡ WE LOVE...

very refreshed' • 'eye area was clearer, less puffy and incredibly refreshed – felt fantastic' • 'roller-ball is very easy to use, and the light gel soaks in easily, gives a moisturising and firming effect as well as brightening and refreshing; very impressive little product that I would buy'.

Clarins Skin-Smoothing Eye Mask

7.7
10

This is akin to a face mask – but just for the eye zone, the idea being you apply lightly, then leave on for 5–10 minutes, removing the excess with a cotton pad to reveal de-puffed eyes. The botanicals in this include decongesting wild rose and saw palmetto,

hydrating rose water and apricot (hence the pretty smell), with chicory and rice starch for a tightening, 'firming' action.

Comments: 'Definite effect on puffiness and dark circles' • 'I'd never have thought of an eye mask other than the refrigerated gel ones you put in the fridge, but I'll use this whenever I need a little extra "help"' • 'eyes definitely looked perkier and more rested – it chased puffiness away' • 'improved crêpiness and eyes look brighter and less tired – really good product which would have passed me by without this trial!' • 'good rescue product after a poor night's sleep – made eyes appear firmer and smoother underneath' • 'a real treat'.

Don't let your eyebrows fade away...

Brows disappear – f-a-d-i-n-g away – if we're not careful. They may just get more sparse or go grey. Whichever, your face will quite simply lose definition – brows are the architecture of the face – if you don't either tint them (your hair colourist may be able to do this, albeit somewhat sneakily), or colour them in

TIP

Lots of clients ask expert Jenny Jordan about cutting unruly brows. She advises investing in a cheap pair of hairdressing scissors for this task. Brush brows upwards first, using a little soap on the brush to make them stick up. (It works a bit like a wax.) Then trim with the scissors – but not too close: brow hairs will fall downwards naturally and if you don't leave a bit, you may create 'huge' holes, she warns. Our advice: proceed with caution, but it can be done.

Brush on a mid-taupe/grey-ish powder shadow to colour your brows. This is most flattering for almost all brows, at this stage, to define them. Too dark and you risk that Cruella look. (Alternatively, use a pencil with a soft chalky texture – read about those which our testers got on with, overleaf.)

Extend the brow outwards, not downwards. Of course you need to follow the natural line of your brow, but by now many of us have lost the 'ends' of our brows (just plain vanished into the ether we guess) and if you need to recreate them with make-up, make sure the line wings out towards your temples, rather than down towards your cheeks. (Also see 'Plot your brow line', right.)

Brush your brows to groom them. By now, for many of us, brow hairs are literally all over the place – it sometimes seems as if they're all making a bid for freedom in different directions. A brow brush – or make-up genius Terry de Gunzburg recommends an old mascara wand that's been thoroughly washed – does the job beautifully. Brush them, apply colour, brush gently again. It makes for a much more natural effect. Legendary Hollywood make-up artist Valerie Sarnelle finishes off with her own Valerie Brow Tamer to keep them in place all day. London's brow goddess Jenny Jordan favours Tweezerman Browmousse, a gel which 'sets hairs in place without them getting crispy'.

And brush them again, if you use face powder. If you powder your face after you do your brows, you need to brush them one more time or (as expert Mary Greenwell notes), 'they can look dusty and dirty. And "clean" brows are really important at this time in life'.

Or you could try a stencil. Go gently because it can create a stronger look than many of us are used to: Valerie Sarnelle (known in Hollywood as the 'brow queen') created such a bold look for us that we nearly had fits at first. But the reaction from onlookers was so positive that we grew to love (slightly trepidatiously) the routine for special occasions. Several brands now offer stencils, including London-based brow legend Shavata. Soap & Glory's Arch de Triumph shaping and lifting pencil comes with pop-out stencils. Choose the shape you like and have a play, we say! Oh, and another tip from Valerie: team 'significant' brows with a sheer wash of eyeshadow and lots of mascara, or even false eyelashes, for a 'gorgeous, wide-awake look'.

Balance your brows with your eye make-up. More on your eyes means subtler brows; less eye make-up means you can play up your brows (as per Valerie's advice, above).

Generally

● Always tweeze in bright daylight, with a hand-held magnifying mirror, facing a window.

● Make sure the brow area is clean and grease-free.

● Use sharp, slant-edged tweezers which grip each hair from the root. Pointy tweezers are difficult to use on yourself.

THE EYEBROW FACELIFT

There's no doubt that 'clean and tidy' brows are essential to a glossy, groomed look. If you have thick brows (lucky you!), then getting them professionally shaped – at least to start off with – can be very helpful, and makes for easier home maintenance. Even if your brows have become sparse, a professional can often improve the shape. (Sarah's were mostly blown off in a gas oven explosion years ago, not helped by over-plucking before that, and they used to skyrocket up at the arch, giving her a rather shocked look. Manhattan expert Eliza Petrescu overcame the problem by carefully plucking hairs above the brows to 'flatten' the arch somewhat, which also worked to create the illusion of widening her thinnish face.)

There's tweezing, waxing, threading, depilatories – a bunch of professional ways of shaping and tidying your brows. Whichever you choose, do talk through what's going to happen and the results you can expect with the practitioner first: it's a bit like a haircut – you can sit like a rabbit in the headlights while your brows are exterminated, which happened to Sarah with threading… (Though Jo swears by it.)

At home, we think plucking – with good slanted tweezers – is by far the easiest way to tend brow shape. We have these tips from Jenny Jordan, whose Eyebrow and Make-up Clinic in London is a mecca for those in search of perfect brows. 'If you want to see the difference that brows make to a face, try putting plasters across your brows. Without them, your face has no shape,' says Jenny. 'As you get older, your brows can literally hitch up and hold your face in place. In the past few years, a new, straighter, upwards-slanting shape has emerged which is as good as a facelift.'

A word of warning: avoid over-plucking. If your brows are scanty, neglect them for a bit; applying olive oil or Vaseline every night may encourage them to grow (OK, that's a folk tale but a lot of people swear by it).

Plot your brow line

● The line slants gently up, starting at a point above the inner corner of your eyes, but with brows never more than an inch apart over your nose.

● It goes out to a wide-angled bend (rather than the old-fashioned extreme arch), above the point where the white begins at the outer rim of your eyeball.

● Then let the line straighten up, winging towards your temples. To find the outer edge, lay a slim pencil (or a slender-handled make-up brush) up from your nostril, past the outer corner of your eye – where it crosses your brow is the natural finishing point.

● The line should be neither fat nor slim, gently tapering to the outer edge – but do avoid the dated 'tadpole' shape.

● Swipe your tweezed brows with a cotton bud dipped in pure tea tree oil, which is a natural antiseptic.

● To fill in the line, Jenny likes to brush on taupe powder so it smudges into the line, and then fixes it with brow gel.

Brow pencils: *our award winners*

Life isn't fair. Just as hairs start randomly sprouting elsewhere on the face (see page 146 for how to tackle that), brows become finer, lighter – and can fade away drastically. Some go grey. Others just get fairer. Or sparser. But a well-defined brow – even if you have to 'fake' it – is near miraculous for helping to accentuate your features and give the face 'structure'. We've three fantastic high-scoring new entries in this edition…

AT A GLANCE

New CID i-groom Eyebrow Grooming Pencil & Brush

Suqqu Eyebrow Liquid Pen

Benefit Instant Brow Pencil

MAC Eye Brows

Although brow powders are now available on the beauty counters, we were interested to find that none of those we dispatched did well enough to be included in our winning line-up. Testers definitely preferred these pencils… NB: do try different shades, and remember that a lighter, softer shade than your natural brows can often work best.

REVIEWS

New CID i-groom Eyebrow Grooming Pencil & Brush

 A truly stupendous average score for a swivel-up propelling brow pencil which boasts a shaped 'rectangular' lead, facilitating thicker or finer strokes, as you choose. There's a built-in brush at the opposite end; several of the award-winners feature these, and they certainly are useful for post-pencil blending, as well as grooming stray hairs. To simplify life it comes in one neutral, suits-all-browtones shade.
Comments: 'Brilliant: the most natural eye pencil I have ever tried; so easy to apply and I felt confident using it as there was control over how dark I wanted to go and I could shape my brows without heavy mistakes' • 'having pale blonde brows I've struggled with pencils, yet dyeing looks unnatural – this is the first pencil in 40 years of wearing make-up that's worked for me!' • 'so easy to use – I am really thrilled with it' • 'stayed put all day' • 'easy to achieve natural results with light, feathery strokes' • 'they say one shade suits all; I tried it on my husband and it seemed to work quite well on him too!'.

Suqqu Eyebrow Liquid Pen

 We'd heard about this fine felt-tip from make-up artist friend Mary Greenwell – though until we tried it, couldn't imagine how the 01 Green shade could possibly work. But it does! (To be fair, it's mossy/taupe – and if you're still not convinced, it comes in an actual 02 Brown). Great for fine feathery strokes – and we'd recommend it for anyone who may have lost their brows through over-plucking or chemo, as with a little practise the results are super-natural and also totally budge-proof.
Comments: 'Produces absolutely perfect, long-lasting brows with the flick of a brush. My brows looked like they'd been professionally tinted – love it!' • 'I have never been much of a fan of brow pencils as they do look unnatural and clown-like – but this is a totally different kind of thing and very natural' • 'far from being the lurid green I'd imagined, the colour is a soft browny-grey which gives a natural appearance; I'm smitten with this little eyebrow marvel and I'll definitely buy another' • 'also tried it as an eyeliner and it works a treat!' • 'no sharpening required and very easy to create a natural shape'.

♡ WE LOVE...

Brow pencils are an essential part of our make-up arsenal: without them, Jo says her eyes 'vanish'. Having read our testers' comments Jo is an evangelical convert to the MAC award winner featured here, but has recently discovered Tom Ford Brow Sculptor (in Blonde) – also a twist-up option (with a useful built-in brush, and a lead shaped to allow for thick/thin strokes. Another long-term favourite include is Dior Sourcils Poudre Powder Eyebrow Pencil with Brush (which gives the effect of a powder shadow, stroked on in pencil format). Sarah is another brow pencil devotee – as a victim of over-plucking plus an exploding gas oven! Her all-time favourite is Arch de Triumph Brow Shaper by Soap & Glory, a double-ended pencil with foolproof soft taupe one end and pink highlighter the other. Plus it comes with three pop-out brow stencils, should you feel like playing...

Benefit Instant Brow Pencil

8.2/10 Benefit resubmitted this for our new edition – whereupon testers gave it an even higher score. In three shades (we tried Light), it's a more soft-textured pencil, transforming from a creamier texture to long-wear powder, with a brow-brush built right in to the other end of the pencil itself. Benefit pride themselves on brow expertise with over 500 brow bars in 22 countries and if you're looking to have yours shaped for the first time, these bars aren't a bad place to start.
Comments: 'Amazing; really, really pleased with the results which give a very professional make-up artist feel to my brows' • 'did a great job of making my brows look tidier and more uniform; loved the attached brow brush – overall, a great product!' • 'very natural, good quick-fix' • 'glided on so effortlessly – great to use! Asked my husband and a friend if it looked natural: both said my brows looked great, not fake at all' • 'I'm a convert, I don't usually use a brow pencil but this was so easy to use and gave me an instant lift'.

MAC Eye Brows

8/10 Probably the slimmest and most streamlined pencil on the market anywhere, this is self-propelling and self-sharpening. (Which means you're never at risk of harming skin with a wooden pencil stub. And yes, we know it happens!) It's super-easy to create fine, feathery strokes, and the initially waxy texture transforms to a budge-proof finish. Six shades to choose from (more than most brow colour options), spanning fair to dark; our ten testers received Lingering, a light taupe.
Comments: 'Very easy to apply, went on smoothly and beautifully, the fine tip is perfect for precise feather strokes and you really can't go wrong with the colour; slight waxiness helped hold brows in place; looked very natural – as if I had no make-up on' • 'the perfect brow pencil – although I have very dark brows, the light brown looked really natural on me, and blended in easily' • 'was amazed how much difference this made to my appearance – very easy to apply, I'm not used to using these but found it a doddle!'.

Your eyes are changing

...and so should your eye-make-up technique

As with foundation, we can't be as 'prescriptive' in this section as we are elsewhere in this book. (OK. Bossy!) That's because eyes present very different challenges. But here are your options, depending on your particular eye make-up 'challenges'. As make-up artist Terry de Gunzburg explains, 'The eyes become smaller and less "defined" as we age – but you can't just add lots of shadow, because the texture of the skin has changed and too much shadow, or the wrong texture (especially shimmer or pearlised products), can draw attention to wrinkly or saggy areas.'

'Of course, you can draw attention to your eyes,' says make-up guru Barbara Daly, 'but in a different way. Aim for a clean, defined look – smoky if you wish, but never that messy, come-to-bed-look of our youth...'

Try applying an eye base under your eye make-up. Then try again, without an eye base. See which looks better on you. Mary Greenwell believes that eye bases can make your eyes look over-done and over-made-up, but some women feel very self-conscious about the redness of their lids and like an eye base (aka eye primer) to smooth out the skintone before shadow. As an alternative, Mary suggests: 'Try going with the colouration. I love seeing a real eyelid. Apply eye cream and allow it to sink in, so your shadow has something to "cling" to; then put a bit of smudgy brown shadow on the lid – soft, warm, even mossy brown – and leave it at that, with light liner at the base of the lashes, and mascara. That may be enough.'

Eliminate dark circles under eyes with a light-reflecting concealer. Apply the concealer in the hollows under your eyes to brighten the area. (Our recommendations for the best products are on page 56.) A great tip given to us by expert Trish McEvoy for correctors and for brighteners is to stroke the product on as a triangle of lines, one under your eye, then the two sides sloping down to meet at a point on your eye-socket bone: then pat in lightly with a finger to cover the area.

A word on puffiness. If you tend to puffiness under your eyes, which Sarah does (often due to various ingredients in cosmetics or foods, also hay fever), first stroke an ice cube round your eye area for a few minutes then try a specific product such as Origins No Puffery (which we think is 'genius'!), or one of the other treats for tired and puffy eyes, on page 60. And don't draw too much attention to your under-eyes; a little mascara winged out to your temples, a fine line under the outer third of each eye and a spot of brightener (as above), under your eyes, high on your cheeks and also on the browbone draws attention away from the puffies.

And some secrets for hooded eyes. If your eyelids are actually drooping over your eyes, the only truly corrective option is surgery. But for less pronounced cases, use a highlighter/luminiser under your brow to 'lift' the eye, a very soft wash of taupe on the upper lid to mute it, mascara to define upper and lower lashes, plus fine eyeliner pushed into the lash-line along the lower lashes to draw the attention downwards.

Define the shape of your eyes differently. 'Using a dark shadow to create the "crease" in the socket, as you might have done when you were 20, just won't work,' says Terry de Gunzburg. She advises this approach to open up your eyes: over the lid try a sheer wash of matt eyeshadow, in a neutral shade (eg, mid-taupe – a sort of mushroomy-pink tone, but nothing muddy), then focus on eyeliner and mascara to frame the eyes. Try a sharpened eyeliner pencil or liquid product with an inbuilt fine brush – in grey, deep brown, aubergine or navy – pushed well into the lashes. (If you like, and have time, 'set' liner with a similar shade of powder eyeshadow on top. We often don't bother…)

Top with two coats of mascara. Apply the second coat before the first has dried to avoid clumping. We think soft dark brown can be more flattering for many women – though Trish McEvoy is a firm believer in black 'to enhance definition', for virtually everyone. (Jo goes for black, always.) Waterproof mascara avoids panda eyes, especially during hot flushes. (For more about eyeliners recommended by our testers, see page 68.)

If your 'socket crease' is unlined and droop-free, use a taupe-y grey or even a pale purple shade to accentuate the socket. We rather like a tip from our smooth-lidded singer friend Lulu, who applies powder shadow to the socket of her eye holding the mirror a good two feet (60cm or so) away, so she can gauge the effect from the distance most people see you from. (But then blend so the edges are seamless using a blender brush, holding the mirror up close.)

Add a touch of highlighter on the browbone. This is universally flattering (except possibly for those who have very high eyebrows, in which case it can make them look loftier). Dot on a touch of ivory or bone-coloured shadow, and if (but only if) the skin is smooth, it can be very subtly shimmering.

If you wear stronger shadow and eyeliner, play down your brows. Terry explains that it's all a question of balance. 'If you're wearing quite a bit of eye make-up, and you add a strong brow, you'll look like you've put on way too much make-up. But if you wear a sheer wash of shadow, and fine eyeliner, you can afford to add a bit more brow definition.' (See page 62 for more brow wisdom.)

There is truly no substitute for analysing the different effects yourself, in a mirror. With a discerning friend if available. Eye make-up is an issue where we can't be psychic and make up your mind for you about what looks best: you're going to have to experiment (do give yourself plenty of time for this), based on the advice above. And, of course, you can go and get free make-up consultations in-store from most brands, which might give you valuable tips and info (even if it's to show you what you don't like).

Eyeliners: our award winners

Mascara is only half the answer for lashes, which invariably become sparser over the years. An eyeliner also works extremely effectively to create the illusion of thicker, longer lashes. There are many options: pencil, gel, liquid, cream – and they all make a big difference to 'eye-oomph'. We recommend you experiment with different textures till you find the formulation that works best for you – and if you've never trialled a gel or cream liner, do give them a go

AT A GLANCE

Bourjois Effet Smoky Pencil

New CID i-gel Long Wear Gel Eye Liner Trio with Brush

Sue Devitt Eye Intensifier Pencil

Estée Lauder Double Wear Stay-in-Place Eye Pencil

Guerlain Eyeliner

Bobbi Brown Long Wear Gel Eyeliner

REVIEWS

Bourjois Effet Smoky Pencil

 An excellent score for this very affordable pencil, which comes in a range of smokily dark shades; we sent out a selection including Dark Purple, Deep Green and Smoked Brown. (We try always to send out identical products but sometimes brands don't play ball!) A creamier pencil for someone who wants a sultry, maybe even smudged effect from their eye definer.
Comments: 'Top marks: pencil goes on perfectly, very easy to apply precisely; smooth texture without being too soft, smudges easily but controllably' • 'comes with a brush on the other end which is ideal for softening and smudging' • 'cheaper than my usual Clinique pencil and just as good for my very sensitive eyes' • 'didn't drag at all • 'I *love* the pointy brush, so you can soften the line precisely as you want it; product wore well all day'.

New CID Cosmetics i-gel

 The subtitle of this tells you pretty much all you need to know – Long Wear Gel Eye Liner Trio with Brush – and our testers had the Bronze, Copper and Stone version. There's a built-in mirror in the lid, while the brush is flat.
Comments: 'Very long-lasting: stayed put from first thing in the morning till I got home from the office' • 'I've tried many liners but have never been able to achieve the clean-lined look before – this takes

away all the hard work' • 'a dream to apply and love the colours (great for green eyes)' • 'haven't used liner in years but am converted: so easy to apply, with no dragging.'

Sue Devitt Eye Intensifier Pencil

 This stubby, velvety-textured pencil is one of Jo's faves, because it delivers quite intense effects very speedily. Like the Bourjois entry, this is one for the Bardot-esque smoky-eye look. But there's a useful 50 seconds to play in before the colour sets: we tried Bangalore and there's a choice of 12 shades.
Comments: 'So easy to apply I didn't even use a mirror; soft creamish texture; excellent sponge tip for smudging but once applied didn't smudge unintentionally – fantastic!' • 'amazingly easy to apply, no skill needed, although it's fat and chunky is better than its slimmer sisters' • 'I use lots of eye pencils from all brands, but this is the best ever, blends like a dream and has real staying power' • 'couldn't draw a very fine line but gives a good smudgy look – an instant eye make-up when you can't be bothered to do the whole eye thing!'.

Estée Lauder Double Wear Stay-in-Place Eye Pencil

 As the name implies, this double-ended pencil (colour one end, blender/smudger the other) comes from a capsule Lauder collection created to deliver specifically long-wear results. It features silicone technology to deliver stay-true colour for up to 12 hours. We normally ask for black or dark neutrals, but on this occasion our testers enjoyed the subtly shimmering Bronze shade, one of seven jewel-rich tones.

Comments: 'Anyone should find it easy to apply precisely, and also very smudgeable – and it stayed like that until I took it off, how refreshing!' • 'very useful and versatile, and lasted well' • 'creamy, easy to apply and sticks to your skin until you remove it' • 'what a dream, perfect consistency for an eye pencil, went on smoothly and evenly, and precisely, as long as I kept it sharp'.

Guerlain Eyeliner

7.94 / 10

Steady of hand? Fond of a kitten flick? Love a touch of Marilyn…? This is your best eye-lining bet: the only liquid-style option to have impressed testers, it offers a long, pen-like lid for calligraphy-style application. Testers had Noir Ebène 01, a black-brown and one of three sultry long-wear shades.

Comments: 'Love it, love it, love it! Compared with other liners (mid-ranged and higher-priced) performed well, lasted all day (and some nights!) • 'gorgeous, stylish product which adds a touch of

old-fashioned glamour to my dressing table' • 'like the way it can be used for a thin line or a dramatic, thicker line – all effects easy-to-achieve' • 'fine line against lashes makes them look thicker; lasted all day but easily removed at night'.

Bobbi Brown Long Wear Gel Eyeliner

7.83 / 10

One of the first gel eyeliners on the market, it's a beauty classic, created to withstand heat, humidity, even rain. As you get to know this product – which glides on smoothly – you'll learn it can be layered easily, for extra intensity. Packaged in a chic little 'inkwell'-style bottle, our testers tried Caviar Ink, which is a deep black brown. NB: it doesn't come with its own brush so you need to acquire one.

Comments: '10/10: perfect for a novice, really easy to do a smooth line, and good for me as a contact-lens wearer; needed a separate brush; lovely creamy, smooth texture which lasted well with no smudging or flaking; really opened up my eyes – they looked brighter too' • 'this is now my desert island product, it survived two weeks in a very humid Florida, including a torrential rainstorm' • 'I thought the colour would be too dark but it made my lashes look a lot thicker, and it's long-lasting if you apply a base or powder shadow first'.

♡ WE LOVE…

Jo is a sucker for a smoky eye pencil, in particular the ultra-chunky Sue Devitt Eye Intensifier Pencil testers rated. But she often layers a gel or cake eyeliner over the top, to enhance the staying power of this soft pencil: Bobbi Brown Long Wear Gel Eyeliner or Laura Mercier Tightline Cake Eye Liner (you need the 'matching' Eye Liner Brush), or sometimes the New CID Cosmetics i-gel (she likes Granite, Graphite and Carbon, a trio of deep grey/blacks). Sarah's eyes just don't look good smoky, so she bucks the pencil trend and loves YSL's liquid Easy Liner.

Cream eyeshadows: our award winners

Cream shadows are easiest to blend on more 'mature' eyelids – and in a pale neutral can also become a fabulous base for other shades. They're also a lazy, 'everyday' option for a fast make-up effect if you swipe on a taupe-y neutral shade. The right formulation is a must, though – because you want to avoid 'creasing'. With that in mind, we've now dispatched over three dozen cream shadow options to our testers – including a new and improved one, which rocketed to the top of the charts – asking for feedback on smoothness, ease of application and endurance

REVIEWS

Clinique Lid Smoothie Antioxidant 8-Hour Eye Colour

We panicked slightly (and we're sure we're not alone) when Clinique withdrew the previously category-winning Quick Eyes Cream Shadow – but we needn't have fretted, because this is a top-notch replacement, available in 12 shades. (Our testers received one of two neutrals: shimmering ivory Cashew Later, or taupe-y Seventh Heather.) With an angled tip (like many lipglosses), it glides smoothly onto the lid with a 'cooling action', and features skin-caring ingredients including plenty of antioxidants.

Comments: 'I've really sensitive skin around my eyes and most products make my eyes water, but this shadow soothed my skin if anything' • 'previous memories of cream eyeshadows is that they're often quite sticky/tacky, but not the case with this, which has a dry, smooth texture and is silky to the touch' • 'LOVED this product: finish even and smooth and both colour and finish lasted right though till evening, despite being out in the rain and wind for the morning' • 'suits my two-minute make-up routine, applying evenly and smoothly with a finger' • 'cream shade brings a touch of flattering gleam to the brow-bone, delivering a bit of "lift"' • 'loved how light this felt on my eyelids; my eyes looked alive!'.

Bobbi Brown Long-Wear Cream Shadow

'At last, a cream eyeshadow that stays on and doesn't crease', promises the Bobbi Brown blurb – and as our testers' comments go to show, this pretty much lives up to that. In a cute small pot (you dip with fingers or use a synthetic brush), it offers a 'breathable polymer technology' (which delivers the long wear and makes it crease resistant), and it's also recommended 'for oily eyelids'. Bobbi is of course known for her super-wearable shades – and there are 20 to choose from, mostly matt but some with a slight shimmer. Our testers trialled Cement, which they found good for daytime on its own, or as a base for evening colours. NB: as some testers pointed out, the little pot is not the most portable.

Comments: '10/10 for the easiest to apply eyeshadow I've ever used, either with brush or finger; the smoothest most velvety texture, matt finish but not flat; have binned all my other eyeshadows and bought several more of these' • 'made the slightly crêpey skin on my eyelids looks as smooth as a teenager's again' • 'long, long, long, long-lasting! Stayed put with great finish and same colour – work means my make-up can be on for 16 hours, this was still fresh at the end' • 'seemed to fill all imperfections; made eyeliner apply easier and last longer on top of it; wish I'd discovered this before' • 'loved the creamy texture

AT A GLANCE

Clinique Lid Smoothie Antioxidant 8-Hour Eye Colour

Bobbi Brown Long-Wear Cream Shadow

Benefit Creaseless Cream Shadow/Liner

Shu Uemura Cream Eye Shadow

which was easy to apply, and the colour, and it lasted! But found the opening of the pot too small for fingers once the contents went down a bit, so you need a brush' • 'gave soft wash of colour that you could build up, didn't cake at all, just a smooth veil of colour'.

Benefit Creaseless Cream Shadow/Liner

 Crease-proof, smudge-proof, offering 'buildable' colour with a choice of 12 shades. Our testers tried Flatter Me, a creamy metallic rose gold colour, with quite a lot of shimmer (some felt too much) but a smooth, flattering finish, they commented. No applicator is provided, so you may need a brush. Benefit may sometimes seem like a young range but pros love their make-up 'Fix-Its' (and so do we).

Comments: 'Can I give this 11 out of ten? Easy peasy to apply, and so simple to layer up if you want to, use both fingers and brush; shimmery but subtle finish, a sheen rather than shadow – yes, oh yes, I would buy, I loved this and so did the other women in my family (had to lock it away) – it gave me so much pleasure!' • 'very easy to use with a brush, spread easily to give a wash of colour and could be built up into stronger coverage; so you could have it subtle or dramatic' • 'lasted about four hours' • 'felt like a creamy powder, if that makes sense! Quite smooth to use, and easy to

blend in and didn't cake' • 'packaging is adorable – glass container, with a large lid in a pretty little box, makes applying it feel like a ritual'.

Shu Uemura Cream Eye Shadow

 Loved by make-up artists the world over, Shu Uemura are known for their bold shades – but search hard, and you'll find some wonderful, more neutral tones within the Shu range, including the Taupe our testers trialled. Again, the shadow's creators promise that it won't fade, crease – and that this comfortable 'stretch' formula is even waterproof.

Comments: 'Great product; never used cream before but I really liked it for a natural daytime look; lovely and kind to small lines and creases' • 'silky finish that glided on, really smooth and crease-resistant, blended beautifully and stayed put all day and into the night' • 'finish improved when I set it with a little powder, which prolonged it too' • 'best applied with a brush and once I'd achieved an even colour it looked great; slight shimmer which looked best in the evening for me, lasted a lot longer than my usual powder shadow, and the overall finished effect was more dramatic' • 'stayed put brilliantly, lasted all night without any signs of disappearing (out late so didn't take off make-up, naughty I know!)' • 'lasted well in a hot climate'.

8 Mascaras: our award winners

Lashes get thinner and sparser over time, so mascara is even more essential to help define the eyes and structure the face. However, there's no such thing as a one-type-fits-all mascara – so here are the top recommendations with details of what they do. On this page, the non-waterproof versions – see opposite for new entries to get you through rain and weepy films!

AT A GLANCE

Non-waterproof

Estée Lauder TurboLash All Effects Motion Mascara

Clinique High Impact Mascara

YSL Luxurious Mascara for False Lash Effect

Lancôme Hypnôse Drama Instant Full Body Volume Mascara

Waterproof

Paul & Joe Waterproof Mascara

Clinique Lash Power Mascara Long Wearing Formula

Chanel Inimitable Waterproof Mascara

Estée Lauder Sumptuous Waterproof Mascara

TIP

Do replace your mascara every three months for best results and to avoid 'bug' build-up.

NON-WATERPROOF MASCARAS

Estée Lauder TurboLash All Effects Motion Mascara

 8.89/10 Suddenly, there's a new category of mascara: vibrating mascaras, which imitate the effect of wiggling the brush from root to tip, for extra curl and coverage. A gimmick? Not according to our testers, who gave TurboLash a really excellent mark. The long, slim brush makes it easy to access all lashes – and a bonus is that once the battery in the LashSonic brush has breathed its last, you know it's time for a fresh mascara. Jo has found that it's the only mascara she's ever used which can be reapplied after a day at the office, as the vibrations break up clumps. (NB: a little D-I-Y is required to install the battery!) This retains its top slot, despite many new contenders trialled.
Comments: 'I laughed when I saw this! What next? But it's just a gentle whirring, then it's magic! You put the wand against your lashes and it starts to coat, separate, curl, lengthen – golly!' • 'I was very sceptical but this is excellent, making lashes longer and thicker with two coats; but had to decode instructions for battery first!' • 'no clumping, good separation of lashes, fantastic lengthening and thickening effect – looked like false eyelashes!' • 'lashes looked longer, thicker, curlier'.

Clinique High Impact Mascara

 8.75/10 We love Clinique's precision: this, they say, gives 'up to a 26-degree curl'. We know from experience there's plenty of 'playtime' while you're applying, but the high-impact brush delivers results with just a few sweeps. This too has lash-conditioning waxes in the blend. (Particularly good for extra length and curl.) As with the Lancôme mascara opposite, this was re-entered and did even better this time round, so we've included testers' new observations for both.
Comments: 'Fantastic staying-power with a dramatic effect on eyelashes, yet felt natural not heavy' • 'Five *****! Best I've ever tried: leaves lashes luscious all day, yet easy to remove' • 'I suffer from blepharitis, which makes my eyes water – yet this really coped well without smudging or running, or irritating eyes' • 'still going strong at 10 p.m.' • 'I'm the world's worst for mascara flaking but this held its own' • 'happy with the glossy, dark-pigmented results from just one coat'.

YSL Luxurious Mascara for False Lash Effect

 8.7/10 A bit of a legend in beauty circles, this: we know lots of beauties who swear by the va-va-voom results False Lash Effect delivers, and this was backed up by our testers. The formulation includes beeswax, carnauba and candelilla waxes plus pro-vitamin B5 for lash-conditioning, nylon micro-particles to boost lash diameter – and the brush is generously fat. Good for volumising. (Also in a waterproof version.)
Comments: '10/10 for the lustrous finish and lengthening plus natural curl; loved the wand' • 'no clumping, excellent glossy, lustrous finish, very good at thickening, excellent lengthening; a new-found gem for evenings' • 'looked realistic but in an exaggerated way! Just what I want in a mascara, one coat was plenty' • 'fat brush was very good for top lashes, a little harder to angle on lower ones, lashes looked longer, thicker and curled nicely – and not false' • 'fantastic lash-lengthening, looked glossy and loved that it was "extra-black"'.

Lancôme Hypnôse Drama Instant Full Body Volume Mascara

Retrialled for this edition (and notching up a higher score even than for its first appearance), this looks wonky when you take the wand out of the tube – but it's specifically curled like an 'S' to follow the lid-shape, allowing for easy access to even the shortest lashes. A smooth, non-sticky formula promises easy glide through lashes for dramatic, volumised results. The original Hypnôse mascara became the world's best-seller after its 2004 launch. (Good for volume, testers say.)

Comments: 'Easy to apply, left lashes longer and silky-looking and looked as good at the end of the day as when applied' • 'will definitely buy, recommend and spread the word to friends: brilliant coverage and lasting effect of long, luscious lashes, with fantastic staying power' • 'a friend even noticed my lashes looked good and asked what I was wearing – I'm a convert!'.

WATERPROOF MASCARAS

As we age, eyes become more sensitive to light, and often to allergens. The result? Eye-wateriness. Our panellists have now put more than three dozen waterproof mascaras through their paces in daily life (as well as the shower and pool). Here are their enduring (!) favourites, with three high-scoring new entries. Those promising curl and length did better than volumising ones. Be warned: you need specialist waterproof eye-make-up remover!

Paul & Joe Waterproof Mascara

From a 'cult' brand better known for fashion-forward shades and gorgeous boudoir-esque packaging, a seriously high-scoring mascara that really stayed the distance! Testers universally loved the wand, the finish, the curling effect and the endurance of this mascara.

Comments: 'Wow – this stuff doesn't budge! I didn't have any trace of a smear after a long, hot shower; gave great length, curl and thickness' • 'truly waterproof – the mascara I've been looking for over 40 years – thank you Beauty Bible!' • 'no clumping, even after a few weeks of use; stayed put all day' • 'I'm not really a fan of waterproof mascaras but this is a cut above the rest: fluttery, coal-black lashes, a perfectly-shaped wand that coats every lash, and a mascara that stays put through hell and high water'.

Clinique Lash Power Mascara Long Wearing Formula

Ideal for the sensitive-eyed, originally created for the ultra-humid conditions in Asia but wowing us in the West, now. Removes with warm water, not make-up remover! (Several testers failed to grasp this essential fact.)

Comments: 'Didn't budge through a five-mile run and only smudged in the shower because I washed my face with foaming cleanser' • 'incredibly easy to apply, and easy to get to corner lashes; now most definitely top of my mascara list' • 'very natural result, no clumps' • 'stayed on surprisingly well yet it was really easy to remove; a great mascara – oh, and it survived a Body Jam class! (Still not a good look with a bright red face, though...!) • 'the brush was particularly good for defining shorter lashes; it flaked a bit but does have incredible staying power'.

Chanel Inimitable Waterproof Mascara

The revolutionary rubber wand (technical-speak: 'soft elastomer') grips lashes beautifully, enabling a real curling action, plus definition and separation. (Great for sparser lashes, we've observed.) As testers observed, you need a really effective remover to get it off.

Comments: 'Fab product, really great performing mascara, which made lashes longer, thicker, more curly and separated, with glossy lustrous finish – and no mascara to be seen on my face in weepy movie or shower' • 'didn't budge through rain and weepy movie, though smudged slightly in shower and swimming pool; didn't flake or crumble; lengthening effect very good' • 'especially good on bottom lashes, made them significantly thicker without glooping together, very pretty: my eyes really stand out – cut onions with no problem'.

Estée Lauder Sumptuous Waterproof Mascara

Lauder promise this 'gives you all the thickening of a brush with the definition of a comb', sweeping 'Micro "Y" Lock Fibres' and 'fumed silica' on to lashes, with mica and kaolin clay to boost volume. There's a 'soft-flex' polymer to prevent brittleness.

Comments: 'Unlike many, this mascara really is waterproof – and not clumpy at all' • 'didn't flake, crumble, smudge – amazing!' • 'I was amazed: this was fantastic at lash-lengthening, swept on and lashes just grew and grew' • 'we should all have this tucked away for holidays, weepy movies etc. – the best I've ever used' • 'glossy and luxuriant'.

♡ WE LOVE...

We have both kissed many frogs en route to discovering our perfect mascara. Jo likes a defining mascara for her somewhat sparse and pale lashes; 'volumising' mascaras skate off her lashes without depositing a molecule of colour. A new fave is Diorshow New Look Mascara with an amazing brush that accesses every lash; she's also a fan of the winner here, Estée Lauder's vibrating TurboLash. Born with Jersey cow lashes, Sarah was in denial for years about thinner 'eye fringe' but can look overdone with volumising mascaras. For day, she loves Dr Hauschka mascara, and for evenings, the Le 2 de Guerlain mascara, ultra-glam with a genius double wand. (There's also a waterproof version.) Jo's long-term favourite waterproof mascara is Chanel Inimitable Waterproof Mascara (see left), which survives her daily summer dips in the Channel without a smudge. Sarah uses the Chanel too but warns, 'do invest in the remover or you'll wake with unattractive panda-eyes'.

Lash-boosting treatments: *our award winners*

This is an entire new treatment category. Just a couple of years ago, there were one or two contenders – and now there's more than a couple of dozen lash-boosting options out there. Do they work? Testers put them through their paces over a period of months, looking out for ongoing benefits as well as instant effects. Sadly, following a reformulation, a previous high-scorer did less well – and most other targeted lash-boosting products got dismal scores. So we're back to recommending more 'cosmetic' lash-boosters, at this stage…

AT A GLANCE

Elizabeth Arden Lash Optimizer – Primer with Conditioners

Lancôme Hypnôse Precious Cells

REVIEWS

Elizabeth Arden Lash Optimizer – Primer with Conditioners

You know about make-up primers. Well, this is a lash-primer (white in colour) to enhance the effect of your mascara so lashes look thicker and longer. Yes, yet another step in your beauty routine – but this is designed to make your mascara stay put and at the same time make lashes softer, healthier-looking and more supple, with less breakage. Our testers awarded it a pretty impressive score; here are their comments. Even after trialling several new products for this paperback, it retains its lash-boosting crown.

Comments: 'Really liked this product, easy to use, didn't flake/crumble/smudge/clump, and made my lashes look longer' • 'mascara-style wand made it easy to coat the conditioner on your eyelashes' • 'lashes considerably longer and seemed to improve staying power of my mascara; as I used this for longer, I started to see more benefits with lashes softer and in better condition' • 'really good at lash-lengthening and lashes were also thicker, just had to make sure I covered all the white'.

Lancôme Hypnôse Precious Cells

We'd categorise this as a 'lash-caring mascara': the cream formula sweeps on to lashes to deliver not just volume and definition, but also a Lash Densifier Complex conditioning ingredient derived from plant cell extract from apples. Lancôme are renowned for their mascaras, and this has been formulated in their labs to boost lash strength. Our hunch is that the 'trickle-down' effect we're seeing will continue – with the result that more mainstream mascaras will promise more than just here-today-gone-when-you-take-your-eye-make-up-off lash benefits. For now this is the best of the bunch – although the lash-enhancing effects testers perceived were (mostly) temporary, lasting only while it was worn.

Comments: 'Lashes not much curlier, but definitely thicker and longer' • 'my new favourite mascara: lashes appeared longer and denser after use – especially after two light coats, almost as if I had more lashes!' • 'very easy-to-use wand: no gadgets or silly features; a lovely, straightforward mascara that's not too wet, not too dry, not too smeary – and I love how "black" it is' • 'I've had my lashes professionally "enhanced" and extended before but the results with this were much more natural'.

TIP

We have supersensitive eyes and have suffered dreadfully from some eye products. The big companies have to be incredibly careful with testing but may we suggest you observe the following advice:

● Make absolutely sure the conditioner is ophthalmologically-tested (it will say so on the packaging), and ideally is endorsed by eye-care professionals.

● Stop immediately if you do experience irritation. It's not normal for eyes to be irritated or for you to experience any form of blurred vision. If this does happen, we suggest you contact the manufacturer immediately, and press for a refund.

● Be careful! Most products are swept along the lash-line using a fine brush; take care not to get the product into the corner of your eyes, and don't apply if you're wearing contact lenses. If you're using lash conditioner in the morning, allow it to dry 100 per cent before applying anything else.

● Have patience. Most lash conditioners suggest nightly application for maximum results. Use as ritually as you would a cleanser, toner or moisturiser.

♡ WE LOVE...

Jo tried quite a few and had to give up because they make her eyes itch, but has finally had good results from Rimmel Lash Accelerator Mascara which really does seem to have had a slight lash-thickening effect. Sarah admits to being too lazy to remember to paint on the longer-term ones daily; of the quick fixes, she agrees with testers that the Elizabeth Arden Lash Optimizer is very effective. And don't forget that Joan Collins swears Vaseline is the best lash conditioner ever!

'Wrinkles don't
scare me;
they are a part
of LIFE and I
will and do
EMBRACE them.
But I look at
surgery and that
scares me'

Christy Turlington

Get glowing – by recharging your skin

A visit to a facialist for a skin-reviving treatment is a rare indulgence for most of us – but in this book we show you the amazing masks, scrubs, creams, oils and transforming techniques that you can use at home to give your skin a real boost…plus insider tips from the experts

There are several ways to wake up your face fast. You can go the professional route: trek to a salon, have your face massaged (or needled as in acupuncture – see page 155), be slathered with creams (and lie there hoping you're not getting a parking ticket). Or you can go the D-I-Y route, which is infinitely cheaper and more accessible. Now, that's not to say we don't love a facial – see a list below for some of our favourite facialists. But realistically, who has the money or, just as importantly, the time to indulge more than once in a blue moon…?

Your daily regime is one thing. But it's easy to be lulled – out of sheer inertia and/or laziness – into doing the same routine for your skin, day in, night out. So we really, really can't encourage you too strongly to try some of the products and the face-transforming techniques in this book.

You can achieve a huge amount – near-miraculous, actually – with a simple, at-home, two-step blitz: a gentle-but-effective exfoliation, followed by a mask. On the next pages, you'll find our diligent testers' top facial scrubs and masks – the skincare wonders that, over the space of 18 months' research for this book, they identified as being the most effective on the market. And on page 212 you'll also find our rundown of the best

'instant face-revivers', packed with glow-getting ingredients that boost skin circulation, and are absolutely fantastic for emergencies (hangovers, jet-lag, or after a cold or flu, when skin can look positively grey). They're as close to eight hours' sleep-in-a-jar as you're going to get.

Throughout this mini-section of the book, we've also included some 'trade secrets': insider tips to try at home, from facialists who we rate and revere – and who, if we had a lunching-lady sort of life, we might see more often ourselves. But even though we're beauty editors, we can't justify that sort of indulgence as frequently as we might like.

But try the products, too, and prepare to be amazed.

5-MINUTE FIX FOR TIRED FACES!

Facialist Suzie Mitchell (who's local to Jo in Hastings) is something of a miracle-worker for tired faces. She has this tip for temporarily 'ironing' away lines from the face and boosting glow.

● Put a little facial oil in one palm and rub hands together, then smooth over face, neck and bosom.
● Rather than fingertips, use the big muscle in the cushion at the base of your thumb, always working upwards.
● Start by fanning out over and round your neck, then work round and up your jaw and cheekbones to the temples, then across and up your forehead to your hairline.
● Repeat, covering the whole face for five minutes. The oil will be absorbed, skin velvety, and your face look rosy and 'lifted'.

'You only perceive the *real* beauty in a person as they get OLDER'

Anouk Aimée

IF YOU HAVE 15 MINUTES OR MORE, TRY THIS!

We adore acupuncturist Annee de Mamiel's facial acupuncture treatment, which she combines with massage. If you can't get to see her (or anyone else), just try this…. Then look in the mirror and go, 'Wow!'.

● Smooth your favourite facial oil over your entire face and neck.
● Cup your hands over the nose and mouth, breathe in and out deeply.
● Tug your earlobes with thumb and index finger. Then with fingertips, use firm, circular movements to massage from behind ears to base of neck.
● From the point of your chin, work up and outwards along the jaw to your ear; then from the corners of your mouth over the cheeks to the ear; then from the base of the nose to the top of the ear. Repeat the whole sequence three times.
● Sweep your fingertips firmly over your eyebrows, then under, then gently pinch along them. Repeat twice.
● Pressing firmly with your middle fingers, circle the eyes beginning above the inner corners and working outwards. Repeat three times.
● From the centre of your forehead, just above the nose, zigzag middle fingers in small, firm motions out to the temples; repeat working up the forehead.
● With the side of your index finger (held vertically), smooth skin from centre of face outwards, beginning with your forehead, then sides of nose, middle of mouth and centre of chin.
● Finish by breathing deeply, hands cupped over your mouth and nose.

OUR FAVOURITE AGE-DEFYING FACIALISTS…

Amanda Lacey
Anastasia Achilleos
Annee de Mamiel (see her massage tips above)
Emma Hardie (not your typical facial – no products, but seriously 'lifting')
Ole Henriksen
Sarah Chapman
Vaishaly Patel
Su-Man Hsu
Plus: Bliss Triple Oxygen Facial

Facial scrubs: our award winners

Dry, dull surface skin cells are the key issue lying between many a woman's complexion and a youthful radiance. When cell turnover slows, the dead surface skin cells don't reflect the light in the same way as a twentysomething's naturally fresh, dewy skin – but the good news is that a gentle exfoliator can go a long, long way towards restoring a healthy glow. Look out below for a new Liz Earle entry in this revised edition of our book…

AT A GLANCE

Darphin Age-Defying Dermabrasion

Liz Earle Naturally Active Gentle Face Exfoliator

Dermalogica Daily Microfoliant

Clinique 7 Day Scrub Cream Rinse-Off Formula

TIP

To avoid overdoing the use of a scrub on the face, use your ring fingers to massage in, using circular movements. The touch of this finger is naturally more delicate than with the index or second finger, all but eliminating the risk of over-zealous application.

G-E-N-T-L-E is our watchword, though – it's important to avoid anything that scratches or over-buffs the skin – so in our quest to discover the most effective facial scrubs, we dispatched several dozen to our panels of testers (ten for each product, as normal). They had truly glowing praise for some. PS Try using a facial scrub before applying a mask for maximum effectiveness.

REVIEWS

Darphin Age-Defying Dermabrasion

Darphin (originally a French brand, now owned by Estée Lauder) promise this very high-scoring product is kind enough even for sensitive skins, with buffing particles of jojoba, silica, pearl and lava to refine skin texture, plus a corn-derived ingredient to target age spots. Gentian and bisabolol have been added for a soothing action, and Darphin say this can be used as often as every other day. (Though we advise: try it once a week first, and assess results. That may be enough to keep you radiant.) Luxuriously-textured and luxuriously-priced.

Comments: 'Love this, the rich, creamy, lush texture and my glowing, cleaner, brighter skin after; you can use it without water but if it dries out a little, just add a touch then you can really massage it in; a small amount goes a long way' • 'skin never felt taut or dry after' • 'very fine grains exfoliate skin gently, lovely fresh smell, skin looks polished and fresh, clearer and brighter after; people say how good my skin looks' • 'super product that does brilliant job of exfoliating in the most gentle way – really lovely' • 'skin felt so soft and smooth and moisturised, it was wonderful, looks brighter'.

Liz Earle Naturally Active Gentle Face Exfoliator

Featured as one of Jo's 'loves' (see right), this is a softly-softly introduction to exfoliants, if you haven't tried one before. As with the whole Liz Earle range, botanicals feature generously (purifying eucalyptus, which also delivers a 'clean' scent, and lashings of cocoa butter), and – crucially – the skin-buffing action is down to rounded particles of jojoba. Gentle by name and gentle by nature – but effective, too, testers reveal.

Comments: 'Skin felt immediately smoother and really moisturised – and I liked the refreshing, uplifting eucalyptus scent' • 'my husband tells me my skin looks smooth and glowing and I think it's because of this' • 'loved this from the first time I used it' • 'just the right consistency to massage around my face without feeling I was stressing my skin' • 'leaves skin feeling moisturised, unlike most scrubs' • 'no redness or irritation – the best scrub I've ever used' • 'zingy scent helps to wake you up in the morning – even helped with blocked nose from a cold!' • 'a real "wake-up effect": thinking of using this as part of a hangover cure!'.

♡ WE LOVE...

Personally, thanks to diligent use of a muslin cloth at night-time, we go easy on facial scrubs – reserving them for an occasional blitz. For Jo, favourites include Liz Earle Naturally Active Gentle Face Exfoliator (yes, it truly IS gentle) and Origins Modern Friction (ditto), which has done well previously in our trials for *The Green Beauty Bible*. Sarah uses a flannel at night and in the morning to remove cleanser and virtually never exfoliates – though reading the reviews here, she's beetling off to the beauty cupboard!

Dermalogica Daily Microfoliant

8.75/10

As the name suggests, Dermalogica tell us this rice-based enzyme powder can be used every day – but please read the comments we make for Darphin about frequent use, above, before you do that. The powder formula – which shakes out of the container into the hand – activates when you mix it with water, releasing papain (a skin-brightening enzyme), salicylic acid and rice to smooth and boost cellular renewal. To add to its brightening power, bearberry, liquorice and grapefruit are incorporated, along with a skin-calming blend of green tea, ginkgo and oatmeal.

Comments: 'Not grainy at all, felt really soft and gentle, very easy to apply; skin looked really fresh and glowing, and felt unbelievably soft and smooth; people say I look very well; after a month skin looks glowing and refreshed' • 'can't believe people spend a fortune on expensive facial treatments when they could use this! I use it twice weekly, which is enough, but you could use it daily – a lovely comforting treatment without any harsh abrasiveness' • 'using this regularly has reduced my fine wrinkles and enlarged pores, made skin smoother and my skin feels so much nicer – a very lovely product, and moisturiser goes on much better' • 'husband says my skin looks brighter and fresher, and he's been trying it too and is very impressed!' • 'after a month, skin looks a lot smoother, brighter and more toned'.

Clinique 7 Day Scrub Cream Rinse-Off Formula

8.57/10

A 'second generation' version of a product that's been a pillar of the Clinique range for years, with gentle exfoliating beads that enliven skin after just 30 seconds of massage. It can then be easily swooshed away with water but may also be tissued off, Clinique tell us.

Comments: 'Quite grainy, gritty texture but not unpleasant; very easy to apply and skin looks glowing and much healthier, much smoother and softer – very gentle on my skin' • 'top marks! Really nice creamy texture, feels like it is doing its job, doesn't dry skin at all, after a month skin looks really great, and there's been a noticeable reduction in spots' • 'my combination skin looks much better and the product lasts ages as you only need a 5p-sized amount' • 'looks rich and creamy – a bit like toothpaste!; pleasant herby smell, and skin looks fresh and smooth, with a lovely healthy glow'.

ℱAnti-ageing face masks: *our award winners*

We love, love, love face masks. The ritual of slapping on a mask once a week can be a rare moment of pampering in a hectic life. But more than this, we like the results that many masks swiftly deliver: brightening, smoothing, plumping and delivering a surge of dewy moisture to thirsty skins. Plus some now feature specific 'anti-ageing' ingredients, such as skin-brightening enzymes. Our diligent panellists lay back and relaxed while trialling an incredibly wide selection of masks – and their top choices, featured here, with the top two award winners both from Elemis (no mean achievement), and two new entries in this new edition of our book

AT A GLANCE

Elemis Fruit Active Rejuvenating Mask

Elemis Pro-Collagen Quartz Lift Mask

OSKIA Renaissance Mask

Ole Henriksen Feel the Difference Perfecting Mask

REVIEWS

Elemis Fruit Active Rejuvenating Mask

8.86/10 The first of two award winners from Elemis in this category, this mask contains strawberry and kiwi for radiance-boosting, macadamia nut oil, shea butter – and kaolin clay, which is deep-cleansing, helping to refine the skin and banish dullness. (Interestingly, they recommend it for smokers – which we don't recommend! – because of the circulation-boosting effect.) It's not tight, but it does 'set' more than the other winning masks.
Comments: 'Top score for a perfect mask! My skin looked fresher, less puffy, more "perky", dreamy texture, smells like a fruit smoothie, my face was rejuvenated – result!' • 'skin looked fresh and smooth, definitely brighter, which improved with regular use' • 'loved this creamy, light mask which felt a little tingly but not uncomfy, skintone improved, definitely healthier, and could actually see the difference' • 'skin softer to the touch and dewier-looking, gives a clearer-looking complexion than my usual nourishing mask' • 'make-up went on like a dream and stayed put so I felt far more confident after just one treatment'.

Elemis Pro-Collagen Quartz Lift Mask

8.78/10 Much richer and creamier than the first Elemis entry, left (and pricier, too), this is from the spa brand's state-of-the-art Quartz Lift collection. Quartz, they tell us, enhances cell communication, while argan offers a 'facelifting effect' – and two other botanicals (padina pavonica and noni) relax and smooth the skin. There's also an 'anti-pollution complex', and Elemis call this 'the take-home facial'. As for our testers…?
Comments: 'Top marks! Instantly lifted and toned my skin, revealing a more radiant complexion, felt glorious and beautiful smell; left with such a soft, glowing skin and fine lines smoothed out, really hydrated and plumped out skin' • 'usually have salon treatments but this could persuade me to do it at home; skin very much rejuvenated, glowing, smooth, soft and tight – seemed to contour it' • 'skin did feel as if I'd had a salon facial – glowing and not taut at all' • 'pleasingly moisturising, left skin very soft and more toned without feeling tight in any way' • 'skin looked brighter and clearer, pores tighter'.

OSKIA Renaissance Mask

British brand OSKIA's formulations all include an MSM-Regen Complex because founder Georgie Cleeve is so convinced of sulphur's skin-saving powers. It also has natural skin-brightening fruit acids (lemon, passion fruit and pineapple), prebiotics, plus papaya enzymes and soothing butterbur and Swiss garden cress. Clever stuff: this skin-brightening pink creamy mask turns white once massaged into skin, so you know it's been correctly applied.

Comments: 'Amazing: brightening straight away and skin felt soft and plumped-out for two days after use' • 'YES, YES, YES! Unbelievable product, really great as a pick-me-up when I was going out (and didn't want to, and it showed in my face)' • 'feeling of complete relaxation when you inhale the fragrance' • 'the first time I tried this I was blown away, results were so immediate; love the healthy glow and fresh look, which lasted for hours' • 'a dream product: lovely to put on, easy to remove and you look in the mirror and think WOW this works; seemed to diminish age spots a little, too'

• 'the scent's fabulous and it works, plumping, refreshing, calming redness – and fine lines reduced'.

Ole Henriksen Feel the Difference Perfecting Mask

We're big fans of LA-based facialist-to-the-stars Ole Henriksen, whose ten-minute award winner here features mega-antioxidants including African red tea, white tea, pomegranate extract, borage seed oil, linseed oil, hyaluronic acid, plus stimulating grapefruit, tangerine and orange extracts. To enhance the oxygenating action, the mask has a special cooling effect (which lasts for up to 20 minutes after application).

Comments: 'Made skin cleaner, brighter, clearer and even reduced size of pores; my face mask of choice from now on' • 'like a mini-spa treatment: divine uplifting smell and cooling action really wakes up the skin' • 'love instant improvement and refreshing feel' • 'a great product that gives you a lift in ten minutes; doesn't feel drying and even seems to moisturise a little, leaving complexion fresher' • 'when you're a bit "bleugh", really wakes up skin leaving it looking fresh'.

♡ WE LOVE...

Jo's bathroom shelf is somewhat crowded with face masks, including lots of new favourites, but top of her charts is the incredible Sarah Chapman Skinesis Instant Miracle Mask: it sets to a rubbery finish which presses the hyaluronic acid into skin – and, she swears, leaves her with a 12-year-old's complexion (albeit only for a few hours...) Sarah loves Les Fleurs de Bach Anti Stress Mask and Liz Earle's mask offerings but her big miracle-worker is Darphin's Youthful Radiance Camellia Mask, which plumps up skin and makes it more even-toned and, yes, radiant!

Facial oils: *our award winners*

The best facial oils sink softly into skin, plumping and nourishing without ever feeling tacky or greasy. Specific ingredients are often chosen for their age-defying properties, helping to brighten skin or lessen wrinkles. We asked our beauty sleuths to help narrow down the choices for you – and here are their top choices, all natural, from over 100 that we've now put through their paces, including what is (still) the highest-scoring product we've ever trialled for any of our books

We love oils, for mature skins. (And yes, they can even work to balance oilier complexions, with the right blend of essential oils.) They're also ideal for touchy skins, which may react to synthetic preservatives: oils are naturally self-preserving, so don't need anything extra to extend their life. As Geraldine Howard, of Aromatherapy Associates, observes: 'Think of facial oils as "food" for the skin, and moisturisers as the water. Skin needs both to keep it soft and supple.'

A few drops is all it takes. While they're sometimes expensive (because of the cost of the concentrated botanicals in the blends), a bottle of facial oil typically lasts for much longer than a jar of cream. Only use as much as your skin needs: usually three or four small drops is enough. It should sink in quickly, so if skin looks greasy ten minutes later, you've used too much.

Try layering, under face cream. We like to apply facial oil under night cream, for a double-whammy of effectiveness. Great for skins prone to dryness at any time – or in winter, when central heating wicks the moisture out of skin. Alternatively, put a little cream into your hands and blend it with facial oil using your fingers, before applying. We're great believers in 'customising' our treatments to deliver what our skin needs at any point in time, and this is a great way to make a not-quite-moisturising-enough night cream a bit richer.

You can make your own blends. (Shameless plug: in Jo's book *The Ultimate Natural Beauty Book* there are many recipes.) Or you can opt for one of the pre-blended oils which are increasingly widely available, many of which we trialled for this book. Once the exclusive preserve of Frenchwomen, who learned early on how powerfully skin-caring facial oils can be, there are now dozens and dozens of options on the market – which is why we've put them through their paces.

REVIEWS

Nude ProGenius Treatment Oil

$\frac{9.65}{10}$ Wow. We have waited 14 years for a product to notch up a mark this staggeringly high – averaged across ten testers (mostly they gave it a ten). Renamed but with the formula unchanged since the last edition, Nude ProGenius Treatment Oil – from the range developed in tandem with Ali Hewson (aka 'Mrs Bono') – has just ever-so-slightly nudged ahead of our previous long-standing highest scorer, Liz Earle Cleanse & Polish, and we have no reason to believe it won't also go on to become one of the great beauty classics. With its blend of active oils (including macadamia, raspberry and cranberry seeds, apricot kernel and kukui), this is super-rich in omegas 3, 6, 7 and 9 and the pump-action bottle is sculpted from eco-plastic. **Comments:** 'Absolutely enhanced radiance, I felt and looked ten years younger – smoother, less lined, brighter, this is serious skincare' • 'makes my dry crêpey skin and flaky patches softer and more dewy, and didn't aggravate at all, which is a miracle in itself' • 'my combination skin was definitely plumper, smoother, more moisturised and younger-looking, within 24 hours of first using' • 'my dry sensitive skin was much smoother, I would absolutely buy' • 'a real anti-age product, a must-have for mature skin'.

Liz Earle Superskin Concentrate

9.15/10 This previously came top of the facial oils category in *The Green Beauty Bible*, but when we sent it out to our mature testers again for this book, they awarded it a micro-mark higher than its previous score (which was 9.1/10, in that case). Which, to us, just goes to confirm what we know: that our trials are incredibly consistent! This is Jo's favourite (see We Love…).

Comments: 'Skin was immediately much smoother and after four weeks the difference was quite dramatic, my skin was more toned and firm' • 'my combination/dry skin looks youthful and I think the aromatherapy oils help me unwind and sleep better' • 'I'm 45 with slight wrinkles, dry skin, tightness, sun damage – and this product makes me look younger! Definitely plumped my skin, made jaw line more toned and helped my lines on my forehead' • 'my sensitive skin is smooth and soft; particularly liked the instruction to inhale the fragrance, which seemed to calm my mind before bed'.

AD Skin Synergy Night Treatment Facial Oil

9.12/10 Therapist and former PR Amanda de Ayala poured years of insider knowledge into her small signature (AD) range, which includes this super-nourishing oil. It's based on £8,000-a-kilo cold-pressed rosehip oil from Chile – an ingredient renowned for its age-defying benefits – together with jojoba, sweet almond, evening primrose and vitamin E. The delectable scent's down to a skilful active blend of essential oils of rose, lavender, palmarosa, ylang-ylang, neroli, frankincense and jasmine.

Comments: 'I've had several people ask if I have been on holiday because of the healthy look to my skin' • 'seemed to replace plumpness skin loses over time, making it look younger' • 'the inclusion of lavender makes it relaxing to wear while going to sleep, and I've noticed a reduction in fine lines' • 'surprised how well this sinks in, and after a few days I received comments on how well I was

looking' • 'my beauty therapist commented on how well-hydrated my skin is' • 'wrinkles less noticeable, skin more nourished' • 'loved this and it lasts for AGES!' • 'skin glowing, but less redness'.

The Organic Pharmacy Antioxidant Face Firming Serum

8.83/10 They call this a 'serum' – but technically, it's a super-rich facial oil formula powered by rosehip seed oil (clinically proven to reduce wrinkles and scarring), antioxidant carrot oil, grapeseed extract, DMAE (another antioxidant which targets sagging), plus grapefruit, lemon and sweet orange. (Hence the comments about its uplifting fragrance…) Organically-certified (by The Soil Association), this new winner is from a Brit brand created by Margo Marrone, a homeopath/pharmacist who specialises in herbal medicine and nutrition.

Comments: 'Fresh orange-y smell puts you in a good mood for the rest of the day – or at least gives a few moments of bliss and relaxation before the stresses start' • 'skin feels soft as a baby's bottom' • 'Wow! Wow! Wow! I never want to be without this again – it's made a huge difference to my skin' • 'slight "lifting" effect, which is a surprise' • 'skin generally plumper and healthier' • 'lovely citrus smell' • 'I had a very pronounced line under each eye that was beginning to run down on to my cheekbone but this has now tailed off and disappeared altogether – fantastic stuff! Pricey but worth it'.

Vaishaly Night Nourisher (Dry/Sensitive)

8.78/10 The Normal/Combination version of this also appeared in *The Green Beauty Bible*, but with our anti-ageing testing panel it was Vaishaly's blend for drier skins which wowed. The skin-cocooning oils include jojoba and macadamia nut, plus Arctic raspberry seed extract and grapeseed.

Comments: 'This is luxurious to use and makes me feel pampered: I followed the massage technique from the leaflet and my skin feels plump and hydrated, soothed and comfy; make-up stays put the next day too' • 'people say my skin is glowing, it feels intensively moisturised and really smooth, also fewer hormonal breakouts' • 'feels wonderful to massage your face with this, even nicer if you can get someone to do it for you!' • 'my dry/normal skin loved this – looked amazing! So soft and plump' • 'I didn't have that sinking feeling when I looked in the mirror in the morning!'.

♡ WE LOVE…

There's only one, for Jo (and apologies if she's starting to sound like a scratched CD here): **Liz Earle Superskin Concentrate,** with its 100 per cent pure plant oil blend, based on argan and rosehip oils – which did so well with testers, too. 'I love the smell: neroli, lavender and chamomile – it's become part of my wind-down ritual before bedtime, with a few drops under moisturiser for extra plumping.' She also found it fantastic for healing scars after an op on a broken wrist. Sarah now relies on acupuncture facialist Annee de Mamiel's handmade, limited-edition seasonal oils, which are incredibly effective (with night cream on top). Otherwise she loves a few drops of La Clarée's fantastic **Radiance Elixir,** which does just that, and the **AD Skin Synergy Night Treatment Facial Oil,** which also won favour with testers for this paperback.

Learn the new foundation rules

As your face changes, so should your approach to creating a flawless canvas…

Throughout this book, we're very prescriptive about what works and what doesn't – because we know what really works, and we're giving you the inside info. (That's what we're about.)

However, there are two areas of make-up – foundation (aka base) and eyeshadow – where we can't be totally prescriptive, and where you'll need to experiment to see which of our various proposed options work for you. Some will, some won't.

We suggest setting aside a little playtime to experiment with the different techniques (and maybe even products), to see which give you the best results. We don't have a webcam on your computer so we can't look and tell you which works, which looks best – but if you use two mirrors (one hand mirror, to get a side view), you should be able to judge for yourself. If you're not certain, ask a friend who you trust.

What we know for certain, though, is that the products you've been using through your twenties and thirties are pretty unlikely to make you look fabulous once you hit forty – let alone beyond…

As Trish McEvoy says: 'As we get older, we lose evenness (principally due to cumulative sun damage), clarity, colour and definition. That's the difference between a young face and an older one. Your aim should be to recreate these as naturally as possible.'

HOW TO APPLY YOUR BASE

The better your skin, the lighter the foundation.
That's the rule – according to Mary Greenwell and other make-up pros we respect. But she adds: 'Every woman over forty has to wear foundation. Ironically, up until that point it can sometimes be ageing.'

Echoes Terry de Gunzburg: 'I could get away without foundation until my forties, but no longer. Skin doesn't look neat – or even clean, in some cases – because the skintone is no longer uniform (which also makes you look tired). Your complexion may be a bit red, or look a little shadowy and grey or sallow. But this doesn't mean just applying more of the foundation you've always worn (if you have). Layers of heavy foundation make all lines look worse. If you have always worn quite a lot of base, you probably need to use less and with a lighter touch. You want uniformity – but you don't want a mask-like effect.' Never use your base as an all-over corrector/concealer. If you have flaws, use a corrector/concealer sparingly, just where it's needed. For the best effect, you need to learn to 'layer' products (as we explain here).

● **So: start your 'layers' with a primer.** (See page 89 for more information, and which ones our testers liked best.) Applied after your moisturiser (and don't forget to let this sink in for at least five minutes) and/or serum, a primer adds softness and luminosity, can go some way towards evening skintone, and helps turbo-charge the staying power of your make-up.

● **Rethink your foundation.** 'Nothing too matt, nothing too heavy,' is Mary's wisdom (she likes cream bases best). Our recommendations for Anti-Ageing Foundations, see page 90, are another good place to start. The 'finish' should not be too matt; a little dewiness or 'light' is flattering, but not so much that you look shiny. If you have oily skin, go for oil-free; dry skin, choose one labelled 'moisturising'. The big new option is mineral powder foundations, which many experts including Trish McEvoy and Jane Iredale (the pioneer of mineral make-up) recommend, particularly for conditions such as acne and rosacea. See page 92 for more.

● **Test the foundation shade on your neck.** 'Just below the jaw is the right place,' says Mary Greenwell. 'Your base should match your neck, not your face or even the jawline itself, and should "disappear" to avoid that tell-tale join line.' Be brave, and check it out in bright daylight, adds Barbara Daly.

● **Try a foundation brush.** We're big fans of these, and so is Terry de Gunzburg. 'I don't like sponges but I do like brushes,' she says. 'You can control the quantity that you apply and you can "layer" the foundation on a little at a time, using the brush to make tiny feathery strokes that tap it into the skin and pores. Apply a little foundation to the back of your (clean) hand, and pick the foundation up from there with the brush, a little at a time. You can always add, but it's harder to take away. Then use the warmth of your fingers to "press" the foundation into the skin, which makes it look natural.' (NB: we're big fans of all the products in Terry's By Terry make-up range: after all, she is the woman who created the legendary Touche Eclat/Radiant Touch for YSL, and there is probably nobody who understands light-reflecting particles and how to introduce radiance into make-up products better than her. She's very funny about her line, insisting: 'I created it for women who want to look as good as their daughters. Or their husband's mistress.' A very French approach…!)

Alternatively, use your fingers to smooth in your foundation, from the word 'go'. Fingers are Mary Greenwell's preferred 'tools', also Barbara Daly's. 'They

Can you fix an open pore? We know these bug you from the number of emails to www.beautybible.com, over the years. Pores tend to 'stretch' as we age, especially for those who've had oily skin in the past. Conversely, they can be very obvious on dry skin. The old advice was to avoid moisturising the affected area – but first, that's not practical and also we'd rather you protected your face with an SPF. And actually we suggest reading the comments made about award winners in our Miracle Treatments, Serums and Night Creams section as many testers observed improvements in tightness of pores as a result of using certain products featured there; ditto, the clay-based mask in our Face Masks section. But do avoid toners which can over-stimulate sebaceous glands. For a quick fix, try patting on a primer or line-filler – they can make pores vanish in a flash (albeit temporarily) and are your fast track to pore perfection.

are warm, and so help "meld" foundation into skin,' Mary says. (We say: try a brush, try your fingers, and see which gives you the best effect. Sarah favours fingers most mornings – with brushwork for dress-up days – but Jo finds fingers take off as much as she's putting on so uses a brush. So the mantra is 'experiment'!) Don't feel you have to apply it all over your face, says Barbara Daly. 'Start from the centre and blend out, so by the time you get to the fine hairs at the side (don't worry – everyone has them), there's nothing there.'

Remember, your base is not a corrector or concealer. So, once you've applied your foundation, stand back and take a look. If you still have flaws you want to hide, such as brown spots, red cheeks, scars or dark circles under your eyes, read on.

COVERING REDNESS, AGE SPOTS AND OTHER FLAWS

While Trish McEvoy believes every woman of a certain age should own a corrector, concealer (see below for the difference) and luminiser, they are certainly essential for camouflaging hyperpigmentation (brown spots), redness and other blemishes. Her advice: 'After you've primed skin, take your corrector (always matt, yellow- or peach-based, with deeper peach for women of colour), and dot it on with a little brush, then press it in. Very important to dot and press, do not sweep it on. If it needs more blending use a little make-up sponge.' You can then apply cream/liquid foundation, or brush on mineral powder base if you need it. Setting with translucent powder over liquid foundation is optional. 'Technology has advanced so tremendously that many formulas today are long wear and don't need powder,' says Trish.

'My grandmothers lived long into old age and they were always BEAUTIFUL to me. They *loved life* and it showed in their faces'

Penélope Cruz

And what's the difference between a corrector and concealer? Sometimes very little: though generally correctors are lighter and aim to correct colour and tone on very red cheeks or rosacea – rather than a concealer which sits on a blemish such as under-eye dark circles or a scar to conceal it. For more pronounced flaws, you might want to use a corrector followed by a concealer. (For more camouflage advice on covering rosacea and acne scarring, see page 168.)

For frown lines, try patting on a silicone-based filler, which will soften the edges (more on page 94).

Brighten up with a luminiser. Aka a light-reflecting pen (see page 56). These magic wands add luminosity to your high planes: cheekbones, upper brow, forehead – and you can dab a tad on your bosom and shoulders. As well as accentuating the positive, they draw attention away from the negative areas.

Set your make-up with face powder. This will definitely make it stay in place longer. (Disappearing make-up is a perennial problem for thirsty skins, and also anyone who's experiencing hot flushes.) But it has to be the right powder – feather-light and barely-there – and it must be used judiciously on the areas that need it rather than all over the face. A finely-milled, translucent loose powder will reduce pore appearance too, says Barbara Daly.

Apply face powder with a fat eyeshadow brush. (Yes, really.) Mary Greenwell advises using an eyeshadow brush (albeit the largest of these you can find) to target powder on the areas of the face that tend to shine: nose, chin, centre of forehead. Also try putting it on very lightly over your eyelids before you apply make-up. Leave the rest of your face naked of powder: you want to see the radiance, and powder may dull that.

One exception to the rule: By Terry Voile Poudre Eclat. This whisper-light, transparent face powder has the subtlest light-reflecting pigments which correct and even out skintone, mattifying while still leaving skin luminous. It also seems to add a veil of 'softness' to the skin. (Like all of the By Terry products it is far from cheap but a pot will last you just about for ever.) Rose Lumière is a colour that works on all skintones except black and Asian. To set your make-up for a long evening out, an all-over dusting of Terry's powder is the key. But this time, use a large round-headed brush, please.

ANTI-AGEING
AWARD
WINNERS
BEAUTY BIBLE

Make-up primers: *our award winners*

We challenge you to discover the difference that a cosmetic primer can make to how well your make-up lasts and how much smoother your complexion appears

REVIEWS

Guerlain Météorites Perles Light Diffusing Perfecting Primer

8.57 10

Delicate petal pink pearls are suspended in this gel primer, and diffuse when massaged into the skin to give a radiant glow without – miraculously – adding shininess. (In fact, there are absorbing powders to neutralise sebum.) It has the usual signature Guerlain violet-y fragrance (which we love, love, LOVE...though some testers didn't.)
Comments: 'Really loved this product, easy to use, fantastic packaging, sank in quickly and made my skin feel like silk; enhanced radiance and an excellent base for make-up, which lasted longer – my skin glowed through the day' • 'gives a gentle, pretty glow which lasts all day' • 'make-up looks satin-smooth on top of this smooth, light serum, which left a sheen on my skin, and my friend said how good it looked; I like the ingenious pearls' • 'gave a much more smooth and professional look, fabulous fragrance, foundation glided on'.

Clarins Instant Smooth Perfecting Touch

8.39 10

Clarins do tell us that this little pot of silky-smooth skin perfector CAN be used all over the skin – over day cream and under foundation/powder – but the dinky size of the jar means you might get through it quite quickly, even though you need very little. (It can also be used on specifically lined areas, as an instant smoother.) Has a 'Line Minimiser Pigment' for soft-focus effect, plus 'Acacia Micro-Pearls' which plump up to fill lines.
Comments: 'Rich, silky texture is very easy to apply and sank in immediately; definitely enhanced radiance and is an excellent base of foundation – the glow lasted throughout the day; this little pot can work wonders' • 'you need to apply just a little then let it sit for a few minutes before applying

AT A GLANCE

Guerlain Météorites Perles Light Diffusing Perfecting Primer

Clarins Instant Smooth Perfecting Touch

Elizabeth Arden Good Morning Skin Serum

Cosmetics à la Carte Rose Dew

♡ WE LOVE...

Somewhat to her shame, Jo often does her make-up on the train, first using a sponge to smooth in Cosmetics à la Carte Skin Veil to turbo-charge the staying power of her make-up. For home use, she likes the Sue Devitt Microquatic Blue Anti-Aging SPF30 Protection Primer: it helps neutralise redness and creates a good base for make-up. Sarah is devoted to Trish McEvoy Even Skin Face Primer, which does indeed even out skintone and helps foundation create a (more or less) flawless finish.

foundation or else it gets mixed in; made skin look brighter and smoother and has encouraged me to use a primer more regularly'.

Elizabeth Arden Good Morning Skin Serum

8.28 10

A slim glass bottle of serum featuring 'energising' botanicals and vitamin A, in what feels like a silicone-rich base. (Silicones do have a fabulously skin-smoothing effect and are widely used in primers.)
Comments: 'Easy to apply, blended smoothly and made skin really velvety; evened skintone and gave complexion a fresh look; make-up did go on more smoothly and evenly' • 'left skin feeling silky and looking quite flawless, am convinced pores looked smoother after applying it; my husband said I looked lovely!' • 'skin was much more radiant; seemed to smooth red and dry patches and give a more even skintone, great base for make-up; I almost lost the "frazzled teacher" look!' • 'had a brilliant effect on my skin, lessened the redness of acne scars and my mum said I looked like I'd had a good night's sleep'.

Cosmetics à la Carte Rose Dew

8.15 10

From a much-loved Knightsbridge make-up school and beauty emporium, this non-greasy primer features aloe and witch hazel for a skin-firming effect. The heavenly rose scent of this makes morning application a total pleasure. They recommend applying after moisturiser, 15 minutes before foundation.
Comments: 'Brilliant base for make-up – mineral foundation and blusher – skin did not shine so I looked better!' • 'wonderful fragrance, worth buying it for that alone' • 'quite runny but rich too, and wonderful; a dream to apply, gives skin a glow; let it dry, apply make-up – and it makes skin look and feel fabulous' • 'enhanced radiance and made make-up last longer; the rose smell is adorable'.

*F*Anti-ageing foundations: *our award winners*

Now there are foundations designed specifically for older skin that give good coverage to hide imperfections and create a more radiant, even tone

AT A GLANCE

Clarins Skin Illusion Natural Radiance Foundation SPF10

Estée Lauder Re-Nutriv Ultimate Radiance Makeup SPF15

Bobbi Brown Skin Foundation SPF15

Clarins Super Restorative Foundation SPF15

TIP

The most important thing with foundation is still the right colour: but don't try it on the back of your hand – the skintone is invariably dramatically different. Use a Q-tip to try it just below your jawline. If it disappears, it's the right shade.

In the past few years, a whole new category of bases has emerged to cater to the wannabe-fabulous-at-forty-plus market. Anti-ageing foundations mostly do double-duty: instantly evening out skintone (one of the most instantly de-ageing tricks) plus moisturising, and some contain ingredients to help perfect skin over the longer term (firming/plumping/damage-limiting, etc). The snag is that foundation should only be applied where you need it – definitely not as an all-over 'mask' – so there's a limit to what can be achieved in terms of serious ongoing improvements. Here are the high-scoring bases which seriously impressed testers, including new award-winners appearing for the first time in this edition. Aces bases, indeed.

REVIEWS

Clarins Skin Illusion Natural Radiance Foundation SPF10

 The secret moisturising 'weapon' for older skins in this antioxidant, anti-pollution foundation is a 'time-released micro-patch', so Clarins tell us, to reduce dehydration. The medium-coverage formula enhances radiance thanks to pink algae extract and (cosmetically) a 'pink opal powder' for an opalescent glow, alongside light-optimising pigments for a soft focus effect. It offers light sun protection (NB only where applied) – SPF10 – and there are also ten shades available. (Our lot were dispatched 107 Beige.)
Comments: 'Brilliant! Amazing a foundation so light can cover so well' • 'my partner asked me what on earth I'd done as I looked so much better after putting my make-up on; he said he wished he could get away with wearing make-up!' • 'just amazing: covered so well, looked so radiant and un-made-up – love, love, love…' • 'helped to cover the dark circles under my eyes well' • 'skin felt softer and looked plumper – the best foundation I've ever used,

smelt divine and a little went a very long way' • 'I have already recommended to lots of my friends following their compliments on how good my skin looks. It is amazing how different you can feel about yourself just by using a different foundation, I absolutely love this product and it would take something very special indeed to make me ever change it – I am converted for life!'.

Estée Lauder Re-Nutriv Ultimate Radiance Makeup SPF15

 Lauder, of course, are known for their anti-ageing technology, and the Re-Nutriv range is their most serious (and luxurious) treatment range. Alongside hyaluronic acid, vitamin E and broad-spectrum UV protection, this contains a 'micro-fine crystal mesh of precious gemstones and crystals' for radiance (and an SPF15). It's fragrance-free.
Comments: '10/10! Gave just the right coverage, not heavy or thick, looked very natural, made skin younger-looking and brighter instantly and improved over time, with fine lines diminishing; made my skin feel lovely and light' • 'sheer coverage but you can build it up; looked glowing and smoothed my complexion, all tiredness disappeared instantly, worth every penny!' • 'could go through all day and into evening without reapplying' • 'balanced skintone very well, made it look more radiant due to light-reflecting particles, definitely evened my skintone, smoothed lines and reduced the look of imperfections'.

Bobbi Brown Skin Foundation SPF15

 If it's a supremely weightless formula you're after, look no further. (We'd almost categorise this as 'foundation for foundation-phobes'.) Though it's super-lightweight in texture, coverage is good and impressively long-lasting, with an SPF15 active where applied. We appreciate Bobbi's acknowledgment that skins come in all tones: our testers received Beige, but there are 16 other shades.

Comments: 'The best foundation I've ever used! Felt weightless and comfortable as if it wasn't there' • 'stayed put all day, without the usual oily patches on my forehead, and the colour was true to my own skintone; no tell-tale lines' • 'more dewy than powdery: it evens skin, blurs light blemishes – loved it' • 'easy and quick to apply for a natural look' • 'over the last ten years I have tried many types of foundation and all have ended up unused and in the bin. They have always felt heavy (even light formulas) and I could feel them on my skin. This has completely converted me'.

Clarins Super Restorative Foundation SPF15

 Two winners in this category from Clarins: testers also liked this velvety, fluid cream, with a 100 per cent mineral SPF (so no chemical sunscreens), and firming pine extract. Created to brighten and 'lift' skin, there are 'Soft Focus Pigments' to blur lines. It's for all skin types (and especially from age 50+) seeking medium-to-full coverage, with an SPF15.

Comments: 'Very pleased with the finish; my sister told me my skin looked clear and smooth – very good product which I would buy' • 'gave lovely dewy finish, very natural sheer coverage, which suited my fair complexion perfectly' • 'lovely thin silky texture, excellent coverage for redness and spots, evened my skintone well – didn't need concealer, more dewy than powdery' • 'this genuinely makes me feel a lot more confident as it improves the look of my skin so much, is really quick to apply and I love the SPF'.

♡ WE LOVE...

Jo's former fave By Terry Teint Lumière Veloutée has been updated to a new incarnation called Cover-Expert: an equally moisturising formulation which offers really good, velvety coverage – just what she needs for an English rose skin somewhat plagued by red veins. For weekends, she's addicted to the very affordable Bourjois Healthy Mix Foundation: serum-based, delivering good, dewy coverage at great price! Sarah favours the finish and coverage of Clinique Even Better Makeup SPF15, which promises to help combat hyperpigmentation and give brighter skin and even skintone, and, for really dry days, the light super-dewy finish of new Lancôme Teint Miracle.

Concealers: *our award winners*

Many cream concealers (usually a little thicker than cream foundation) we've tried are not suitable for under-eyes, as they can look cake-y – but the top scoring products here (with two new entries) do claim to work well for dark circles. So, depending on your needs, you may only have to invest in one double-duty concealer for your make-up bag.

Benefit Erase Paste

 A seriously spectacular score for a product from a pretty light-hearted brand – which actually does serious products. This concentrated creamy formula principally targets discolourations and flaws but can also be used on dark circles, as the three shades are specifically 'brightening'.

Comments: '10/10 for thread veins, small blemishes and pigmentation, also made wrinkles look less obvious – but not enough for scars; blends in very well and looked natural' • 'I used it on moles, blemishes, scars, wrinkles, pigmentation and it covered them. I also used it on my daughter who has acne – it was incredible to see the difference'.

Jemma Kidd i-Rescue Bio-Complex Cover

 A little Lucite pot of creaminess to pat on to skin (or use with a brush/corner of a cosmetic sponge). Make-up artist Jemma also proposes it as an eyelid primer.

Comments: 'Very light in consistency and blends easily to a very, very natural finish' • 'I'm SO going to buy this instead of my old concealer; you can't tell I'm wearing concealer (unlike others which flake and are a different colour); also covered a two-inch scar from childhood so it's barely noticeable' • 'a miracle product; fantastic on eyelids to prevent make-up fading'.

Crème de la Mer The Radiant Concealer SPF25

 A ritzy silver palette with a mirror in the lid accompanied by the perfect synthetic brush for application. Don't rely on the SPF, though, as it's applied so sparingly (but useful for age spots, we'd say).

Comments: 'Very easy to apply and blend, it sort of melts into the skin; brilliant for dark circles' • 'great on pigmentation' • 'covered thread veins and age spots completely, and blended into wrinkles: I was very pleased overall'.

♡ WE LOVE...

To erase redness, Jo dips her finger in the product that collects around the neck of her foundation tube (By Terry Cover-Expert) – which makes for a perfectly matched shade, in a slightly thicker and more covering format (because some of the water's evaporated from the formula). Sarah doesn't use much concealer but for the odd blemish, pigmented spot/patch and redness is delighted by By Terry VIP Touch-Expert Advanced, which does the trick beautifully.

Try a mineral foundation

Mineral make-up has been a huge beauty buzz over the past few years, and many women around our age are converts. But it does require a new set of make-up skills, so if you're going to try a mineral foundation, we want to ensure you optimise your chances of great results

Two things we'd say: the first is that provided you use a good product and follow this advice, you will get great coverage – one friend used Susan Posnick's ColorFlo to camouflage the flaming redness after she had her face lasered (and went out dancing, she was so confident). Second, mineral make-up need not look dry or caked if you start here…

Moisturise your face first. The mineral powder will adhere to the natural oils of your skin, but as there's no natural moisture in a mineral foundation you need to add some extra. If skin's too dry, the powder will end up looking just like that – powder. (As usual, wait ten minutes for moisturiser to sink in before applying make-up.)

Use a specific mineral foundation brush. Some of these are 'kabuki-style': stubby and short-handled. Because they're almost circular, they work for the 'swirl and buff' movement that's best for applying this type of make-up (see below for details). Some brands – such as Susan Posnick – have the powder in the handle of the brush, so of course you use that.

Tip a little of the powder into the lid of the jar. If the powder is loose (rather than contained in the brush handle), never, never dip your brush directly into the mineral make-up – you'll pick up way too much. A little is all you need. If you require more, gently tip a tad more into the lid, and swirl your brush in that. But all you'll need is a pinch or so.

Then tap the brush. This dusts off any excess powder.

Swirl and buff. You apply mineral foundation by holding the brush at right angles to your skin, not at a sloping angle. Then rub the brush on to your skin using circular movements, particularly focusing on areas you want to conceal. You can gradually build coverage this way, until it's the level you want. This isn't like normal face powder where you want to skim it over the surface: you're really aiming to buff and push the powder into the skin. As with all foundation techniques, it takes a little practice, but is worth persevering.

Spot-target any veins, etc, with a fingertip dipped in

powder. This is a great tip we picked up: rather than continuing to layer on mineral powder, you can put a dab on the end of your finger and press it on to something you want to conceal (a broken vein, an age spot). The heat of your finger helps the powder to meld into skin.

Try a setting powder if you find your mineral make-up disappears. In general, women report to us that mineral make-up lasts for longer than regular foundation. But if that's not the case with you, try a specific mineral setting powder (such as BareMinerals Mineral Veil). Do not, however, try setting mineral make-up with your regular face powder: the textures don't work well together.

Mineral make-up: *our award winners*

Mineral make-up appeals to women for two reasons: in powder form, it's easy to swirl on to the face (though you may need a bit of practise, see our how-to, left), and many users like the fact it's 'natural'. All mineral foundations aren't created equal, though. If you are looking for a truly 100 per cent natural product, check out the daisy rating of the award winners listed here (for more about this see page 7). NB: we list other excellent mineral make-up products in our book *The Green Beauty Bible*, but not all those were tested on mature skins – unlike these winners. Look out for a surprise new entry below, for this updated edition…

Comments: 'My first experience but it was easy to apply with my own sponge; gave sheer coverage which you could build up without looking overdone; concealed open pores and small blemishes but needed concealer on thread veins; brilliant product' • 'lovely sheer natural finish which covered well without looking cake-y' • 'used my own brush which gave a sheer natural finish, minimised the open pores on my cheeks' • 'loved this fine texture, fantastic at evening out my skintone'.

Youngblood Mineral Cosmetics Natural Mineral Foundation

8/10 From California, an attractively-packaged mineral range (they aren't all!), which is 100 per cent pure mineral powder and no 'fillers'. Comes in a wide screw-top plastic jar, which is helpful when it comes to swirling your brush in the lid, and there's a clever dispenser which releases just the right amount of powder at the tap of a finger. In 16 shades – from pale to Mahogany (great for black skins); our testers received Neutral, one of the light-to-mid tones. Testers were a bit mixed in their reactions – mainly novices, because they needed time to practise.

Comments: 'Once I got the hang of using this, it wasn't messy, and lasts well: after years of using liquid base, I'll always use mineral powder now for great natural coverage' • 'once blended it looks good, and I felt like I was wearing no make-up – but it did take me a quite lot of work' • 'looked sheer but covered well, especially open pores and small blemishes; I would buy' • 'concealed my open pores and gave a dewy glow' • 'very impressed, but I had to learn how to apply'.

MAC Mineralize Skinfinish Natural

7.95/10 This does well for sheer ease – it's a pressed powder compact (eliminating any risk of spillage, which can be a factor with some mineral powders) – but it's not 100 per cent natural if that's a concern for you. (No mirror in the compact, or sponge, which lost it marks.) The powder delivers a matt radiance, and would also be good for 'setting' a liquid foundation. Eight shades (we had pure golden beige Light/Medium) – and be sure to go for the Skinfinish Natural option, as the original Skinfinish is seriously frosted.

AT A GLANCE

Youngblood Mineral Cosmetics Natural Mineral Foundation

MAC Mineralize Skinfinish Natural

Keromask Mineral Rich Finishing Powder

Cosmetics à la Carte Cover Tint

♡ WE LOVE…

For sheer ease, Jo chooses Susan Posnick Colorflo – less messy than most, because the powder's contained in a see-thru tube with a built-in brush, which makes for easy swirling while gradually building coverage. And she's very impressed with the way this can easily cover her red veins. Sarah's a recent (pretty evangelical) convert to BareMinerals, meanwhile.

Keromask Mineral Rich Finishing Powder

7.75/10 The Keromask range is just brilliant – but better known to women who have serious skin challenges. Its camouflage products can prove life-transforming for women with vitiligo, birthmarks, port wine stains, etc – so we were a little surprised when Keromask submitted their 'finishing powder' (used more often to 'set' the concealing base) for our general mineral make-up trial. But it did great! In a lidded compact with an accompanying brush, it features blackcurrant seed oil, which may also help heal scars.

Comments: 'Coverage better than my usual foundation; took down redness and covered the thread veins on my nose' • 'hats off to whoever designed the compact: you "grate" the amount you need, so there's no mess in the pot' • 'the best powder I've come across: sheer coverage and natural finish' • 'made skin soft as velvet without drying it out' • 'made skin look much better than usual even without foundation but I now use it over my regular base and it's made a huge difference'.

Cosmetics à la Carte Cover Tint

7.71/10 For easy application, the mineral powder in this 100 per cent natural powder features a built-in sponge; you swipe it over the surface of your skin for the lightest coverage, and 'press' it into your complexion where more help's required. Again, spill-proof – and we like the built-in mirror on the lid. Nine shades and we trialled Vanilla.

Comments: 'Ten out of ten! Fantastic to use, blended really well and no mess; natural even finish that balanced all redness – a powder that felt like a cream foundation' • 'felt like silk and covered all flaws without concealer' • 'gave a warm glow, even coverage, balanced skintone, covered small flaws'.

*F*Wave a magic wand over your lines

Fact: most of us are cowards when it comes to physical invasion of our one and only face with a syringe. (And we say: that's no bad thing.) But as an alternative to Botox and line-filling injections, there is a new generation of cosmetic wonder products which make lines vanish in a flash

You may have decided, like us, that doctor-administered fillers aren't for you. But after a certain stage can there be a woman among us who hasn't glanced in the mirror and wondered what we'd look like if a magic wand was waved over this furrow, or that laugh line, or the annoying little groove – or 'marionette' line – that's just started to run from mouth to chin? Yes, we've all been there…

Which is why we are very, very, VERY excited about the latest trend to hit the beauty scene. Call them 'faux fillers', if you like – but what they really amount to is Polyfilla for faces: products that you apply to your lines and hey, presto! They're gone. Of course, it's all an illusion. But who really cares? Because isn't that what make-up is actually all about? (And personally we love them!)

Bear in mind, of course, that topical fillers will never be as effective as those applied with a syringe by a cosmetic doctor. True volume can only be created when the 'volumiser' is applied deep in the skin's fat layer, and that's not going to happen when you merely pat something on. (If you really want to go down that route, see page 46 to arm yourself with all the right questions to ask before anyone comes waving a syringe in your direction…)

Choose your product. There are two categories of these products (known to insiders as 'optics'). The first is purely cosmetic: the Polyfilla-types – called 'line-smoothers' or 'line-fillers', which have a temporary effect only. As well as delivering those blink-of-an-eye results, the second category of these line-diffusing fillers also offers anti-ageing benefits, which claim to work with regular continuous use to fight those pesky grooves.

Essentially, how do they work? According to Steven Hasher, Vice-President of Research and Development for GoodSkin Labs (an exciting and somewhat hush-hush new division of Estée Lauder Worldwide), 'Imagine a cloaking device – similar to the technology used to make planes invisible to radar.' He goes on to explain in more detail that by taking different sizes of spherical particles – including nylon, talc and silicones – and matching them to the skin's own 'refractive index' (that's the way light naturally bounces off the skin), you can hide and veil the wrinkles… We would add that although this type of line-concealer has anti-ageing benefits, we'd say you also need a 'miracle' cream, or

an eye treatment product – rather than relying on a faux filler alone to treat lines and wrinkles.

Remember: practice makes perfect. Unlike a face cream, there's a little bit of extra work involved in applying these fillers – and just maybe, a bit of experimentation, while you establish which technique works best for you. (Persevere. It's worth it.) Here's our advice:

● Most of these products have tiny nozzles or pen-style applicators which dispense just a little product – and with those, we've found that squeezing the product along the length of the line, then patting it in lightly with the ring finger, delivers the best turn-back-the-clock results.

● Try this over make-up, but also underneath: some fillers won't shift if you apply foundation over the top, although we recommend leaving the 'filler' for a minute or two before applying base. There's really no way round it: you need to experiment.

● Carry the product round in your kit for on-the-go touch-ups since our experience is that none of them – yet – endure from breakfast to dinner without a little repair work.

So which to choose – 'Polyfilla' (for instant results only), or with the addition of precision-targeted anti-ageing ingredients…? We can't make up your mind for you. So we suggest you read our testers' comments on both types of line-filler, opposite.

Line-fillers: *our award winners*

AT A GLANCE

Benefit Porefessional

Cosmetics à la Carte Skin Veil

Nuxe Visible Expression Lines Serum

♡ WE LOVE...

Jo went into something of a decline upon discovering that TRI-AKTILINE Instant Deep Wrinkle Filler is no longer available in the UK (although it is still on sales in the States...). That was until she tried **Benefit The Porefessional**, which has also rocketed to the top of the line-smoothing charts here, converting our panellists (she likes the fact it's skin-toned, so it really does look natural when patted into lines, blurring them quite astonishingly). Sarah is still eking out her tube of TRI-AKTILINE: the good thing about line-smoothers is that a little really does go a heck of a long way...!

For anyone troubled by lines, wrinkles and grooves, these are utter magic. We've even managed to dissuade women from opting into Botox treatments by demo-ing the instantly line-blurring power of some of these 'line-fillers', which work by depositing optical pigments, silicones and synthetic ingredients like nylon into lines to minimise (and in some cases, even eliminate) their appearance. As a bonus, some of these also contain anti-ageing ingredients which target the lines themselves, over time. There are now dozens of options, of which our testers rated these highest (including a new top-scorer and another new entry). Most others, they observed, performed far less well, with plenty languishing in the line-filling doldrums...

Benefit Porefessional

8.11/10 We have a new and conclusive winner at the top of the line-smoothing charts for this edition – and don't be misled by the name. Although The Porefessional does a fab job of minimising the appearance of open pores (something we know bothers many of our mature readers, since the pores stretch over time), the other well-kept secret action of this lightly skin-tinted silicone-rich product is to blur lines.

Comments: 'Went over make-up really well; made face look softer and dare I say it...? Younger – and husband said I looked "fresh"' • 'goes onto skin effortlessly and leaves you with a completely flawless complexion; I am amazed somethng so easy to use produces such dramatic effects that last such a long time' • 'perfect product to put on my pores and fine wrinkles, knowing they'd be smoothed neutralised in close-up situations' • 'skin looked even and fine lines dramatically reduced; lasted all day without the need for touching up' • 'other fillers I've used have looked white and chalky, but the tint gets rid of this – Benefit should definitely do more to market this as a line-smoother as it truly does the job well' • 'will be adding this to the Christmas list – it's a winner!'.

Cosmetics à la Carte Skin Veil

7.87/10 A product that Jo, too, rates highly: a sleek silver mirrored compact, this is super-easy to use: it features a velvety sponge which you can swipe over lines and wrinkles, under or over make-up (most testers preferred the latter). The optical pigments also work to minimise the appearance of open pores (great around the nose), and it can also be used all over the face as an under make-up primer. Skin Veil comes in three shades: Original (untinted for any skintone, which our lot received); Vanilla (for paler complexions) or Honey (for medium-to-dark skintones) – although none deliver actual coverage. Very easy to use.

Comments: 'The texture is like a creamy/satiny foundation which goes on invisibly and gives a fabulously smooth, luminous quality, with the illusion of flawlessness; I am totally addicted!' • 'I applied with fingers, and my foundation went on easily over it; all seemed to blend together to cover and plump' • 'fine lines seemed to disappear, worked best under mineral powder foundation, made my skin look air-brushed! Loved it as a primer' • 'this really gave a very natural look that lasted all day'.

Nuxe Visible Expression Lines Serum

7.21/10 In a hefty glass bottle, this treatment serum isn't something to lug around for on-the-go touch-ups, but testers who used it in a home setting liked the way it tautened, tightened and smoothed wrinkles, melting to a velvety finish. From a French brand founded by Terry de Gunzburg (formerly of YSL and creator of the By Terry line), with her sister Aliza Jabès, this has a gorgeous scent – a touch of frangipani, we'd say – as well as anti-ageing oak serum.

Comments: 'First time I used the serum my skin looked amazing, healthy, radiant, almost like a soft-focus effect; an hour or two later I glanced in the mirror and was literally stopped in my tracks – stunned that the face staring back was my own' • 'tried this on one half of my face: gave skin a more smoothed and plumped look, with wrinkles filled out a bit' • 'wrinkles diminished; not a miracle cure but does seem to help in making face look a little younger and clearer' • 'loved the smell of this – also very refreshing and light on the skin' • 'fine lines seemed to disappear; not a dramatic difference but my "number 11" lines between my brows, and my marionette lines, definitely less prominent'.

Be very, very nice to your feet

…every single day. We put more stress on our feet than any other part of the body. And, as leading podiatrist Margaret Dabbs says, 'Foot pain shows on your face.' (Like any pain actually)

Feet are the foundations of the body: when they go wrong, it impacts on our whole being. Plus we want our tootsies in the best possible shape, not just to look good but to take us walking, which is nature's greatest medicine – good for our heart and lungs, and for improving bone density (of our lower half), doesn't strain the joints – and gets us from A to B absolutely free. Walking can also work as a weight-loss technique, if you put in the miles regularly and vigorously.

All of which means that after about 35, we need to think of our feet in terms of much more than ways to show off fabulous shoes and glam nail polishes. Foot problems before that aren't unknown, of course – though they're usually shoe-related (corns and bunions, in particular). But as we age, feet become more problematic. And our experience is that whenever we stop walking regularly – because of illness, injury or simply painful feet (Jo was once almost crippled by an allergic reaction to MSG, Sarah by an ingrowing toenail) – then it's not long before everything feels like it's falling apart.

Remember: foot 'wellbeing' is vital. Overleaf, you'll find answers from one of the most respected 'foot pros' that we know, to help you tackle specific foot problems. Because unless feet are happy, the rest of you is going to be miserable – and that's going to add ten years to how you look. Give them some daily 'foot love' and you'll float along, looking like a spring chick!

Treat yourself to some sexy, comfy shoes. Once upon a time, comfy shoes equalled 'old lady' shoes. Well, baby, look at the comfortable shoe selection NOW! The reason's simple: as the population ages, we're just not giving up on fabulous shoes. We're both absolutely fetishistic about shoe/foot comfort because we walk wherever we can, and we now have a wider-than-ever choice of shoes which look great – but, very importantly, cushion our feet. (This is crucial because the collagen in the sole of the foot dwindles, along with the collagen in our faces.)

Look for these brands we love: Taryn Rose, Clarks (don't write them off because they've been seriously jazzed up), Ecco (ditto), Terra Plana, ShoeTherapy pumps (with posture-correcting soles), Aerosoles, FitFlops and Chie Mihara, a fantastically funky but wearable Spanish brand Jo recently discovered, which is increasingly widely available. And Sarah adores her Ugg boots! All these have extra 'padding' beneath the ball of the foot. (NB: we find those 'party feet' gel insoles squish your toes, putting pressure on the top, so aren't ideal for everyday wear – although fine for the occasional cocktail *soirée*.)

Buff, buff, buff. One of the basic but avoidable ways feet become painful is through the build-up of hard skin – on the balls of the feet, the big toes, and/or heels. A minute of daily exfoliation is literally all it takes to prevent this. (See below for our thoughts on medi-pedis, to get you started.) Lightly whisk a foot file (see page 101 for recommendations) across areas of hard skin. Do not use pressure because this 'compacts' the layers of skin, making the problem worse, according to medi-pedi guru Bastien Gonzalez. NB: we like to buff dry or slightly damp feet, rather than wet ones – on a towel to avoid unalluring 'foot dandruff'.

Massage, massage, massage. Bastien's other critical piece of advice is to use a moisturiser every single night to keep feet soft and comfy. And really, really work that balm or butter into hard skin areas with your fingers like a deep-tissue massage so it breaks down any 'compacted' skin.

Treat yourself to a medi-pedi. This isn't about polish and paint (though you can sometimes tag those on to the end): it's about ultra-efficient removal of hard skin, correct trimming of toenails (to avoid ingrown nails), nail-buffing, cuticle TLC and diagnosis of any problems, which can then be professionally addressed. Once you've had a medi-pedi (we have them every couple of months), it is much, much easier to do the maintenance at home. In fact, given the choice between having our face and our feet attended to, we'd choose feet every time.

Go mad with a nail polish. This is one area where you don't have to worry at all about being 'age-appropriate'. So go a little wild: crazy metallic jade; pillar-box red; Chanel's classic vampy burgundy/black Rouge Noir. It'll make people smile. Especially you. (And that takes ten years off.)

'Give them some daily *foot love* and you'll FLOAT along, looking like a *spring chick!*'

Put your best foot forward

... and treat any foot woes. Podiatrist Margaret Dabbs's London clinic is where beauty editors (and many other foot-aware folk) head, when feet need not just a treat but actual treatment. So we turned to Margaret for some sole-searching advice on how to stop common foot problems in their tracks

Actually, the biggest problem that Margaret sees in older feet, she says, is dehydration. As we age, the skin thins, we lose subcutaneous (just-under-the-surface) fat, and our tootsies become as dry as the desert. Fascinatingly, that's partly a side effect of the circulatory system preferentially looking after the female organs, and directing blood there. 'Your feet are the end of the road,' explains Margaret. The rest, though, is down to us not looking after them – so, if we may repeat earlier advice, it's vital to moisturise every night.

What's more, it's important not to wear closed-in shoes without socks or tights: 'The moisture from your feet drains into the shoes, drying out the skin – and your feet and shoes are liable to get a tad whiffy, too,' says Margaret. (Open sandals with bare feet are fine because they let your feet breathe.) Now deal with…

Calluses and corns. A callus is a thickening of the surface layer of the skin – hard skin, in other words – which usually forms in response to pressure, often on the ball of the foot, the heel and/or the underside of the big toe. Well-fitting shoes, plenty of moisturising and regular buffing should keep calluses in check, while seeing a podiatrist for regular treatments is also a boon. For corns, professional attention is vital – ideally, as soon as you get one.

A corn is a tiny, cone-shaped mass of

hard skin with a visible centre; it can be excruciatingly painful. The key is to consult a podiatrist who's experienced in biomechanics (the action of how you walk) to find the cause – which could be tight shoes, toe deformities, sticking-out bony bits or an unbalanced gait. As well as treating the corn, you should get advice in order to prevent a reccurrence; they may suggest supportive inserts called orthotics, which can be individually made (expensive) or, increasingly, off-the-shelf (much cheaper).

Warts. These small, rough lumps on the skin, caused by a virus, occur mostly on feet (where they're called verrucas) and hands. Most clear up spontaneously in time (could be a long process though). But since they're contagious and unsightly, treatment is worth exploring. Margaret Dabbs uses a 'holistic' combination of cryosurgery (freezing) and acupuncture: 'It's really successful over about three sessions,' she reports. Pharmacist Shabir Daya, who specialises in natural remedies, recommends this regime: twice daily, apply Manuka Paint, which contains a powerful antifungal and antiviral herb called horopito plus antibacterial manuka (tea tree). Cover with a plaster. Also take L-Lysine 1000 mg, one tablet twice daily on an empty stomach, to help prevent the virus multiplying, plus the herb astragalus (an effective immune enhancer).

Thick toenails. This is a perennial problem for Sarah, again due to horses stamping affectionately on her toes! Medically called 'onychogryphosis', it's also known as Ram's Horn Nail. It's safe to file thick toenails down with a sturdy emery board or foot file, advises Margaret, adding that podiatrists can reduce them speedily with a diamond file. But the damage to the nail bed is likely to be long-term, so don't expect nails to grow back quite normally.

Morton's neuroma. Women over forty sometimes get a shooting pain in one foot

THE BEST EXCUSE WE KNOW TO BUY NEW SHOES

It's not just the pointy-toed and heeled Jimmy Choos that may be putting pressure on your feet. (Actually, we're rather keen on wearing flimsy, pretty shoes because it means you have to keep your feet looking good.) Supportive footwear – from Birkenstocks to trainers, via FitFlops and MBTs – may all cause problems if you don't replace them annually. 'They definitely benefit your feet, building to an optimum in about six weeks,' says Margaret Dabbs. 'Then you need to wear them to maintain the improvements. But be aware that the footwear itself will wear down over time – so you'll begin to notice hard skin building up. The bottom line is: don't over-wear supportive footwear – and buy a fresh pair regularly.' Experts also recommend not wearing the same shoes two days running – both for your feet's sake and because leather needs a rest.

when they get up in the morning. This may be down to a condition called Morton's neuroma, where a nerve is compressed, usually in the space between the third and fourth toes. Acupuncture can help, but in some cases surgery may be necessary.

Plantar fasciitis (PF). Inflammation of the plantar fascia, a band of tissue that stretches from your heel to your middle foot bones, causing intense pain. One thing we know: FitFlop sandals help this foot condition (and many others). Among fans is Olympic long-jumper Jade Johnson who had PF; she was given foot exercises to do in sand by her physiotherapist but found she got 'the same effect from wearing FitFlops for 20 minutes daily. They were really helpful in getting my feet working and pain-free quickly.'

Bunions. These inflamed and painful bumps on the side of your big toe joint afflict about one woman in three in the West. The moment you notice a problem, consult a qualified podiatrist specialising in biomechanics and human movement. The underlying cause is usually the foot shape you inherit, but looking after your feet – and in particular wearing roomy, softer, foot-shaped shoes (eg, trainers) – may help. Wearing toe separators round the house may also be helpful (check out Beech Sandals, which are a specific type of footwear that separates the toes). Avoid high heels and pointed toes except briefly

for glam occasions, and don't wear flip-flops continuously. If you need surgery, make sure the surgeon is really experienced: we've heard horror stories of general orthopaedic surgeons (who do just a few bunions a year at most) taking out too much bone. Sometimes, says Margaret, the problem is actually arthritis on the joint: this can be cleaned out via keyhole surgery, but may need repeating.

TIP

'Always cut toenails straight across: don't curve and dig down into the outer corners,' advises Margaret. A poor pedicure resulted in a sore toe for Sarah when the therapist dug down one side of the nail, causing a small but very painful build-up of hard skin. It was only diagnosed when she had a pedicure at the fantastic Beverly Hills salon of the 'Hollywood queen of nails', Jessica Vartoughian. We think it pays to invest in your feet: good shoes, good pedicurists and podiatrists, top-notch salons.

Foot treats: our award winners

First you buff (see opposite for foot files), then you slather. That's our mantra for soft, supportive, supple feet. After a certain age, feet cry out for richer emollients to deal with cracked heels and hard skin, which can ultimately have a wider impact on health, affecting how we walk. At the same time, we want products to put the spring back into our step – that's where reviving botanicals (think camphor, rosemary, mint) can work mini-miracles. So, good news: the foot treats listed here – all but one brand new entries for this edition – had our valiant testers skipping with delight.

AT A GLANCE

Aveda Foot Relief

CCS Foot Care Cream

Elemis Treat Your Feet Foot Cream

Champneys Spa Treatments Cracked Heel Balm

Bliss Softening Socks

REVIEWS

Aveda Foot Relief ✿

 Already a seriously high-scorer in our books, we dispatched this to a fresh panel of ten mature testers who awarded it similarly stellar marks. The lavender and rosemary oils deliver instant welcome refreshment, there's a moisture surge from castor and jojoba oils, and all the while, salicylic acid (from willow bark) and lactic acid help gently soften calluses and rough patches.
Comments: '10/10! I've used this product on my very dry feet twice daily; it's creamy and I love the fragrance; worked exceptionally well, feet feel refreshed, cool and silky soft; the most amazing cream I have ever used' • 'I get a lot of hard skin on my feet, leaves them soft and smooth, as well as cooling and refreshing; it's expensive but you only need a little dab: I'm a reflexologist so I know about feet!' • 'a really refreshing effect – lovely cooling sensation that lasted a long time – and liked the faint menthol fragrance; left skin soft and moisturised'.

CCS Foot Care Cream

 To be honest, foot products don't come more – well, pedestrian than this… Used by professionals, it's richly-textured – packed with glycerine and urea (though lanolin-free) – and has a somewhat clinical eucalyptus aroma.

Though this cream may never get your beauty-hound's heart beating overtime, testers nevertheless gave it a really high score!
Comments: 'The most effective foot cream I've ever used: deeply hydrating and the effects are cumulative and long-lasting' • 'this thick lotion works really well on hard skin: my tootsies are going to be in tip-top condition in sandals this summer!' • 'skin on feet has lost its scaliness'.

Elemis Treat Your Feet Foot Cream

 Lashings of shea butter and jojoba power Elemis's luxurious winner in this category, which also boasts a particularly nice (non-camphor-y) smell – down to patchouli, lemon and an understated eucalyptus note – more akin to a body than a foot treat scent, we'd say.
Comments: 'Feet soft, really much softer, even on dry heels – and feel revived' • 'just love it – an instant 10/10; after just one application, feet refreshed and soft' • 'sumptuous, rich, divine: after just a week my midwinter feet (with their hard skin) were much improved and I could have started to wear sandals – thrilled!' • 'I wouldn't mind being massaged all over with this cream!'

Champneys Spa Treatments Cracked Heel Balm

 Almost Vaseline-thick in texture, this ultra-smoothing cream features 25 per cent urea (renowned for soothing dry skin), plus shea butter, jojoba, orange, peppermint and a little touch of anti-fungal, antiseptic tea tree.

Comments: 'Noticed a 95 per cent reduction in hard skin on heels' • 'fantastic minty fragrance; feet still fresh at the end of the day' • 'gave this to my stepdaughter who has the worst cracked heels I've ever seen; she loved it and found it really helped to reduce the soreness she suffers' • 'refreshing, uplifting fragrance' • 'significant improvement in cracked heels'.

Bliss Softening Socks

8.14/10

For the foot-carer looking for something different: turquoise rubbery gel-lined cotton socks actually infused with foot-caring, heel-smoothing ingredients. Alternatively, turbo-charge their action by applying an extra cream before slipping these on.) Fab for feet, if not your sex life...!

Comments: 'If I hadn't tried them there's no way I'd consider buying them, but they're worth every penny: my feet are as soft and conditioned as if I've had an expensive pedicure – I now pop these socks on for 20 minutes, put my feet up and relax while they do all the work' • 'loved them: feet relaxed, softer, less ache-y' • 'excellent for reviving tired, overworked feet, which are less swollen' • 'couldn't believe these would work – but they did: after 20 to 30 minutes feet felt soft, moisturised and no hard skin!' • 'my feet get rough and sore – not quite the feet of a camel, but almost; these transformed them although the postman got a bit of a shock when I opened the door to him wearing them!'

♡ WE LOVE...

For Jo, a new 'find' is Kate Logan Shea Salvation Balm: hand-made from a small British 'boutique' skincare brand, wonderfully rich and nourishing, unctuous with evening primrose and lavender oils. She is also a convert to just about all of the many, many products in a targeted range called All About Feet from a (slightly-strangely-named) company called Upper Canada Soap. The whole ritual takes some time, but is very foot-perkifying. Sarah revives her feet with a scrub such as Yes to Carrots Feel the C Pampering Hand & Nail Spa, then massages in (really important to do this thoroughly) a butter or balm; currently it's Neal's Yard Remedies Rose Body Cream – which leaves them baby-soft and delightful.

Foot files: *our award winners*

Hard skin is Public Enemy Number One when it comes to happy feet. Rather than an occasional blitz, we prescribe a nightly buffing session when that day's skin build-up can be lightly scuffed away. (For serious hard-skin removal after a long period of neglect, there's nothing to beat a professional pedicure, or a visit to the chiropodist – or a medi-pedicurist, those brilliant hybrids of the two.) The key with a foot file is to find one that is hand-friendly, so it's comfortable to hold and allows for the perfect 'angle' when you access your soles and heels. These award winners were several steps ahead of the competition, and read on for a new top-scoring entry. NB: if you have diabetes it's always best to consult your health professional before using anything like this.

Diamancel Diamond Foot Buffer

9.25/10

A wowzer score for this classic, top-of-the-range foot buffer. Like a giant, raspy metal nail file, it's thin and quite flexible (washable, too), making it easy to buff feet with almost no pressure.

Comments: 'Most effective on the balls of my feet where I tend to get hard skin build-up; definite improvement in condition and smoothness' • 'love it, love it, love it! Even used it on my parents' feet (please note I hate feet) as it's so brilliant for instant results; also removed a callus' • 'just a couple of swipes leave you with baby-soft skin'.

Tweezerman Pedro Callus Stone

8.87/10

Tweezerman recommend using this wet for best results; first the rough side (for removing calluses), then the fine side (for smoothing).

Comments: '10/10 for this double-sided rough pad, which whisked away rough skin so it was soft and smooth with no irritating bits left!' • 'resounding yes to this: the smoother side was also excellent for rough elbows'.

Marks & Spencer Miracle Foot File

8.87/10

This tied with Tweezerman's. It also has two sides: the top for hard skin zones, the underneath for general sloughing.

Comments: 'Exceptionally well designed, left skin lovely and smooth' • 'easy and comfy to use and removes all dead dry skin quickly'.

♡ WE LOVE...

In our opinion, Alida's Foot File can't be beaten, for three reasons. First, because it was designed for elderly and disabled people, it's incredibly ergonomic – so fits in the hand beautifully making it easy-peasy to access the soles. The two sides – coarse and fine – really do subtly shave away even the toughest hard skin. And last, the holes make for easy cleaning (we think that's rather important for anything to do with feet...). It is, in fact, almost identical to the Marks & Spencer Miracle Foot File, but we prefer the feel of Alida's own handle: a soft, cushiony rubber.

Maybe, just maybe, switch your fragrance

Most of us by now have acquired a 'perfume wardrobe' (as a couple of scent-o-philes, ours are more walk-in closets, actually). Or maybe you're one of those women who've worn a 'signature scent' all these years. Well: don't be surprised if gradually your favourite fragrance smells different on your skin. Or, which is also very common, fades faster...

You are not hallucinating. There's a reason. As Roja Dove (the oft-quoted *professeur de parfums*, who is an old and valued friend of ours) points out, 'Skin tends to become drier from perimenopause onwards and that affects fragrance – because it interacts with the oils in your skin. Less oil means there's nothing for the fragrance to "grip" on to.'

As a result, evaporation is speeded up, which also fast-forwards the process of the fragrance's development. So the base notes swoop in much sooner, and you'll get a more fleeting encounter with the top and heart notes.

But you should also be aware that there's another reason why fragrance may not smell on you as it once did: the formulation may have changed. New laws and guidelines governing fragrance ingredients have led to many ingredients being withdrawn – either for reasons of potential irritancy or for environmental conservation reasons – which has forced fragrance brands to tweak some legendary confections.

We do suggest trying Roja's tips, right. Then you may well find that your favourite fragrances smell 'right' on you again. Or if not, then he's come up with a shortlist of scents (which we echo) to explore now you are *d'un certain âge*. (You can feel a little bit smug that on younger women, most of them smell way too grown-up and elegant – a bit like a little girl trying on mummy's shoes.)

ROJA DOVE'S TIPS FOR HELPING FRAGRANCE

Use a pH-neutral body wash. This won't strip away your skin's natural oils, which are already in shorter supply than they were. (Many body washes trumpet their pH-neutrality on the label, but as a short cut, you'll find them in ranges including Dr Hauschka and Garnier.)

Apply moisturiser before you apply your scent. This gives the scent something to 'cling' to. On your body, use either a totally unscented lotion (or oil), or the 'matching' body lotion to your usual fragrance. (Most neck creams aren't so scented that they'll interfere with your fragrance choice, but they will help by counterbalancing dryness.) 'Layering' the body lotion or oil that matches your scent, in our experience, actually 'time-releases' the scent during the day as you warm up (which you may well do quite a lot!) and cool down.

Try something new. If the advice above doesn't help with your current scent, look for something different – it could be a wonderful discovery! Don't rely on scent-strips in stores (except for eliminating things you really aren't ever going to like); it's crucial to know how something's going to smell on your skin. Apply to your well-moisturised pulse-points, allow a few hours to develop – and don't be rushed. Which means that duty free is not the place to find your new 'signature scent'; go to a department store, an independent perfumery or a specialist fragrance store – there are more and more of these, showcasing fabulous 'niche' brands in which there are some truly sublime creations.

N°5
CHANEL
PARIS

10 *FABULOUS* FRAGRANCES FOR *FABULOUS* OLDER WOMEN

This list – compiled by Roja Dove – features some of the most divine fragrances, which, if you don't already know them, are worthy of at least a brief encounter, but we suspect might have you falling in love…

GUERLAIN *Shalimar*

GUERLAIN *Mitsouko*

JEAN-CHARLES BROSSEAU *Ombre Rose*

LANVIN *Arpège*

CHANEL *No. 5*

HOUBIGANT *Quelques Fleurs*

YSL *Rive Gauche*

ESTÉE LAUDER *Private Collection*

CHRISTIAN DIOR *Diorella*

NINA RICCI *L'Air du Temps*

SEM

'ATTITUDE
is *everything*'

Diane Von Furstenberg

Get a great hairstyle

(And if you like, tear up the rule book into a million pieces)

We may be bossy about how to clean your face or apply foundation so that it takes years off you, but we don't feel that anyone should be prescriptive about what hairstyle suits who at what age. That's because – as legendary Manhattan stylist John Barrett says – today, almost anything goes for older women. Pixie short-cuts. A bob. A funky-chunky textured cut. Long hair. Think: is Julianne Moore cutting her hair short and getting a perm? Is Daryl Hannah or Joanna Lumley? No way. And nor do you have to. But there is *one* absolute rule: you've got to keep it in fantastic nick.

What we've done is to create a montage of some fabulous-looking hairstyles. Use it as your inspiration if you don't feel your current style is working for you and you need ideas. You might also want to keep your own cuttings folder of women whose hair you think looks fabulous. Tearsheets aren't just for teens: they're a great communication tool at any age. Don't be shy to take this into your present stylist – or to a new one: please don't be afraid to divorce your current hair beau if they can't give you a good hair year – and workshop the ideas with them. (Actually, at this age, you really don't need to be shy about anything, any more…)

Personally, we recommend opting for the very best cut you can afford (also colour, see overleaf). We prioritise hair over clothes, because unlike even the most favourite jacket or pair of shoes, your hair is something you wear every single day of your life. Going around with good hair makes you feel amazing, whatever else is iffy. And it can make such an impression on other people.

If you've had the same hairstyle for years, think about this: is this your 'signature' style? In which case that's absolutely fine. We know plenty of women who've had the same style for-flipping-ever, and we can't imagine them any other way – think Goldie Hawn, for instance. With those visual markers in place, your actual age can be almost unnoticed. What may need to change, however, is your colour.

If you spot someone with a great haircut, ask them who looks after their hair. We do it. Our friend Lulu does it. Honestly, that person will just be flattered.

Don't decide on a new cut while you're wearing a salon robe. The style should suit the type of clothes you wear, and your stylist should always, always see you in your 'everyday' clothes before cutting your hair for the first time. They should also take into account the texture of your hair, which is the ultimate deciding factor for any style. Never trust a stylist who decides on how to cut your hair having only ever seen you after a shampoo; Jo once walked out of a New York salon – with dripping hair – when this happened to her.

Which means: ideally, schedule a consultation before you get your hair cut. Use this face-to-face (which you should never be charged for) to give your stylist a potted history of styles you've loved – and hated – so they can get an idea of your favourite looks. Let them run their fingers through your hair, and feel its weight and texture.

Be truthful with your hairdresser about the amount of time you have for upkeep. Can you wash and blow-dry it every day? If you opt for a short, precise cut, have you got time and funds to have it trimmed every three to four weeks? If you want to dedicate your life to your hair, that's your call, but if you want low-maintenance hair so that you can get on with everything else you want/have to do, you're going to need a style that can be tousled dry with some styling product, or tied back, or pinned up simply. Honesty pays. What do we do? Jo takes her shortish layered style to the hairdresser once a week, and has a blow-dry, then goes again a week later. Sarah mostly does her own (she does live in the wilds) with an occasional 'treat' when she's going out. She actually finds long hair's easier (except for the time

it takes to condition and dry) because she can tie it back for riding, etc – and it only needs trimming every six weeks.

Avoid razor cuts like the plague. Sarah spent months in recovery after an attack! Always, always talk through with your hairdresser how they're going to 'texturise' the ends, if that's part of the look you're going for, or thin out very thick hair. Razors can roughen the cuticle and the tips; the hair appears more dull because you've disturbed the reflective surface, and it can go as flat as a crêpe Suzette. That's our experience (and that of others) – and if anyone comes within 20 paces brandishing a razor in the direction of our hair, we're outta there.

If you have very curly hair, go very short – or go very long. Anything in-between is unbelievably high-maintenance and can have a massive 'broom' effect. (Or you could consider a Brazilian keratin hair-straightening treatment, though be aware that in tandem with banishing the frizz, it can flatten your previously fulsome hair. The results can be temporary – but one friend nearly had a nervous breakdown; nothing gave her back the volume she'd taken for granted, not rollers, not thickening lotion, not backcombing – nuffin!)

And for more on which cut suits which face shape… Visit www.beautybible.com/faceshapes. We have archived on our website some drawings from our previous book, *Feel Fab Forever*, which offer guidance about cuts and styles that suit particular face shapes. You might find it useful.

Learn to speak the language of hair colour

If it sometimes seems as if your colourist is speaking another language – well, he (or she) is. So here are all the key terms translated into real-life words – which should help you achieve the look you want, whether you're having your hair coloured in a salon or doing it yourself

TIP

After colouring, never shampoo before 24 hours. This will help the colour to 'set', so it takes perfectly.

We truly, truly recommend, though – if at all possible – that as you start to develop grey, you have your hair coloured professionally at least once, and then at least occasionally. We know that hair colouring can be pricey and can carve huge chunks out of your diary to maintain. A sympathetic colourist, however, will be able to advise you on the best shade for your skintone. If they're really generous-spirited, they may be able to point you in the direction of a particular shade in a drugstore/chemist brand that might work for you, or at least tell you where on the Hair Colour Level Charts you are (see right), and what level of shade would work best with your (undyed) colour.

HAIR COLOUR GLOSSARY

Baliage (aka balayage) The technique of painting highlights directly on to the hair without using foils (see Highlights, right); this can enable a colourist to get closer to the parting/roots with the bleach. Can give a 'beachy' look and lessens the occurrence of unwanted regrowth lines sometimes associated with foil highlights or those pulled through a cap – but best left to true hair colour artists.

Demi-permanent colour Lasts up to 28 shampoos. Contains lower levels of peroxide (which means it's less harsh and drying) than permanent colour. It's great for creating natural-looking tone changes (such as taking brown hair to a rich auburn shade) and will cover grey. Gradually fades back to the underlying shade.

Double process A technical term for having single process colour (all-over colouring of the hair, see single process, below), at the same hair colouring session as having your highlights done.

Glaze (aka Gloss) A pigment-laden or clear liquid used to enhance a hair colour temporarily.

Highlights Streaks or chunks of lighter colour (created through the use of ammonia/hydrogen peroxide), applied through the hair – usually using foils or pulled through a cap.

Permanent colour This doesn't wash out, and requires the roots touching up every four to six weeks. It contains both ammonia and peroxide, so it can lighten, darken and/or completely change your hair colour; it can also cover grey.

Peroxide Otherwise known as hydrogen peroxide, extensively used in hair colouring as a 'developer' or 'activator'. Its role is to open up the cuticle and allow bleach or colour into the cortex of the hair.

Rinse See temporary colour, below.

Semi-permanent colour Washes out after six to 12 shampoos. This enhances natural hair colour but won't lighten it and won't cover grey, although it can soften its appearance. (NB: the reason hair colouring companies cite the number of washes rather than a time-frame is that some of us wash our hair every day, others as occasionally as once a week.)

Semi-temporary Not to be confused with semi-permanent: this colour lasts from four to six washes, contains no ammonia and isn't mixed with a 'developer' such as hydrogen peroxide.

Single process All-over colouring of the hair, from the roots at the scalp right through to the ends, in one step.

Temporary colour Simply coats the hair shaft and rinses out after one shampoo. These cannot lighten hair, but only temporarily brighten or darken.

Tint May sound subtle, but this is an alternative phrase used by hairdressers to describe permanent colour.

Tone-on-tone colour Another phrase for demi-permanent, see left.

HAIR COLOUR LEVEL CHARTS

Now you've mastered this, get your head around Hair colour Level Charts. This is why so many women head for the salon to have colour done (and that includes us). There is an absolutely fiendish system for numbering hair colour: there are 12 levels, with one representing black and

TIP

Home hair colouring can be incredibly messy. We are very, very impressed by some new innovations – including Precision Foam Colour from the John Frieda brand – which are 'mousse-like' once they have been mixed, rather than liquid. This means they are drip-free, don't wreck all your towels and there is no need to cover every surface in the bathroom before applying – because unlike most, they don't splatter all over the place. A truly welcome haircare revolution.

12 representing ultra-light blonde. As a general rule, the first number on the label of a box of hair colour will tell you the colour level of that product. However, your own base colour – and where it falls in that spectrum from one to 12 – will affect the final shade on you personally. This is why colourists advise that you don't stray more than one or two shades lighter or darker than your current natural hair colour, for optimum results.

But remember: no matter what the language of hair colour, one picture speaks a thousand words. It's all very well being able to speaka da lingo when it comes to knowing your semi-permanents from your demi-permanents – but in our experience, the biggest challenge can be successfully communicating actual shades and colours to a salon colourist. So: you say 'brown'. Your colourist could be thinking: anything from milk chocolate to dark chocolate. At the same time, what's 'red' to you might be pillarbox to a colouring professional. (Yikes.) This, we think, is where photographs truly come into their own: brandishing a cutting torn from a glossy of the colour that you are hoping for, in front of your hairdresser, can save an awful lot of confusion. (And, potentially, tears.) We recommend keeping tearsheets of anyone whose hair colour you'd love to emulate. You can then talk through what's actually achievable and – crucially – what the upkeep would be.

HAIR COLOUR LORE

The golden rule of hair colour is this: don't stray more than one or two shades from your natural colour. It won't suit your skintone, and will be a nightmare of upkeep. Now read on! When it comes to covering a whole head of grey, don't go darker. Not only does it showcase greys and regrowth, but it can look opaque, like you painted your head with shoe polish. Generally, you should request a single process (see our GLOSSARY) and highlights that bring your natural hair colour one shade lighter, because it will add dimension and disguise the greys, and flatter your complexion. If you're thinking of going blonder, a shade or two lighter can be very flattering – especially because skin gets sallower with age, and a few fine streaks can wake it up. But going too light can be just as ageing as going too dark. Here's a quick way to tell, from Manhattan colour maestro Louis Licari: 'If you have to put on more make-up to make your new colour work, you've picked the wrong shade. The one colour you should absolutely avoid when you're over 40 is raven black. It will sap life and colour from your face.'

H Coloured haircare: our award winners

Statistically, most women colour their hair from mid-life onwards (and many of us, of course, start much earlier). But we know that many of you don't take advantage of the growing number of products specifically created to put back some of the shine and life that colouring can take out, as well as preventing colour fade

It's a fast-growing section of the haircare market, and our testers trialled shampoos and conditioners for different shades of coloured hair, including many new options (with several new entries in this edition). You may like to choose a product that targets your specific haircolour – or go for one of the other, suits-all-hairtones products.

SHAMPOO REVIEWS

Aveda Camomile Shampoo

8.78/10 Aveda's high-scoring colour care products feature deeply conditioning babassu oil, which leaves hair silky and helps to revive colour. The formulas are infused with plant-derived ingredients to refresh colour naturally – in this instance, chamomile and calendula, enriched with beta-carotene to enhance golden tones. It was trialled by blonde testers, who loved both this and the 'matching' conditioner (opposite).

Comments: 'Great product, left hair feeling light and clean, helped brighten and freshen up my blonde highlights' • 'good gloss on my ashy-blonde hair, and made it more manageable and a bit more golden' • 'made my dry blonde hair blonder, softer and more shiny: I would buy' • 'great shine – best for golden blondes rather than grey blonde'.

Aveda Clove Shampoo

8.71/10 Well, well, well: when Aveda put forward a brunette shampoo, it scored a few micro-points behind the blonde Camomile option! Definitely a go-to brand for coloured hair, then – and with that signature Aveda scent to revel in, throughout. Here, find detoxing clove, brown-enriching coffee plus antioxidants, to shield from environmental challenges.

Comments: 'Really enhanced my colour – delighted' • 'gave colour a new lease of life and fantastic shine' • 'after three weeks my grey is usually starting to show through but with this it lasts another week' • 'hair has so much more shine and looks incredibly healthy; colour richer' • 'couldn't see re-growth and emerging grey as much after using this' • 'no itching, dryness or soreness on my scalp, unlike with most shampoos' • 'improvements in manageability I'd never have thought possible'.

Pureology Hydrate Shampoo

8.19/10 Pureology – a new-ish botanically-rich vegan colour-care range under the L'Oréal umbrella – has done well in our anti-ageing hair categories, here with a highly concentrated shampoo (each bottle is said to last 80 washes), which is zero-sulfate and delivers their 'anti-fade' complex, to optimise colour protection for any shade of coloured hair.

Comments: 'Prolongs the brightness of my colour, delivered a beautiful gloss and shine, improved manageability and the overall look of hair, so yes, it's anti-ageing!' • 'no problems with scalp irritation which is important because I occasionally get psoriasis on my scalp; helped to keep colour "truer" for longer and hair is in much better condition' • 'very impressed, this nourished my hair so colour became brighter and lasted longer'.

Liz Earle Botanical Shine Shampoo

7.8/10 This gentle, SLS-free shampoo – enriched with vitamin E, aloe vera, West African shea butter – and with a divine scent, from eight essential oils plus orange and apple extracts – breaks all the rules, since it's pitched as being ideal for every hairtype, including those who tint/dye/highlight their hair.

Comments: 'Colour hasn't faded as fast' • 'have to hide this from my family as they all think it's fantastic' • 'fantastic zingy grapefruit smell – great first thing in the morning!' • 'used the shampoo with matching conditioner and my hair has never looked better' • 'improvement in shine so highlights look better' • 'hair glossier than usual'.

CONDITIONER REVIEWS

Aveda Camomile Conditioner

 The 'matching' conditioner to the winning shampoo (for blondes and lighter shades of hair). By popular demand, Aveda's colour-care range also comes in one litre bottles.

Comments: 'Works best if used as instructed! Leaving in for five minutes or longer gave great shine to my grey-blonde hair' • 'excellent for brightening and freshening blonde highlights/colour but probably not rich enough for people with very dry ends' • 'gave good gloss and manageability to my ashy-blonde hair' • 'easier to get a brush through, and made my dry hair softer, more shiny, easier to straighten' • 'pleased that my hair colour was more even and the grey-blonde is brighter'.

Pureology Pure Hydrate Conditioner

 For more about the range, see the shampoo write-up; meanwhile, here's the feedback from testers.

Comments: 'Hair looked really shiny and healthy after first use, definitely brightened hair, easy to comb through and didn't dry frizzy before blow-drying; hair felt great, not heavy, and in far better condition despite using hair striagheners etc' • 'I used these products just after having my hair coloured and I do think they have improved the colour for longer, very impressed by gloss, shine, manageability – hair seemed to stay cleaner for longer too' • 'seriously noticeable defrizz effect, I have dreadfully frizzy hair and while using this I could omit my usual leave-in conditioner'.

Lee Stafford Blinding Brunette Conditioner

 This contains what Lee Stafford refers to as a 'Pro-Brunette System Pigment' (oh, how we love beautyspeak), with a rich texture and a slightly caramel tone to the conditioner. It

actually enhances brunette warmth and colour with ingredients like walnut and henna, plus moringa seed extract (a.k.a. 'Miracle tree') to enhance depth and shine, and create 'reflections' of hazel, mahogany and cocoa.

Comments: 'Not really glossy but did seem to enhance and deepen the colour' • 'friend said my thick, extremely coarse hair looked shinier than usual and was much softer, which my husband agreed with; think it did slow down the fading process a bit' • 'high gloss and much more manageable, but slightly weighed down my fine, flat hair' • 'delivered a super gloss and shine, hair felt softer and was easier to style, brought out highlights and I would definitely buy it'.

Liz Earle Botanical Shine Conditioner for Dry/Damaged Hair

 Once you've shampooed with the 'one-size-fits-all' Liz Earle botanical award-winner opposite, then you choose the appropriate hairtype-matched conditioner. So our tinted testers trialled the Dry/Damaged version, which features blue seakale (for colour protection) and lashings of yangu oil, sustainably harvested by a Kenyan forest community.

Comments: 'Amazing! I have long, thick wavy hair and this not only moisturised my highlights beautifully but there's a huge improvement in manageability' • 'without doubt the best conditioner I've ever used on my hair, which looks smoother, healthier and in lovely condition • 'only need a small amount as it's very rich; took good care of fresh highlights' • 'lovely fresh, natural and clean fragrance, and left hair lovely and smooth'.

TIGI Bed Head Colour Combat Colour Goddess Conditioner

 Warning: blondes need not apply! From the bestselling, much-loved TIGI brand, this is specifically formulated using 'Colour LockDown Technology' to keep rich, dark chocolate and cherry hues fresh and fade-free. (NB: The toffee scent proved a bit divisive.)

Comments: 'Made colour more vibrant, with extra gloss' • 'rich burnt caramel fragrance, which I liked' • 'haircolour seemed to last longer and hair was more manageable after use' • 'healthy hair with a good colour can take years off a woman, and this is impressive: have already bought more, plus the matching shampoo' • 'gloss-enhancing, which made hair look younger'.

WE LOVE...

Of the haircare out there that's specifically targeted at coloured hair, Jo has always liked the John Frieda Sheer Blonde range and is particularly keen on the Sheer Blonde Colour Renew Shampoo and Conditioner, which rise to the challenge of keeping her very, very highlighted hair shiny and soft. But we're both converts to the Liz Earle range which did well with our coloured-hair testers here – to the point where (ssssh, don't tell!) we've been known to sneak tubes into the aforementioned West End salon, having found its moisturising, glossing action brightens our highlights and prolongs colour.

TIP

To camouflage grey roots on dark hair, dust on a dark powder shadow with a blusher brush.

Moisturising haircare: our award winners

We get so many emails from readers concerned about dull, dry hair. The dryness can be linked with hair colouring, or simply be a manifestation of the fact that as we get older, everything seems to desiccate a bit. A mini-revolution in the haircare market has seen a raft of haircare products calling themselves 'moisturising' – so we wanted to know: how hair-quenching are they, really…?

AT A GLANCE

Shampoo

Sebastian Professional Strengthening and Repair Shampoo

Matrix Biolage Réjuvathérapie Age Rejuvenating Shampoo

Aveda Dry Remedy Moisturizing Shampoo

Percy & Reed Splendidly Silky Moisturising Shampoo

Conditioner

Matrix Biolage Réjuvathérapie Age Rejuvenating Conditioner

Aveda Dry Remedy Moisturizing Conditioner

Sebastian Professional Strengthening and Repair Conditioner

Alterna Caviar Moisture Conditioner

Kevin Murphy Luxury.Rinse

Here's the low-down, on both shampoos and conditioners, with quite a few new entries. (NB: normally we're cynical about the need to use 'matching' products, but it does seem to have paid dividends for some of our testers, as with coloured haircare.)

SHAMPOO REVIEWS

Sebastian Professional Strengthening and Repair Shampoo

Sexy, sleek packaging – but that's not what swayed our testers, who highly rated this shampoo, designed to repair, strengthen and protect hair. It's also 'colour safe', Sebastian tells us, so could have been trialled in that category – but was primarily judged by our ten-strong panel for its moisturising qualities.

Comments: 'Hair looks better than it has in years; I thought I would always have greasy hair and scalp but not any more' • 'very easy to apply, delicate fragrance and user-friendly packaging, lathered well, and got hair clean with one shampoo; left hair really shiny and manageable, tangle-free and easier to style; I could leave it for a day or two longer than usual' • 'left hair clean but not stripped of natural oils' • 'fab rich product which made hair a bit shinier, lighter and softer than usual'.

Matrix Biolage Réjuvathérapie Age Rejuvenating Shampoo

Promising 'optimal suppleness, resilience and renewed radiance, all without weighing hair down', key ingredients in this specifically anti-ageing range (also recommended for long hair) include antioxidant lycopene, elasticity-boosting rice protein and 'weightless' omega-3 fatty acids from camelina flower seed.

Comments: 'Rich product that gave glossy, easy-to-manage, healthy-looking hair' • 'I would seriously recommend this product; it kept my coloured hair from going too dry and didn't leave any residue; could leave it for two days instead of washing daily' • 'made hair look glossy and hydrated without being heavy, so I guess this counts as anti-ageing' • 'made my slightly coarse hair feel very sleek and soft and easier to style'.

Aveda Dry Remedy Moisturizing Shampoo

Aveda have risen fabulously to our anti-ageing haircare challenges, with several new entries in this edition. This mega-moisturising shampoo offers meadowfoam oil, jojoba, sunflower, buriti and soybean oils, which all work to lock in hydration without weighing hair down – and Aveda groupies will love the signature scent. Testers loved the 'matching' conditioner, too (opposite).

Comments: 'Smoother, healthier hair – didn't always need conditioner if I was in a rush' • 'my normally dry, coarse hair felt lustrous and silky, with a subtle sheen; I washed hair every other day instead of every day but it didn't lose its bounce (unlike with my normal shampoo)' • 'my hair's been manageable and in great condition ever since I've used this – and my scalp wasn't irritated, itchy or dry, a problem I've had in the past' • 'on bad days my hair can resemble a Brillo pad, but this has really helped with the dryness'.

Percy & Reed Splendidly Silky Moisturising Shampoo

 Percy & Reed's 'celeb hairdresser' tag perhaps doesn't do their products justice: this dynamic duo (as nice a team of hairstylists as you'll ever meet, FYI) deserves to be taken seriously for creations like this new award-winner 'hair pick-me-up'. It's infused with blueberry extract, grapeseed oil, sweet almond oil and aloe vera gel, and prettily-scented. (That went down well with most testers.)

Comments: 'Love the smell of this shampoo – fresh and fruity/floral – and it left my hair looking sleek and shiny' • 'I don't think I'd ever need to use a conditioner with this shampoo as it left my hair in such good nick, nothing else was necessary' • 'can't praise this shampoo enough: I had problems with dry hair and manageability but they're all in the past; it's resulted in so many compliments on my hair – brilliant!' • 'hair was less flyaway with this shampoo'.

CONDITIONER REVIEWS

Matrix Biolage Réjuvathérapie Age Rejuvenating Conditioner

 In the conditioning category, the Matrix entry nudged slightly ahead of Sebastian. The key ingredients in the Réjuvathérapie shampoo and conditioner – used as a duo – are the same. Really high scores and delighted reviews.

Comments: 'Amazing to see such a visible difference in my coarse hair; it shines, is definitely smoother and keeps its shape well; a noticeable improvement in condition – a real stand-out product' • 'gave my hair a good shine, and it's healthy and moisturised-looking, improved my colour too' • 'really impressed with this conditioner which works well with the matching shampoo'.

Aveda Dry Remedy Moisturizing Conditioner

 Here, the 'sister' product to the Dry Remedy Shampoo opposite: a rich, penetrating hair treat we've used ourselves over the years, to glossy effect. Aveda groupies will love the signature scent.

Comments: 'My hair really needed some TLC and I was surprised to see the difference after just one wash' • 'hair felt thicker and lustrous' •

'gave hair much-needed body/condition and helped to tame very dry "tufty" short sections'.

Sebastian Professional Strengthening and Repair Conditioner

 The conditioner which 'matches' the top-scoring shampoo in this moisturising category (see that review for more info). Again this attracted several top marks and made for very happy, glossy testers.

Comments: 'Getting a glossy result outside the hairdressers is a challenge on my thick, coarse, coloured hair but this worked! Impressive manageability!' • 'creamy and easy to apply, fresh fruit fragrance, this transformed my hair: my daughter couldn't stop touching it and saying how shiny it looks; also bouncy, full and manageable' • 'I needed a minimal amount to get my very fine hair glossy, shiny, frizz-free and manageable'.

Alterna Caviar Moisture Conditioner

 Caviar by name, caviar-ish by price: a specific range created to counteract the ageing, damaging effects of blow-drying, heat-styling and environmental stress. It's rich in marine botanicals, omega-3 fatty acids, proteins, vitamins and minerals and a 'Color Hold' technology, designed to soothe the scalp.

Comments: 'There is always one miracle product in the Beauty Bible testing packs and this was it! Quite expensive but I will definitely buy it as it transformed my hair. Amazing! Gave lovely shine, so soft it was a miracle' • 'worth investing in as the ensuing boost to self-esteem is priceless!'.

Kevin Murphy Luxury.Rinse

 From Oz's top hair guru, a chic (rectangular-packaged!) moisturising conditioner packed with buriti and kukui oils, murumuru butter, plus antioxidant vitamins – ideal, so he tells us, for frizzy and coloured hair. Our inner hippies are wild for the patchouli in the exotic coconut/orange/tangerine scent.

Comments: 'Left my air-dried hair looking as if I'd used a hairdryer, when it was dry, as there was no frizziness' • 'Loved it. Sister loved it. Mother loved it. Miracle product!' • 'left hair feeling soft and looking smooth and shinier than usual – less frizzy, too' • 'nice fragrance stays with you all day – a little like a creamy vanilla pudding…'

♡ WE LOVE...

We're both newly enraptured by the stupendous and natural Phylia de M. range, from California, which restores a child-like softness even to our very thirsty hair. Jo has also had some amazing, gloss-boosting effects from Philip B's Russian Amber Imperial Shampoo. 'It really delivers an extraordinary radiance,' she says of this deluxe shampoo, which has been dubbed by some magazines 'the Fountain of Youth for hair'. (One for the Dear Santa list?) Liz Earle Botanical Shine Shampoo and the Botanical Shine Conditioner for Dry/Damaged hair are also faves and for Sarah's very thick coloured mane, Liz Earle Botanical Shine products work well, too.

TIP

When your hair looks really dry and thirsty, add a dab of moisturiser to the palms of your hands, distribute over your palms and fingers and run your fingers through your hair. It will do just a little to quench hair's thirst until you can wash and re-moisturise with one of the conditioners here, or apply a mask.

Give yourself more hair

– by pumping up the volume. Hair 'oomph' is a real issue. In general, it becomes a little thinner as we age – and with less of it, volume's even more important if you don't want your locks to look skimpy...

Thinning hair is a very common beauty woe shared by women from forty-something-plus. We're not necessarily talking full-blown, hormone-related/stress-related hair loss: simply the fact that over time, there seems to be less to play with – and most of us could do with a little extra oomph in the hair department.

So we asked stylist Andreas Wild (from the John Frieda salon in Mayfair, London) – who looks after both our mops quite wonderfully! – for his advice on dealing with fine and/or thinning hair.

Have your blood checked to see if you're missing any nutrients. If thinning is associated with the menopause, it could be that you're missing some nutrients – in particular, iron. Women often lose hair around the hairline in pregnancy but it grows back – whereas menopause-related hair loss seldom does.

Work with what you've got. Talk to your stylist about the best cut for your face and shape – and the amount of hair you have. Take pictures with you of styles you like (as with any haircut, frankly), but in particular talk to your stylist about how practical that style might be for you, with your individual volume of hair (or lack of…).

● Shorter hair is almost always easier to manage – and looks younger and fresher; in addition, length weighs the hair down, so shorter may equal bouncier. Shorter-than-chin-length bobs or more gamine cuts may suit heart-shaped faces with a 'right-angled' jaw-line (think Judi Dench), but won't suit anyone with a longer face.

● Actually, there is a simple equation to see if short hair will work for you (see illustration, left). If the measurement from your ear lobe straight down to the level of your chin is more than 5.5cm/2in, you probably won't suit shorter hair. Truly!

● A chin-length bob often works well for women with finer hair (but do remember hair will 'lift' when it's dry, so it should be a good centimetre below your chin when wet).

● If you are tall, broad-shouldered and anything less than slender, bear in mind that you need enough hair on your head to balance your body shape.
(PS Look on our website – www.beautybible.com/hairstyles – to find drawings of which styles work best for which face shapes.)

Camouflage any hair loss at the hairline. The hairline is the first thing people notice about you, so if your hairline is receding, try a soft, graduated fringe – side-swept if you like. Damp hair down in the morning and pop a couple of big rollers in it to keep the oomph up (or use heated rollers).

Don't try to put too much volume in. On some heads, all that extra va-va-voom will just go flat after a couple of hours; better to choose a sleeker, lower-maintenance style requiring less wrist action.

Prep hair for styling with a volumising shampoo and conditioner. We trialled some of these (see overleaf), to help you identify those which work best. Then use a specific thickening lotion or volumising mousse.

Apply a regular strengthening treatment. Kérastase has a dedicated 'Extreme Strengthening' range which many stylists (including Andreas) recommend.

Never overuse heated hair appliances. Dryers, straighteners, curling tongs, etc will damage and weaken hair. When drying, towel hair to damp then lift the roots with a smallish brush or your fingers. Put medium-sized Velcro rollers on and around the top, let hair dry while you do your make-up. Remove rollers and finger-comb or brush smooth.

Try Mason Pearson Sensitive Pure Bristle brushes. These were specially developed for people with thinning or very fine hair.

Between washes, use a dry shampoo. It gives extra volume.

Consider colouring your hair. Colouring your hair tends to make it thicker because the processing actually swells the hair. A good option for non-grey or partially grey hair is an overall tint – no more than a shade or two from your natural colour (VERY important), with balayage (highlights) to lift the effect and make it look more natural.

Discover the upside to grey hair. Grey hair is naturally coarser and thicker than pigmented hair – so don't fight the grey, but instead concentrate on keeping it in great condition. Depending on your skintone, consider adding soft blonde highlights. NB: if you have grey hair, never have a 'mumsy' cut, and remember: make-up (applied as per our make-up chapters) helps stop you fading into the background.

Back-combing can be helpful. But again don't overdo it: ask your stylist to show you how to just tease the roots before you put in Velcro rollers, or when you take them out.

Try a quick fix, when hair's flat. Turn your head upside down, and vigorously rub your scalp with your fingertips. It won't last long but you'll get a welcome instant lift. (Long enough for a lunch or a meeting, anyway.)

Volumising haircare: *our award winners*

For hair that's starting to look thin, there are formulas to help create greater fullness...

Happily, the haircare industry recognises this and is lavishing hundreds of millions of research dollars (and euros) into creating products which give hair extra body, bounce and root-lift. Our more flat-haired testers trialled more than three dozen shampoos and conditioners in this category, and got pretty pumped up about these – which are mostly new entries. The shampoos tended to score higher than the conditioners – which may reflect that conditioner can sometimes weigh hair down a tad...

SHAMPOO REVIEWS

Gielly Green Volume Shampoo ✻

 From a small, boutique, eco-minded London hair salon, Gielly Green's signature haircare is more natural than most, without SLS, parabens or synthetic fragrances. Thickening, strengthening (herby-scented) botanicals here include argan, neem and sea buckthorn oils, plus Dead Sea minerals and mud.
Comments: 'I have the limpest hair ever and this really made a huge difference – my hair didn't feel weighed down at all, and if I styled it, it stayed like that without any extra product like hairspray' • 'this shampoo is amazing, made my hair lovely and bouncy, not heavy and limp and definitely not as greasy as before, it looks great all the time, even in damp weather' • 'top marks for squeaky clean, glossy hair with nice volume – although it doesn't last more than a day, it's much, much better than my normal shampoos' • 'really easy to apply, foamed up quickly, washed out perfectly and left hair squeaky clean; didn't sting my eyes – a big plus and my hair looked and felt fabulous' • 'refreshing unisex/green/citrus scent which could be used by

partner, bit solid/gloopy but works through fine with plenty of water, and lathers well: hair was glossy, kept condition well and it gave some improvement in volume' • 'great product: hair was very glossy and manageable and it did give volume and hair felt thicker'.

Lee Stafford My Big Fat Healthy Hair Shampoo

 Previous testers have highly rated Lee's de-frizzing products; now he's won an Anti-Ageing Beauty Bible Award for this gloss-enhancing shampoo which (as he puts it) 'cleverly banishes dulling deposits that cause hair to go limp'. It also features what he calls a 'Pro-Volume complex', plus strengthening panthenol.
Comments: 'My hair felt fuller and easier to style from the first time I used it; a great shampoo that really did improve my fine hair' • 'nice runny texture and lathered easily; I have lots of very fine hair and it felt much bouncier, was reasonably glossy and had swing and body – it was easier to blow-dry and behaved a bit better, not as flyaway: a really good result' • 'my hair is quite thin and this makes it stand out more from my head but still leaves it soft to the touch; it looked better and bigger with more volume' • 'left hair shiny and fresh-looking, easier to brush and more manageable' • 'great lather and it does feel as if it's reaching deep into the hair and scalp but rinses out easily and no stinging of the eyes'.

Pureology Pure Volume Shampoo ✻

 The Pureology range is actually a colour-care range (it did well in our specific trials for that category, too) – but they offer a volumising option, with a protein complex from soy, oat and wheat, all fragranced very sophisticatedly with amber, mandarin and ylang-ylang. It's sulphate-free, with an 'anti-fade complex'. Your best choice if you have coloured hair that needs oomph.

Comments: 'I love this product, good smell and made my hair feel clean and soft, I use it every wash and my hair is noticeably better and fuller' • 'like this product very much, made hair soft and full, without being flyaway; it's very concentrated and lasts for ages' • 'hair was bouncy and I was very pleased with this, lovely lather, hair felt clean and looked shiny after use; also I usually get slight itching and/or dandruff after having my colour done, this was the first time for ages that I didn't'.

Aveda Pure Abundance Volumizing Shampoo ✿

 Aveda – who have so many different haircare options available – have done well across our hair trials (and we did test LOTS of other brands!). Key ingredients here are acacia gum, babassu, calendula, honey and marshmallow, with a signature Aveda-esque aroma from organic peppermint, ylang-ylang, palmarosa and jasmine.

Comments: 'Gloss was very high and people commented; worked the product into roots and scalp and it really plumped up my hair quite significantly, which lasted approximately three days after washing – fab product' • 'gave some extra volume, both with the first wash and over time; no irritation at all and hair felt good' • 'my hair was immediately abundant – I couldn't stop admiring it; very manageable and easier to style: I used both shampoo and conditioner and have never been more surprised! The shampoo really is the 'amber nectar' of the hair world'.

CONDITIONER REVIEWS

Bumble & bumble Thickening Conditioner

 Silk powder, apparently, features in this formula, which B&b tell us 'adheres to hair strands and separates for fullness'. Moisturising ingredients, too, but it's the testers' comments which as ever are more important to us than PR-speak.

Comments: 'You only need a little and the lovely soft texture goes through hair easily, giving definite volume and lift at the roots and through the length – hair seemed fuller' • 'definitely left a shine/gloss to my hair, and made it feel much fuller, also noticeably reduced my frizz; I felt so happy with it on the days I

used it that I bought some more' • 'my hair was noticeably fuller smoother and had a lovely shine which lasted through the day – that pleased me as I usually come home looking like a mop head…' • 'volumised without weighing hair down; my fine hair felt thicker and looked more defined, with better texture – so much better than any other volumising conditioners' • 'top marks: gave shiny glossy hair with no residue and then definite volume when I blow-dried it, which lasted for two days'.

Lee Stafford My Big Fat Healthy Hair Conditioner

 Testers trialled this in tandem with the high-scoring shampoo, opposite, and it features the same key volumisers. NB In general, scores for conditioners are lower than for shampoos – because by their nature, conditioners tend to weigh hair down a tad. Still, Beauty Bible recommends everyone – even the flattest-haired babe – does use a conditioner, for manageability and hydration. Testers rated this highly for general condition, less for volume.

Comments: 'Really easy to apply daily, and would leave it on for longer once a week for a more intensive conditioning; very impressed that it made my hair shiny and glossy and it didn't weigh my hair down, indeed gave it a little boost though it didn't last long' • 'gave my hair good condition, my hairdresser asked if I'd changed products because I had less split ends' • 'I would buy it for the improvement in condition alone'.

Aussie Aussome Volume Conditioner

 The Aussie range has won many awards and plaudits over the years. Super-affordable and with an unmistakeable fragrance (we're long-term fans), it's 'reincarnated' here in a volumising conditioner boosted by Australian hop extracts to build body from the root.

Comments: 'Very easy to work this thick product through my short hair and made it soft and so much smoother than usual, gave volume without making it feel greasy or heavy – I was really impressed!' • 'my hair is softer and more manageable so I didn't need to use as much product as I did before I used this' • 'hair was fuller and softer with a nice deep shine, and looked better than usual' • 'hair looked good and shiny, and helped give my fine quite thick hair the volume I like – great product!'.

♡ WE LOVE…

Jo has many, many beauty angsts but the volume of her hair (touch wood) is not among them. However, if it was, on the strength of rapturous reviews from her friend Stephanie (who is light in the hair volume stakes), she'd be heading straight for Lulu's Operation Glam range, created by Joe Cincotta, the R&D man responsible for the legendary John Frieda Frizz-Ease range. It is, Stephanie raves, 'a miracle'. Sarah has a mane: the last thing she needs is more volume.

TIP

Legendary London hairdresser Daniel Galvin (founder of the Galvin dynasty) says: 'It's an old trick, but using beer as setting lotion gives tremendous volume and no smell. Light ale is best.'

Hair masks: our award winners

File this under 'essential weekly maintenance', whatever your age. Packed with replenishing oils, nourishing botanicals – and sometimes shine-boosting silicones – we've long believed that hair masks are a must for every woman. More and more women agree with us, and in response the hair industry now offers multiple mask choices. Our testers trialled several dozen (and several dozen more for this paperback), using once a week over a period of time. Alongside their feedback on instant and longer-term benefits, they awarded some pretty stellar scores – and there's a new entry…

AT A GLANCE

Kérastase Masquintense

Gielly Green Repair Mask

Louise Galvin Sacred Locks Treatment Masque for Fine Hair

Kiehl's Olive Fruit Nourishing Conditioner

TIP

Any hair mask will work better if you apply some heat. Wrapping hair in a hot towel is one way. The only problem is that the heat doesn't last long – so instead, our friend Philip B applies conditioner to hair and then blasts it with a hairdryer for 15 minutes, 'twisting' the hair. This is particularly good with oil treatments, though these are best applied before shampooing.

REVIEWS

Kérastase Masquintense

 9.37/10
Kérastase are renowned for their salon treatments, which are now more widely available (via websites) for the at-home user. This is something of a beauty classic, and scored incredibly well: the key re-glossing, strengthening ingredient is their 'GlucoActive Complexe', with lipids and proteins to overcome dryness. It comes in a version for fine or thick hair (our testers had the latter). If you have time though, we can't recommend too highly an occasional Kérastase treatment in a salon, where the stylist will prescribe the exact mask in the range for you. Hair bliss.
Comments: 'Simple to use and delivered a healthy gloss; hair looked full-bodied and shiny, became more silky and easier to shape and style, I would buy' • 'massaged two hazelnut-size blobs through my hair, and it did give a shine and gloss to my blonde hair – which is very hard to do; hair so silky it was much easier to blow-dry, and gave a super-smooth result' • 'definite de-frizz factor with this wonderful conditioner; didn't weigh hair down, it was lighter, softer and more swingy!' • 'one of the most effective hair conditioners I have ever used'.

Gielly Green Repair Mask

 8.81/10
This eco-minded London hair salon and spa in London's Marylebone have two deeply nourishing masks in their boutique haircare line: this new entry's based on mud, alongside neem oil, sea buckthorn oil and what they describe as 'ancient minerals' from the Dead Sea. Argan oil (used for millennia by Moroccan women) is a buzz ingredient in hair circles – and in this lavish formulation certainly worked its re-glossing magic here.
Comments: 'Thick, creamy product: I used a shower hat after applying and kept it on for 20 minutes, and was delighted with results' • 'my hair has not looked this good since I was a teenager; I kept saying to my family "feel my hair!" because it was so soft – gave bounce, volume, brought out highlights and smells divine' • 'after a few weeks of use am happy with improvement in softness, volume, depth of colour and subtle sheen – definite anti-ageing effect' • 'this product has a real "wow" factor and I could see improvements from the very first use'.

Louise Galvin Sacred Locks Treatment Masque for Fine Hair

8.75/10
This luxurious winning mask targets fine hair, which can so often be weighed down by conditioning treatments. Louise's products have done very well in our previous books, including *The Green Beauty Bible*, as they use naturally-derived ingredients in place of synthetics/polymers/petrochemicals/silicones, etc. The treatment masque deploys a form of honey combined with wheat proteins, with twice-weekly treatments recommended.
Comments: 'Very easy to work through wet hair; on first use, hair was glistening!' • 'helped keep my colour bright, hair stayed conditioned rather than becoming dry and brittle, definitely helped with

smoothing and making it manageable' • 'loved this product, so easy to apply and divine smell; left hair squeaky clean, easy to manage and thicker – the first product I've found that really works well on a consistent basis' • 'hair much more manageable, smoother and nice shine'.

Kiehl's Olive Fruit Oil Nourishing Conditioner

8.75/10

There's an even richer Hair Pak in this range, but our testers actually trialled this lavish conditioner as a hair mask, since it's designed for dehydrated, damaged hair. Replenishing ingredients include avocado oil, olive fruit oil and lemon extract, which gives an uplifting zestiness.

Comments: 'My coloured, rather dry hair was shinier and manageable – usually a wet bird's-nest after washing, really tangled and difficult, but this was one of the best conditioners I've used, it was easier to comb out, and left hair light and smooth' • 'delivered an incredible shine; the first time I used it hair was noticeably greasy but definitely a case of less is more for good results; tangle and static-free hair, light and shiny' • 'simple to use, sensible plastic tube, lovely product and very economical; my once-dry hair was softer and more shiny, easy to comb through and to style, which left me more in control'.

♡ WE LOVE...

How much space have we got...? Coloured hair is thirsty hair. So we follow our own slavish advice to use a hair mask once a week, and in Jo's case, that could be generous lashings of the Liz Earle Botanical Shine Conditioner for Dry/Damaged Hair, Christophe Robin Masque au Germe de Blé (that's wheatgerm), which she lugs back from Paris, created by one of that city's leading colourists, or new John Frieda Full Repair Deep Conditioner Mask. And a truly extraordinary intensive treatment she uses once a month is Philip B Katira Hair Masque, based on an ingredient well-known to Persian women, which seems to 'fill in' the cuticle to reflect shine back. Sarah has two favourites: Ojon Restorative Hair Treatment, which is a solid oil that needs warming – a bit messy and takes time but gives great shine – but for speed and fantastic results, she loves Jason Intense Moisture Treatment Mint & Rose which really, really works on her superdry hair.

Hair shine sprays: *award winners*

We don't necessarily advise using these all the time, but for an instant boost when hair looks less-than-glossy, they're a boon. Long term, however, hair masks, moisturising haircare – plus hair-nourishing foods and supplements (oily fish and omega-3 supplements) – are more effective for improving the shine factor. The challenge is that some of these sprays make hair appear greasy rather than shiny. (Start off by using a little, applied to the ends of your hair from the back, so if it's too heavy for your hair, you'll get through the day without it all going lank.) Although there aren't a gazillion options out there, some did go down reasonably (if not spectacularly) well.

A word of warning: do use these sprays before getting dressed in anything you care about – one tester found three spots of shine spray on her T-shirt, and as she says: 'If it had been a new expensive outfit I would have been heart-broken.'

Moroccanoil Glimmer Shine Spray

7.87/10

A new winner: you physically pump the argan-rich shine spray on to hair (so do make sure to keep your distance, even though it's 'non-greasy'). Moroccanoil have taken the hair world by storm with this range, here with a new entry which guards against frizz and environmental damage, adding 'luminosity' to brunette hair.

Comments: 'Created gloss rather than shine on my medium-length fine hair; very light so didn't weigh down my hair or make it greasy' • ' I sprayed some on my hands too, and applied to ends after blow-drying, which made hair look sleek and reduced dry ends' • 'controlled the short fine new hairs in my parting and gave very effective shimmery shine'.

Aveda Brilliant Spray-On Shine ✿

7.44/10

Aveda have done exceptionally well in the haircare department in our book, here with a shine-boosting finishing mist which also tackles flyaways. For all hair types, there's vitamin E as well as Pro-vitamin B5 (to 'temporarily mend split ends').

Comments: 'Made my long hair – thin but lots of it – look good, nice and shiny with no flyaways; no greasiness and no residue at the end of the day' • 'shine lasted a long time; I would definitely buy. Brilliant' • 'amazing shine on my thick coarse grey/white hair which lasted all day'.

Paul Mitchell Soft Style The Shine Spray-On Polish

6.83/10

As well as instantly delivering gloss, this is recommended for use before straightening irons, with a protective shield offered by jojoba, aloe, henna and rosemary, plus silicones. (You can also apply it to bare skin for 'a touch of glamour', Paul Mitchell tell us.)

Comments: 'Gave my fine, wispy baby-like hair a natural sheen/gloss that I liked and lasted through the day' • 'surprised how light this spray is, hair wasn't damp/limp after use, and did stay in place longer' • 'good for my thick coarse coloured hair, which is dry and not responsive to my usual shampoo/conditioner'.

'I've been living
in this EXCELLENT
body for over 60 years.
I *LOVE IT* so much.
As long as it doesn't
get too fat, or too thin,
doesn't break –
I just think,
"*Thank goodness!*"'

Joanna Lumley

Treat your hands with

the same care as your face

Every time Madonna's photographed with her hands on view, bitchy tabloids rush to point out that they haven't aged as well as her face. (Good tip: she often covers them up in gloves, long and lacy for evening, soft leather for day.) We don't go in for bitchiness, but if Madonna's hands are a better clue to her real age – fiftysomething-ish – than her very famous *visage*, she's not the first woman that's true for. There's a very, very simple rule to ensure ageing isn't fast-forwarded when it comes to hands. It is this: lavish them with the same attention as your face. (They are equally visible, after all, though that's so easily forgotten.) Which means…

Shield them from sun damage. Either use a body sunscreen on the backs of your hands and forearms, or a hand cream formulated with a built-in SPF. (There are still too few of these on the market for our liking. Ole Henriksen Hands Forward SPF15 is one of our top choices.) Remember to reapply after washing – so the tube needs to be neat enough to carry in your handbag. Basically, get in the habit of putting an SPF on your hands as part of your morning beauty ritual – post-sleep cleansing, moisturising, SPF-ing, etc. (Apparently it takes 16 to 21 times of performing a task to make it a habit. That's less than a month, for something which is truly going to keep the years at bay.)

Scrub, every week. Just as a once-a-week exfoliation does wonders for facial dinginess, so the same is true for hands. When you're exfoliating your face (and your body), scrub the backs of your hands. It helps treatment products penetrate quicker, while also instantly brightening by buffing away the surface cells. We'd also like to tell you about a product which is frankly a bit of a party trick of ours: Yes to Carrots Feel the C Pampering Hand & Nail Spa. Testers for this book have trialled it and love it too, now (see page 127 for their comments) – and quite rightly so, we say. It's a tub of Dead Sea salts blended into a skin-nurturing oil mixture, which you use as if washing your hands. We have yet to try this on anyone who isn't blown away by how bright, moisturised and incredibly soft hands are, in about 15 seconds flat. (One friend said she couldn't stop her beau holding her hand.)

TIP

Please don't forget the obvious: wear gloves whenever you're washing up, gardening, and maybe even handling paper – it makes nails as dry as the Sahara. If you can't bear to wear gloves while you work with papers (we can't), make sure you slosh on really oily hand and cuticle cream before and after. And don't use your nails as staple removers, to tighten Phillips screws, or dig out stones from horses' hooves…they were not designed for those purposes.

Slap on a mask. When you put a mask on your face, put it on the backs of your hands. Couldn't be simpler. (If you're in the bath, that means keeping them above the water-line. Er, obviously…)

Slather on a rich hand cream overnight. Last thing at night before switching off the light, uber-moisturise your hands with lashings of hand cream. For a shortlist of those which our testers found had anti-ageing powers, turn to page 126. Conventional beauty wisdom says that it helps to apply cotton gloves over the top, but we're not convinced: the cotton 'wicks' the cream off the hands, and they feel frankly odd to us. (Not to mention being total passion-killers.) In the same way that night creams and facial oils applied at night harness the body's skin-repairing mechanism, this is true with hand creams. Where the cotton gloves can be useful is if you're slathering on a cream while, say, watching a movie on telly; stops your greasy paws from getting all over everything.

Hand and nail problems – and the fixes...

Dry and ragged cuticles. This is just another manifestation of (not to put too fine a point on it) the gradual dessiccation of the body. A cuticle oil massaged into nails overnight will go a long way towards fixing this problem, while boosting blood flow to help encourage nail growth (yet another thing that slows with age). For specific recommendations of cuticle treatments, see page 128.

Flaking/splitting nails. The oil treatment mentioned above will help prevent flaking – not immediately, but over time. Submerging hands in water isn't helpful – but it's what rubber gloves were invented for (if you really can't bear the feel of them, try surgeons' latex gloves – provided you're not sensitive to latex – which feel like there's nothing there). Avoid acetone-based nail polishes – the only exception to this rule being the slightly-unlikely-at-this-stage-in-life event that you have fallen for a glitter nail polish: a quick blitz with an acetone-based polish remover is preferable to endless, endless rubbing and soaking with a regular polish remover to get the glitter off. And NEVER, EVER buff if your nails are weak. Oh goodness no, no, NO! – and don't let perfectionist manicurists do it either: shriek, jump out of your chair, run, whatever it takes to stop them, or your nails will suffer for months.

Nails that snap. Over-dry, brittle nails will simply break. Again, oil treatments help. Our testers review nail strengtheners on page 128, but the chemical types should be used for short bursts (not more than a month) – otherwise nails become over-strong, and prone to snapping rather than bending flexibly when challenged.

Ridges. Very, very common, these. Length-ways ridges can respond to very, very gentle buffing; your nails need to be naked for this (although again, as above, you can oil them first). Buff lengthways, but never to the point where you create 'heat'. (And note our caution about buffing above…). The quick-fix is a ridge-filling base coat; we recommend the excellent Diorlisse Pastel Ridge Filler, which comes in two pretty tones – one pinky and one apricot – that can be worn instead of polish (although you'll need a top coat); another good option is Essie Ridge Filling Base Coat. Occasionally, a ridge becomes a split, for which the best solution is a 'patch' applied at a nail salon, while it grows out, or a false acrylic nail. Yet again, you need to boost nail health while it's growing out with stimulating oil massage of the nail bed.

For all these, try nutritional supplements. Sarah is a bit of an oracle on weak nails – her weak spot – and sadly notorious with the manicurists at John Frieda, who are practically as relieved as she is when they grow at all. (Think horses, gardening – and, simply, fragile nails…) The thing that really, really works for her is Sun Chlorella (tiny pillules of food state green stuff, see page 176). Pharmacist Shabir Daya also recommends taking a magnesium supplement at night (as important as calcium for bones, nails and teeth, plus it keeps you calm!) and, if budget permits, silica (aka horsetail), also an important compound for nails.

And eat good food. Try to consume oily fish (salmon, mackerel, sardines, tuna, etc) two to three times weekly for the omega-3 essential fatty acids, which help nails, skin and hair (not to mention brain and pretty well everything else…). If you don't like fish, try a supplement with fish oils, or plant oils if you're veggie. Also make sure you get enough protein for the iron content – iron deficiency is a common cause of flaking nails as well as thinning hair (Sarah finds a steak a week works a treat; veggies should consume lots of wholegrain cereals and flours, leafy green vegetables, blackstrap molasses, pulses such as lentils and kidney beans, dried apricots and figs). And everyone needs lots of multicoloured veg for the vitamin C which is vital for iron to be absorbed.

Camouflage sun spots on the back of hands. Try self-tanner on hands and forearms as this reduces the 'contrast' and thus the visibility of sun spots. Medical peels and lasers are a pricier – and potentially riskier – way to deal with sun spots: we suggest reading the advice on page 186 before you go there.

Veins. Ah, the Madonna problem. Many of us develop large, bulging veins on the backs of the hands, partly to do with the skin relaxing and thinning with age (as well as the gradual loss of fat), so they become more visible. It is, technically, possible to have the veins on the backs of the hands 'stripped out'. The surgery is akin to the way varicose veins are treated, but in general only one hand is operated on at a time as hands can be painful and swollen for the first few weeks after surgery and tender for some time after that. (For more advice which covers all forms of cosmetic surgery, see page 46.) Personally, we'd counsel an attempt at Zen-like acceptance of veins. Gratitude for the miraculous tasks our hands perform on a daily basis – from typing to texting, writing to playing the piano – helps, we find.

TIP

Taupes, oranges and frosted nail polishes can be desperately unflattering to older hands. (No matter how hard Chanel try to persuade us that they are this season's must-haves, and no matter how long the subsequent waiting-lists…) Ironically, mature women often choose taupes because they think this will distract from hands they feel self-conscious about, but instead pale pinks, soft crimson – and even deep berry/wine varnish, which has become a modern classic – will bring nails (and hands) back to life.

Anti-ageing hand treatments: *our award winners*

Because hands give your age away faster than a glimpse in your passport. Because hand-creaming is one of our favourite (and most frequent) beauty activities. Because there is now a raft of creams which promise that as well as soften and moisturise, they help eliminate signs of ageing, by harnessing many of the same ingredients as facial care. For all those reasons, we assessed dozens of hand creams for specifically age-defying actions, rather than just something to leave hands smooth and velvety. Were our testers wowed…? You bet. And for this new edition, there are four really high-scoring new entries, all but one entirely natural

AT A GLANCE

Dr Lewinn's Restorative Hand & Nail Cream

Barefoot Botanicals SOS Barrier Hand Cream

Melvita Bio-Excellence Extraordinary Hand Cream

Yes to Carrots Feel the C Pampering Hand & Nail Spa

Balance Me Super Moisturising Hand Cream

Jurlique Purely Age-Defying Hand Treatment

REVIEWS

Dr Lewinn's Restorative Hand & Nail Cream

 We weren't familiar with 'Canadian Rumex' which dermatologist brand Dr Lewinn's claim as the key ingredient in this 'intense anti-ageing treatment' – so we looked it up: rumex is a form of sorrel. We certainly do know and understand the hand-smoothing action of shea butter, also featured here to deliver its luscious texture. This also promises to reduce splitting and breaking of nails, as well as diminishing the appearance of ageing – so if you're looking for a stellar all-rounder for hand challenges, this incredibly high-scoring product is your no.1 choice in every way.

Comments: 'If I could give this 20/10 I would: easily the best thing in hand creams – dare I say perfect? – anti-ageing effects good' • 'this is brilliant: loads of hand creams that say they're age-defying don't last longer than when you wash your hands – I can't rave about it enough and would give it 13/10 if I could!' • 'hands definitely look better when holding steering wheel (that's usually when I note how old my hands look!) • 'sinks in fairly quickly, leaves hands soft and smooth and nails nourished' • 'I'm a student at the Royal College of Needlework and my hands get very dry where needles pierce the skin – this is better at combating the problem than any I've used' • 'reduced dryness and wrinkles, leaving hands super-soft with fewer lines – amazing!'.

Barefoot Botanicals SOS Barrier Hand Cream

We were a teensy bit surprised when Barefoot put this forward for our anti-ageing category, as we think of it more as a super-moisturising 'barrier' cream for dry/sensitive/eczema-prone skin. But part of the reason hands look 'old' is that they're dry and papery, because of moisture loss – so the shea butter, macadamia/sunflower/jojoba oils, chickweed and mallow extracts work to trap the skin's own hydration, soothing and smoothing at the same time. Very, very light lavender scent to this.

Comments: 'Skin looked smoother, fresher and younger and felt comfortable for hours' • 'lovely hand cream – hands are super-smooth, just wonderful' • 'improved dryness and nails less prone to breaking' • 'lovely hand cream with gorgeous fragrance that worked on my "nurse's" hands; cuticles less ragged' • 'recommended to anyone looking for a "natural" hand cream that works – it does what it says on the box!'.

Melvita Bio-Excellence Extraordinary Hand Cream

8.65/10   Melvita is the all-organic 'sister' company to L'Occitane and Bio-Excellence is their top-of-the-range anti-ageing collection. This rich offering not only targets dryness with prickly pear extract and cocoa and shea butters, but features extracts from lily oil, papaya juice, lemon and olive, known to be effective on areas of uneven pigmentation (and several testers commented on this action). Last but not least, hands wallow in silkifying essential fatty acids from apricot kernel and hazelnut oils.

Comments: 'Loved this product and was disappointed when it ran out; age spots are fading and hands look smoother' • 'age spots less prominent; hands moisturised for ages after use' • 'smell is YUM: lemon sherbets!' • 'age spots have lessened slightly and the dry brittleness of my nails has improved' • 'age spots definitely improved on the hand I specifically tried this on' • 'age spots (and there are lots of them!) much less noticeable' • 'smooth hands definitely look younger'.

Yes to Carrots Feel the C Pampering Hand & Nail Spa

8.56/10   This product's become a bit of a party trick of ours (see also WE LOVE…). The Dead-Sea-Salt-and-oil scrub, massaged into literally anyone's hands, has an instantly rejuvenating effect. It beautifully buffs away dead cells to reveal brighter skin underneath, nourishing at the same time with olive and almond oils. Not a hand cream – but an instant rejuvenator, yes.

Comments: 'Really impressed: not something to use daily but as a regular treatment: hands looked and felt incredibly smooth and soft' • 'a revelation: hands look cleaner, fresher and more youthful than I could ever remember' • 'this product is to hands what a "face base" is to foundation: fabulous

brand and new, happy hands!' • 'transformed my sore, grubby gardener's hands into lady's hands – effect even more pronounced with regular use' • 'a miracle treatment which worked where hand creams have failed'.

Balance Me Super Moisturising Hand Cream

8.4/10   Shea butter, beeswax and sweet almond oil give Balance Me's organically-certified hand cream its mega-moisturising power, in a rich blend that also features healing benzoin and yarrow, patchouli for 'weathered skin' and kukui nut oil for suppleness. As we've come to expect from this niche aromatherapeutic brand, this also smells wonderful.

Comments: 'Fantastic: my hands felt and looked years younger, and my nails became less brittle; perfect creamy texture' • 'very quickly absorbed but hands felt hydrated for a long time; after overnight application they looked amazing, extremely smooth and silky' • 'loved the smell and other people did too; hands looked younger every day I used this' • 'my wrinkly hands look noticeably smoother and it worked wonders on my cuticles' • 'hands more supple and less crêpey, very soothing after weeding or cutting conifers!'.

Jurlique Purely Age-Defying Hand Treatment

8.39/10   Beauty Bible testers have previously awarded Jurlique hand creams very high marks, and this specifically anti-ageing addition to the range continues the winning streak. The non-greasy cream harnesses the anti-ageing power of botanicals such as liquorice (to combat redness and fade discolourations), turmeric extract, softening marshmallow and sunflower oil – and many ingredients are biodynamic, produced and harvested in rhythm with nature. It's lightly rose-scented, and we know from countless previous comments that many of you are enraptured by rose fragrances.

Comments: 'Thick, rich cream which is very easy to smooth in and not too sticky; after a month small age spots have almost gone, my nails are growing very quickly and hands are silky smooth until their first dunking in water' • 'fabulous results: hands instantly went several shades lighter and look five years younger' • 'wonderful, far better than anything I've used before – love this'.

♡ WE LOVE…

We keep tubes of hand cream in our handbags and by every tap, but late-night slathering is best for age-defying hand treatments, allowing them to get to work overnight. On Jo's night-stand are: **Balance Me Super Moisturising Hand Cream**, which played so well with our testers here, **This Works Perfect Hands** (heavenly rose scent), as well as so-affordable **Crabtree & Evelyn Hand Therapy** (comes in lots of pretty scents). As well as her favourite **Seven Wonders Miracle Lotion**, Sarah loves **Lanolips Rose Balm Everyday for Dry Hands & Nails**, and for an instant miracle we both adore **Yes to Carrots Feel the C Pampering Hand & Nail Spa** – a new favourite with testers, left.

TIP

Right before bedtime, slather on a few drops of sesame oil, sunflower oil or sweet almond oil (or any body oil, come to that) and massage into skin. Layer your hand cream over the top and by morning, hands will be baby-soft and smooth.

Nail treatments: our award winners

There are different formulas for nail-boosting treatments. Oil treatments soften the cuticle area and help to nourish nails at the base, making for stronger and more flexible nails. Specifically nail-strengthening (chemically-based) products are painted on like nail varnish, and work to harden nails. (We don't counsel the use of those for more than a month as they can make nails brittle and likely to snap.) Some of these were trialled as cuticle treatments, some nail strengtheners (with plenty more tested for this edition) – and here's the low-down

AT A GLANCE

Nails Inc Vitamin E Oil Pen

Liz Earle Superbalm

Orly Cuticle Oil

OPI Avoplex Cuticle Oil To Go

Essie Millionails Ultimate Nail Strengthener

Nails Inc A & E Treatment Base Coat

REVIEWS

Nails Inc Vitamin E Oil Pen

 9.4/10 A sexy-looking beauty accessory, this: a shiny silver wand-style product with a brush at one end, which you 'prime' by twisting to deliver nourishing vitamin E. It was trialled as a cuticle treatment but used over time you should also observe strengthening benefits, with nails becoming strong but flexible. You'd do well to keep it in your handbag – to put bored moments to beautifying use…

Comments: 'Brilliant having the pen because I have no excuse now! Glides on with no mess, trialled it on my left hand, and the difference is clear: moisturises immediately so cuticles are less obvious instantly, and now soft enough to push down; nails look much stronger and healthier: thanks to this I have now started taking much better care of my hands' • 'nails and cuticles now look uber-glossy and in good health: would absolutely buy' • 'fantastic for strengthening my dry, brittle nails, cuticles softer and easier to push back, easy to do on the move – I am addicted!' • 'I really love the sheer convenience of this brilliant nail wonder'.

Liz Earle Superbalm ✿ ✿

 8.38/10 A seriously multi-tasking product (it glosses lips, smoothes heels, etc) – but here we trialled it principally as a cuticle treatment.

Superbalm's rich texture comes from avocado, rosehip and shea butter oils, plus beeswax, fragranced only with pure natural essential oils of chamomile, lavender and neroli.

Comments: 'After a few weeks nails and cuticles much, much better' • 'also brilliant as a softener for dry, cracked heels' • 'nails have a lovely sheen after use – almost like a clear polish' • 'I was surprised: after a few weeks, nails have grown quicker and are healthier – no mean feat in a cold winter' • 'even after two days I noticed a difference between the treated and untreated hand; I'm glad I could compare as I wouldn't have believed how good this is!'.

Orly Cuticle Oil

 8.12/10 This was tested as a cuticle treatment, not a specific nail strengthener – but again, if applied nightly, we believe it should be good for nail durability. There's a deliciously sweet, slightly citrus scent, thanks to orange blossom.

Comments: 'My dry, slightly brittle nails looked much healthier, did make a difference' • 'great product: very easy to apply, made my really dry, flaky nails and bad cuticles much stronger and healthier, and looked very hydrated' • 'I'm a nurse so wash my hands a lot, then put on lots of hand cream; this helped make my nails stronger so they don't break so much; you only need a drop per nail, so it lasts for ages' • very easy to apply' • 'my dry, scruffy cuticles are softer and in better condition,

Essie Millionails Ultimate Nail Strengthener

 7.83/10 This is part of a three-step nail-strengthening system – but used on its own put on a very good show. 'Positive results for weak, fragile nails are visible within days,' promise Essie. Ideally, paint on a fresh coat of this nail base every other day to benefit from the toughening effect of silk amino acids and iron.

Comments: 'My sad, neglected, flaky nails improved markedly, no breakages and the quality vastly better, but no discernible benefit to cuticles'
• 'with this level of improvement, I became more interested in my nails; I even liked the look with just this on'
• 'very easy to apply, dries really quickly and I had to start using it on both hands instead of the trial one, as the nails on the first hand grew so much longer and it looked weird!' • 'a miracle for nails, only downside is when you remove it and the surface looks stripped'.

Nails Inc A & E Treatment Base Coat

 7.57/10 A second winner from the successful British nail empire started by an ex-Tatler journalist, this nail strengthener is designed to be used either as a protective base coat under colour. Their advice for absolute tip-top results from this 'emergency' nail-fixer treatment is to remove after a week and continue the 'programme' for four weeks altogether for optimum strength, without brittleness.

Comments: 'Easy to apply and happily not nail-breaking to unpack! Fairly quick improvement in my snappy nails' • 'my slightly brittle nails were less prone to flaking and splitting' • 'very practical and straightforward to use, and I noticed a difference in strength within about ten days, and it lasted' • 'nails were 100 per cent stronger after two months' usage' • 'my nails are stronger and longer than I've ever managed to grow them before'.

though nails no different' • 'love, love, love it! So easy to apply and splitting, breaking nails are soft and shiny, and raggedy cuticles look moisturised and very healthy'.

OPI Avoplex Cuticle Oil To Go

 7.87/10 Kept waiting for a meeting? Stuck on the tube? Twiddling your (slightly raggedy) thumbs? Squeeze a little of this avocado-rich gel/oil (you can smell the avo!) on to cuticles via the built-in brush, to nourish them. Avocado is super skin-compatible, but sunflower, sesame, kukui nut oils (and vitamin E) also feature.

Comments: 'I work in a hospital and wash my hands a lot, but this made nails stronger and less easy to break' • 'brilliant around toenails where I had very hard cuticles' • 'loved it – nails much better, flexibility and strength improved' • 'so easy to carry in my handbag and use anytime; got me through winter with fewer chaps and dryness'
• 'luscious oils blend in beautifully leaving nails gleaming'.

♡ WE LOVE...

Nail nourishment really works. Jo has an armoury of products that have defeated her previously flaky nails: divinely-scented Cowshed Apricot Nourishing Cuticle Oil and Body Shop Almond Nail & Cuticle Treatment (with its so-useful built-in hoof stick), plus her new discovery – inspired by testers' comments – OPI Avoplex Cuticle Oil To Go, which now goes everywhere in her handbag. (NB Remove before security at airports: she had the first one confiscated!) Sarah relies on Seven Wonders Miracle Lotion, a hand and body product with sweet almond and olive oils which has transformed her dry, flaking nails – they take time to grow but look better instantly. And please don't forget to eat well – nails need lots of food as much as the rest of you.

'Never stop
your *passion*.
Just keep going.
Be useful.
Stick up for what
you BELIEVE in.
Get *angry* about
what you
CARE about'

Jane Birkin

Learn a few lip tricks that put a smile on your face

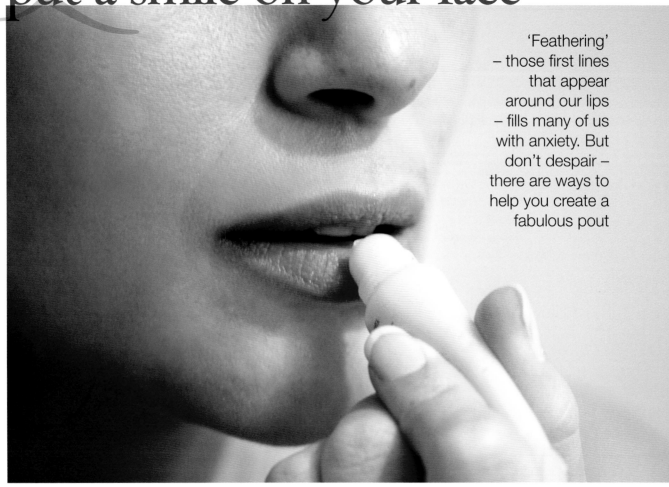

'Feathering' – those first lines that appear around our lips – fills many of us with anxiety. But don't despair – there are ways to help you create a fabulous pout

We speak, we laugh, we eat, we kiss! – so the lip zone gets a lot of action. No wonder, then, that fine lines and wrinkles – starting off with 'feathering' – develop around the lip contour not long after they show up in the eye zone, often causing women we know quite some distress (and beware, it happens earlier – much earlier – if you're a smoker. Skin really doesn't like the free radicals contained in smoke, or that puffing action). Over the next few pages you'll find your 'lip action plan': the treatments, the make-up, the tricks to make your pout fuller, smoother, sexier – and, in turn, maybe just a little smilier. So your lips won't tell the world your real age…

Brush lips with a toothbrush to remove any flakiness. For perfect lip colour, you need a smooth base. To achieve this, we suggest regularly using an old, soft toothbrush – which you keep for this purpose – dabbed in balm: make gentle circular movements to buff away flakes and really push the balm into the lip skin, because it has no natural moisturisation of its own.

Give lips back their natural, rosy hue. Lips – like so much else – tend to fade as we age, and naturally rosy lips are rare. (Though if yours are really pale, do get your iron levels checked.) So we believe in giving them some help. 'As you get older, slightly brighter lips are important,' advises Trish McEvoy, 'but they shouldn't be opaque or matte. Outline the lips [see lip liner tips below], then fill in with sheer or semi-sheer lipstick.' Mid-rose toned lipsticks are, most make-up artists agree, the most flattering for women of forty-plus – think of the colour that lips naturally are, only a tiny, tiny bit stronger. If you choose a really sheer lipstick, you can go a bit darker – it'll just leave a slick of colour.

Use a nude lip pencil for a crisp, youthful outline. Choose a rose-y nude, not a brown-y nude, which should be as close to the natural colour of your lips as possible – and then, explains Terry de Gunzburg, 'You can draw your lipline at the outer edge of your lips and actually increase the apparent size of both the top and bottom lips.' (You have to make sure the line dovetails perfectly at the corners of your lips, though. Otherwise the ghastly spectre of Ronald McDonald swims into the imagination…) There should, of course, never be a gap between the pencil and your actual lip – but you can use the pencil to 'extend' the contour of the top and bottom lips.

Lip pencil will help prevent 'feathering'. The waxiness helps stop moisturising or lubricating ingredients in a lipstick formulation from travelling into tiny lines around the lip line (and we all have those too…).

Try lip pencil and gloss, or sheer/semi-sheer lippy. No matt lipstick ever. Outline lips, then fill in with pencil; top with gloss or balm (tinted if you like).

Feel free to use your daughter's lip gloss. (Or your goddaughter's.) When it comes to many make-up items, we're recommending that you 'shift' your buying habits towards make-up ranges which specifically target more mature skins. But lip gloss? You can get away with pretty much anything, so long as it's not over-shimmery, or too intense in colour. (Or too sticky if you have longer hair – that awful feeling of strands being glued to your lips.)

Having said that, try adding just a touch of

shimmer to the centre of your bottom lip. This really does help make lips look fuller. Apply the shimmer (or gloss) with your finger, and pat it in. (Terry de Gunzburg's By Terry Or de Rose balm is also perfect for this, as well as for an overnight lip treatment: it has tiny shimmering particles of real gold, which look super-flattering.)

Between 45 and 60, give up the statement red lipstick, says Mary Greenwell. Mary remembers the time when she was walking down Fifth Avenue in Manhattan and saw a pair of red lips on legs coming towards her. Then she realised it was a mirror, and that's the moment she gave up her red lipstick. For now. 'Somehow, on a woman at that stage in her life, a geranium or poppy or pillarbox red lipstick is all you see when you look at the face – and it doesn't look sexy. After sixty, you can take it up again – it becomes a glamorous "statement", a bit eccentric and rather divine.'

Also avoid shrieking orange or fuchsia, and very pale lipsticks, advises Barbara Daly, 'although pale gloss is fine'. But, says Barbara, 'bright, rich colour can look very chic at night'; she created silver-mopped fashion designer Betty Jackson's trademark soft, clear crimson especially for her. NB: the word is 'soft'…

Lip gloss: our award winners

Ah, lip gloss. Gorgeous, glamorous, makes-you-feel-girly-at-any-age lip gloss. What's more, it's possible to use lip gloss not just for a slick of sexy shine, but to create the illusion of a fuller pout. At this stage in life you're almost certainly looking for something that stays put that bit longer than the rest. Look no further, say our panellists

AT A GLANCE

New CID Cosmetics i-gloss

Lancôme Juicy Tubes Ultra Shiny Hydrating Lip Gloss

Clarins Colour Quench Lip Balm

Clinique Vitamin C Lip Smoothie

TIP

Applying lip gloss generously all over is fine for 15-year-olds, but there's a more age-appropriate technique for this stage in life. Add a dab to the centre of the bottom lip, swipe it side to side with your finger, and don't rub lips together – smack them like you're saying, 'Ma! Ma!' If you need more, repeat the process. (See our tips for applying lip pencil, page 133, as this gives gloss a base to 'cling' to and prevents gloss and lipstick travelling.)

REVIEWS

New CID Cosmetics i-gloss

 An awfully clever gizmo, this: at the touch of a button it lights up so that you can apply in the dark using a mirrored panel on the side of the wand (very useful for taxis). The colour which our testers received was Moonstone, a sort of holographic, crystalline pink, which is very fetching when lightly applied over a lipstick – but a bit too 'disco' if applied generously on its own.
Comments: 'Would I buy this? Yes, yes, yes and YES! It's easy to apply, very glossy, not sticky, moisturising, colour is just right and I love the shimmery finish – my lips looked like Angelina Jolie's!' • 'blown away by this glam glossy girlie high-tech product, wonderfully moisturising yet sheer; I've bought it for five girlfriends' • 'gorgeous, gorgeous, gorgeous! Loads of comments from girls asking what it was, and men saying how lovely my lips looked' • 'inbuilt light and mirror are one of the most ingenious fab inventions for lippy lovers!'.

Lancôme Juicy Tubes Ultra Shiny Hydrating Lip Gloss

 With their angled tip (for ease of application), Juicy Tubes have become a cult, with limited-edition shades and fragrances. Our testers had Melon 22, a classic sheer rose pink with a melon-y scent. Super-shiny – and often fruit-scented – Juicy Tubes are a love-'em-or-hate'em product; for our testers, it was a Juicy love-in… (Though some did find the stickiness a problem.)
Comments: 'Lovely sheer flattering colour, and it's so moisturising – gave dry, flaky lips immediate relief, also helped plumpness a little' • 'I like how instantly glam it makes me look' • 'impressed by the suitably scrumptious range of shades' • 'lasts well for a lip gloss: I'm never without it'.

Clarins Colour Quench Lip Balm

 Cherry-scented, cherry-flavoured – and available in plenty of sheer and shimmery shades (our panellists received Strawberry Sorbet). Skincare brand Clarins position this new entry as a lip-conditioning 'balm', to repair, nourish and moisturise.
Comments: 'Just by applying this and mascara I look and feel bright for the school run!' • 'thick, comfy and moisturising; tastes like an old-fashioned sweetie' • 'moisturising and comfortable to wear as well as giving the illusion of fuller lips' • 'lips looked fuller when wearing it due to shimmery finish' • 'glam and glossy without being glassy' • 'the tapered "nozzle" makes it easy to apply – a new favourite "weekend" product'.

Clinique Vitamin C Lip Smoothie

 A particular favourite of ours – and another new entry: twist one end and the luscious, non-sticky gloss flows through the brush, conditioning lips with shea and cocoa butters. Although pomegranate and acai berry pack a powerful antioxidant punch, it's not 'fruit-flavoured' or scented. Tons of shades available but testers received strawberry bliss.
Comments: 'With one sweep of the brush I was transformed from dowdy housewife to foxy lady!' • 'a dream to apply: a couple of quick slicks and Bob's your uncle!' • 'amazed at my little lips appearing more "pout-y"!' • 'very moisturising: glossy, glam and enjoyable' • 'I'm converted by this gloss after years as a lipstick girl'.

Lip pencils:
our award winners

A must for the more mature make-up kit. As we've said, lip liner defines the lips (which become more 'blurry' as lines arrive). It helps prevent 'bleeding' by creating a waxy barrier that stops lipstick travelling and gives any lip colour something to 'cling' to, helping it stay put. These were all sent to ten women and had them beaming

AT A GLANCE

MAC Lip Pencil

Inika Mineral Lip Liner

Sisley Phyto-Lèvres Perfect

Revlon Colorstay Lipliner

REVIEWS

MAC Lip Pencil

 8/10

The shade Spice, which was sent to our testers, is an absolute legend in the make-up world, probably the best-known lip liner of all time, as used by supermodels, super-make-up-artists, you name it… A perfect brown-y/pink lip colour, with vitamin E to condition lips, it glides on smoothly and stays put, too.

Comments: 'Soft creamy pencil which lined and filled in lips very easily, I loved using it all over lips with lip gloss, lasts for ages and makes the gloss last twice as long as normal' • 'smooth and easy to apply, looked good, and made other lip products last longer so saving me money – always a bonus!' • 'delighted with this pencil and how natural it looked – I used to dread the dark line around lips but this was excellent as liner and base colour'.

Inika Mineral Lip Liner ✿ ✿

 7.89/10

This is a clever design: there's a pencil sharpener in the lid, so you push the pencil in, turn the cap – and hey, presto! One sharpened pencil. It's the most natural option that our testers rated, with a blend of certified organic plant waxes and oils, from an Australian mineral-based make-up brand which is vegan-certified. It was dispatched in Sugar Plum, a pink-y nude.

Comments: 'Really good texture and I was very pleased with outline; impressed with it as a base for lipstick, lasted several hours although I sip water or coffee all the time' • 'loved the sharpener in the lid, wish I had eye pencils like that: a very good idea'.

Sisley Phyto-Lèvres Perfect

 7.66/10

From the luxury end of the make-up spectrum comes Sisley's winner: a deep rose/nude pencil (Rose Thé) enriched with kokum butter, aloe vera and jojoba oil for softness and hydration, plus beeswax for a long-wear finish. There's a brush at one end for softening the line you've smoothly created.

Comments: 'Simply the best lip liner I've ever tried; slightly creamy and goes on smoothly and precisely for a realistic outline; I used it as a lip liner, base and lipstick; the lip brush applicator at the other end was an excellent tool for blending' • 'nice smooth-textured soft pencil that went on easily and didn't smudge, the outline was not too hard so you don't look like an old woman!' • 'looked good all over my lips; didn't dry out lips'.

Revlon Colorstay Lipliner

Beauty Steal

 7.63/10

Revlon's Colorstay range is designed to be especially 'budge-proof' – which, with a lip pencil, is a terrific boon, as it really will lengthen the lifetime of any lipstick applied over the top. The SoftFlex technology, which achieves this, means that while this twist-up pencil should be durable it's not uncomfortably hard or drying (though some testers pointed out that it's best to apply it on top of balm, as we always suggest). It comes in ten 'full coverage' shades, also five sheer and one clear. Our testers trialled Nude.

Comments: 'Very easy to apply smoothly and precisely, didn't drag' • 'great base for lipstick and really helped my usual colour to last; even when that faded, the lip liner lasted and looked fine' • 'I had a long lunch and my lips still looked great at the end – in my book that's pretty good going' • 'a good beauty "steal"'.

♡ WE LOVE…

Jo has a wide selection (Chanel, MyFace, Benefit) and is fairly unfussy about the brand, so long as the shade is right – a truly nude tone, since she's almost as afraid of VLL (Visible Lip Line) as VPL (Visible Panty Line) from a too-dark liner. Sarah favours Putty Lipliner by Valerie Beverly Hills, a creamy long-wearing pencil in a perfect neutral, both as lip liner and over well-conditioned lips.

TIP

Do condition lips before applying lip liner: even the creamiest can be a bit drying on dry lips! Apply balm and leave to sink in for a few moments before putting on lip product. (Actually do keep lips conditioned anyway, lip liner or not; see page 137 for lip treatments.)

Lip-plumpers: *our award winners*

Nothing in a wand is going to give the plumping effect of something that comes in a cosmeto-dermatologist's syringe – but for millions of us who are happy to help nature along purely with cosmetics, a lip-plumper can be a useful addition to the beauty arsenal

AT A GLANCE

MAC Plushglass

L'Oréal Paris Glam Shine

♡ WE LOVE...

The one that really works for Jo (so much that the tingle's almost painful!) is Valerie Beverly Hills Bee Sting Lip Plump, in a chic little silver mirrored compact which she can now (annoyingly) only pick up in the States. It's a cosmetic effect, rather than a long-term treatment – but definitely does make lips a touch more Bardot. She's also a fan of the wondrously-named Soap & Glory Sexy Mother Plucker Lip Plumping Gloss. Sarah almost never remembers to do it, but the Valerie lip-plumper certainly works – and it's fun!

True 'lip-plumpers' offer ingredients which actually increase the volume of the lips temporarily (such as capsicum, which works by bringing blood to the lips accounting for the tingle in the million or so nerve endings in the lips) – or for longer-term plumping contain ingredients to encourage the production of cushioning natural collagen in the lip area. Sad to report, this proved probably the most disappointing category in the book – and nothing we trialled for the new paperback edition knocked our socks off either (though there is one new entry, from L'Oréal Paris). Of more than 30 products we've now dispatched to our testers, just a couple proved worthy of inclusion – and reading testers' comments this was more to do with an instant optical illusion than any longer-term change. But do also see We Love…, left, and Lip Glosses on page 134: the message is that you can achieve a bee-stung look, albeit temporary (and rather a small bee…but better than a large trout we think).

REVIEWS

MAC Plushglass

A sheer lip colour with a high-shine finish, MAC describe this as delivering 'a cool-warm vanilla buzz to the lips'. It features vitamin E and lip-conditioning ingredients, and is available in 13 shades (our testers received Ample Pink, a soft neutral). As we said above, although this was popular and gained a few high marks, the effect was transient. Testers differed widely on what they felt about the tingling!
Comments: 'Very effective for instant illusion of fullness – gave my lips a plump shimmery, sexy look – and stays on for ever' • 'instant tingle but not unpleasant, I re-applied every two hours and felt my lips were genuinely fuller and looked plumper within minutes of applying' • 'pale pink shade was very natural and youthful, subtle and beautiful; I re-applied every two hours' • 'the tingling made me think it was plumping out my lips and I think it did make them look a little fuller, but I wasn't keen on the "thick" feeling of the product' • 'created a genuinely puffy lips look but I found the "stinging" sensation uncomfortable' • 'pleasant sensation and I think the gloss made my lips look and feel slightly fuller and more youthful: a make-up bag staple'.

L'Oréal Paris Glam Shine

This is also definitely a 'mere' lip gloss rather than the type of product which works by stimulating the nerve endings to 'pump up' the lip tissue – but it, too, out-performed designated lip-plumpers, in terms of results. Glam Shine is an enduring 'classic' within the extremely affordable L'Oréal Paris make-up range, with what they tell us is a high proportion of light-reflective, ultra-glossy oils – plus 'Crystal Shine' particles, to catch the light in all directions. Glam Shine comes in a really big portfolio of shades, finishes and textures: our lot had 400 Juicy Rose Glow (the sort of rosy neutral we always request from participating brands, as it matches almost everyone's colouring).
Comments: 'This is a comfortable gloss to wear which definitely made lips look shiny and full – although the results, as with most lip glosses, are pretty fleeting' • 'deliciously moisturising – feels like a balm, looks like a volumising gloss' • 'overall, I've enjoyed using this' • 'not exactly Brigitte Bardot or Angelina Jolie, but definitely my normally thin lips (which have further deflated with ageing) look a bit fuller' • 'comfy texture compared to most other lip glosses – not too sticky'.

Lip treatments: *our award winners*

For lips and the surrounding skin, a treatment product can be a boon. The winners here are mainly uber-lip balms, which condition lips (and some plump them out). Use them on your lips for daytime hydration and at night on your lips and lip zone to target feathering

Among the many, many lip treatment options out there, these earned the biggest smiles from our panellists (we've now trialled over 30 entries, in this growing category)…

REVIEWS

Rodial Glam Balm Lip

8.4 / 10 A high score for this new category-winner: a lip-targeted version of Rodial's cult Glam Balm, featuring special spheres to fill fine lines and imperfections, alongside antioxidant vitamin E, a pomegranate extract and nourishing rose wax, which imparts a subtle rosy scent, too. **Comments:** 'The perfect lip balm: gave lips a great boost of moisture and kept them supple and soft' • 'gorgeous natural pinky gleam, and has a tingle that gives you the feeling of plumper lips' • 'love it, love it, love it!' • 'lips feel and look softer, smoother and more defined – less lined and crêpey' • 'lovely packaging: small round plastic jar with silver lid, and tastes of roses' • 'any excess did wonders for my nails!'.

Clarins Moisture Replenishing Lip Balm

8.35 / 10 Ingredients in this little tube of lip magic from the Clarins HydraQuench collection include essential rose wax, ceramide 3 (a super-moisturiser), shea butter and rice oil. It's not specifically designed to be 'anti-ageing', but Clarins submitted it for this category and the responses from our testers show it rose to the challenge. **Comments:** 'Felt good and really delivered on performance: lips are smoother, softer and look more fulsome' • 'quite sticky to start with but soon absorbed and lips look healthier, plumper and more youthful' • 'healed my son's trumpet-playing sore chapped lips in 24 hours'.

Clarins Extra-Firming Lip & Contour Balm

8.31 / 10 Unlike the Clarins product above, this comes in a glass jar that's more bathroom- than handbag-friendly. Silky-soft and lightweight, the balm features Clarins's lip-plumping Maxi Lip Complex, to help boost production of collagen and plump and smooth fine lines, plus vitamin E. The fragrance is attractive, with star anise, cardamom, cinnamon and vanilla. **Comments:** 'Lip-plumping, moisturising and really hydrating – fab, fab, fab!' • 'my lips look plumper and healthier and there is a slight reduction in feathering around them' • 'a soothing balm with a velvety texture which improved the condition of my lips 100 per cent; lips moister and more kissable!'.

Institut Esthederm Cyclo System Lip Contour Youth Cream

7.86 / 10 This cream formula – from a French brand with over 30 years of skin research under their belts – incorporates 'plant-based filling spheres' for an instant effect, together with shea butter, centella Asiatica, vitamin C and lipopeptides, plus what they call 'Cyclanol', to 'reactivate vital skin functions and compensate for hormonal deficiencies' (!). Don't just use it on lips: they recommend smoothing into the expression lines that go from nose to mouth, too. The pretty pot comes with its own spatula, which testers liked. **Comments:** 'Excellent product. I applied night and morning as directed and it helped to alleviate the vertical lines between my nose and lips; lips are softer and fresher and skin around them softer and less lined' • 'oozes luxury and dermatological care: slight reduction in fine lines around lips'.

AT A GLANCE

Rodial Glam Balm Lip

Clarins Moisture Replenishing Lip Balm

Clarins Extra-Firming Lip & Contour Balm

Institut Esthederm Cyclo System Lip Contour Youth Cream

♡ WE LOVE…

Ritualised several-times-daily use of a balm (our very own Beauty Bible Lip Balm, a real steal too!) goes a long way towards keeping our lips soft and supple, and Jo also applies Liz Earle Naturally Active Superskin Lip & Eye Treatment around the lip area, which she feels helps with any incipient 'feathering'. She also loves By Terry Or de Rose, a pink-tinted balm shimmering with 24-carat particles of gold (yes, it's a lip luxury). Sarah adores lip balms but isn't yet evolved enough to use another treatment – but she does smear her night facial oil over her lips, so perhaps that counts!

*L*Moisturising lipsticks: *our award winners*

Don't know about you, but we like our lipsticks dewy, comforting and lip-replenishing. (Since they lack oil glands, lips are prone to dryness.) However, at this stage in life a moisturising lipstick offers more than a mere feel-good factor: its softly sheeny appearance is infinitely more flattering than any matt lip look

Which to choose? You'd do well to start with these top-scorers, from almost four dozen we've now sent out to testers, with three new top-scoring award-winners appearing in this edition. (NB: the one downside of moisturising lipsticks is they often need more frequent slicking, as the richer and creamier a formulation, the faster it slides off lips. But we think it's worth it, for sheer comfort and flatter-factor.)

REVIEWS

Clinique Chubby Stick

 We did slightly punch the air when this big fat lip-slicking pencil triumphed here, because at Beauty Bible Towers we each own an indecently large number of shades. We personally love the fact they're completely goof-proof: so sheer in texture you can literally apply in the dark, as well as the lip-quenching texture – like a balm, really. Now available in an equally chubby number of shades (our testers received Mega Melon, a warm neutral).
Comments: 'Really easy to use and very moisturising: my lips didn't dry out at all during cold weather' • 'had a cold when I first tried this and lips were cracked, but this has made them feel soft and they look better than with my normal lipsticks' • 'loved the giant crayon design' • 'very easy to use, natural finish and no "clogging" feeling you get with some lipsticks' • 'a great invention for when you want a pop of colour – love the fact it's so moisturising and sometimes wear it when I don't have any other "face" on; it's always going to be on my wishlist now'.

Guerlain Rouge G Exceptional Complete Lip Colour

 At the really 'luxe' end of the lipstick spectrum: a hefty silver bullet which you slide the lipstick out of, so it flips open to reveal a double mirror. (Very Hollywood glam, this.) It offers lip-plumping vitamin A palmitate, hydrating wild mango butter, hyaluronic acid and wrinkle-filling Ayurvedic guggul resin – 25 shades, and we trialled 04 Gentiane, a subtly shimmering tea rose.
Comments: 'Left lips feeling soft; didn't dry them out as some lipsticks do' • 'smooth, rich and moisturising; I don't normally wear lipstick as I'm concerned about appearing too "done up" but this has changed my mind' • 'fantastically comfortable – really moisturising and stays on your lips giving the feeling it's continually delivering hydration – the nicest-feeling lipstick I've ever used' • 'using it made me feel I should have been on a movie set in the 1920s – wonderful, feminine packaging' • 'gorgeous!'.

Bobbi Brown Treatment Lip Shine SPF15

 You've an option of 12 shades in this hydrating, lightweight, soft-shine lipstick by our beloved Bobbi, which features cocoa and shea butters, apricot kernel and avocado oils, vitamin C and collagen-stimulating paracress, plus an SPF15. (Wish all lipsticks had that.) There's a clear version, too – but our lot had Desert Rose.
Comments: 'Very moisturising and easy to apply, like a balm' • 'lovely creamy, smooth texture goes on easily with no dragging – a joy to use, my current lust-have/must-have!' • 'feels silky and moisturising' • 'I tend not to use lip colour as everything dries my lips out but this silky, smooth lip treat has got me

AT A GLANCE

Clinique Chubby Stick

Guerlain Rouge G Exceptional Complete Lip Colour

Bobbi Brown Treatment Lip Shine SPF15

Clinique Colour Surge Butter Shine Lipstick

♡ WE LOVE...

The ranges Jo likes best offer a wide shade choice of lush-textured lipsticks: **Clinique Colour Surge Butter Shine Lipstick** (favourite shade Berry Blush, a terrific neutral), **Bobbi Brown Treatment Lip Shine SPF15** in Rosy (a warm pinky-brown), and the wondrous new winning entry here, **Clinique Chubby Stick** – which Sarah's also addicted to – in a rainbow of pinks and reds. For daytime, lazy Sarah usually wears a tinted lip balm (such as **Lanolips Lip Ointment** in Rose) or the aforementioned Chubby Stick, above, over a natural-coloured lipliner. She's also a big fan of **Clinique's Vitamin C Lip Smoothie Antioxidant Lip Colour** in soft rosy-brown Strawberry Fudge.

back into the idea of wearing it sometimes' • 'soft and moist yet not glossy or sticky – just what I've been looking for!'.

Clinique Colour Surge Butter Shine Lipstick

One of Jo's faves, this: really lip-quenchingly comfortable, with a beautiful glossy finish that lasts longer than most lipsticks, she finds. Its secret: special butters, moisturisers and modern waxes that melt at body temperature for a silky texture, plus high-shine 'gellants'. (A new word in beautyspeak!). Fifteen flattering shades (testers received 426 Perfect Plum, a soft mauve-y nude).

Comments: 'Really liked the glossy sheen; moisturising like a balm but with reasonable coverage and no lip gloss stickiness! Really pretty packaging. Not particularly long-lasting though' • 'very moisturising and creamy with a nice sheen' • 'smooth, velvety texture is absolutely lovely on lips, didn't leave my lips dry at all' • 'tube is gorgeous to whip out at a party and colour goes with almost everything in my wardrobe and I don't feel overdone: *love* it'.

FINDING YOUR PERFECT LIP SHADE...

On younger women, paler-than-real-lip colours can look fantastic – but not now! And too dark shades can make an older mouth look harsh. Soft pinks, subtle corals and rosy-browns are the safest bet, subtly putting back the colour that disappears with age (because pigment decreases). Avoid opaque lipsticks: as you get older, solid colours can make the mouth look mean, while the drier matt formulas make lips look tiny and show every line. (That's why we've chosen specifically moisturising lipsticks here.)

Love your life

You can't freeze-frame life. It changes all the time, sometimes slowly, sometimes with chaotic speed. But what you can do is to adopt strategies to help you cope with the rollercoaster. How does that fit in with anti-ageing? A calm mind and taking joy in life make you look beautiful and live well. So laugh as much as you breathe and love as long as you live

Here are some of our favourite strategies, many of which are now used in healthcare.

Be loving to yourself. Sometimes loving and valuing yourself are very hard. That's when we're likely to cause ourselves grief, rely on others for our self-esteem, and make decisions – big and small – based on other people rather than what we really want for ourselves. You could start by just saying to yourself that you are a good person, not perfect – no one is (and please do give yourself permission to get things wrong, make a muddle, be imperfect in everything) – but you try your best. If you believe in spirituality, try thinking of yourself as 'a spark of the divine'. And above all, when you're faced with a decision, ask yourself what you really want to do. (And, of course, extend this loving way of thinking to everyone else too.)

The day starts better after a good night's sleep. We find we sleep soundly when we're glad and grateful. So when you go to bed, write down – or just list in your mind – at least three nice things that have happened. They can be as simple as hearing the birds sing, seeing the sun, or a phone call from a friend. Or praise at work. Or a great cup of coffee. A funny TV show… Then send blessings to the people you love. (And the world in general.)

TIPS

Make things fun: wear a tiara when you're hoovering (try accessories or toy stores for gorgeous bargains); brighten tedious chores with your favourite music; trade help with a friend. Reward yourself with flowers, a movie, a good cup of coffee or tea with a friend.

Keep a Happy Box: collect mementoes of joyful times – letters and cards, emails these days! – inspiring photos, tickets from planes, boats, trains and concerts – and leaf through them when you're having a doleful day.

Don't make decisions in the middle of the night. Around 4am (when women tend to wake if there's something on your mind) is the dark hour of the soul, according to psychiatrist Dr David Servan-Schreiber, the late author of *Healing Without Freud or Prozac*. 'There's a fragile moment at the end of the first long period of deep sleep (about four hours into the sleep cycle) when we cross over into the lighter REM sleep [dreaming time]. Underlying anxiety – especially separation anxiety where we feel a threat to important relationships or a lack of fulfilling ones – manifests then.' Your brain can't process things then, he says, so please don't try: do the breathing exercise right, and if you don't fall asleep read a novel, do the ironing, listen to the radio or even watch a dotty DVD on your laptop.

When you wake up, decide that just for today your intention is that you will be as happy as you can be. Whatever happens. This doesn't mean you won't notice difficulties – of course you will. It does mean you will try to live in the solution, not the problem.

Breathe. Inhale for a count of four, hold for seven, then exhale very slowly to a count of eight. Repeat four to six times, feeling your breath go in and out of your body. If you like, imagine your breath is like a wave coming up a beach, hovering at the top, then ebbing slowly out to sea. Do this whenever you can during the day, but morning and bedtime at least.

Think of someone you love and stretch out your arms to them – literally. (If they're there to hug in person, so much the better.) You will find you're smiling and your heart is warm. Carry that feeling through the day.

Stretch some more. Do some yoga poses if you know them (for more on yoga, see page 204). Or just stretch your arms and legs out, shake your feet and hands – feel the fizz of energy.

Make yourself look as gorgeous as you can. Especially if it's a grey day – weather- or mood-wise. Wear colours, put on make-up, brush your hair.

If you have a wobbly moment of any kind, do the breathing exercise again. Bring your attention to the centre of your chest and widen it – don't cave in. Feel your shoulder blades sinking back, down and together. Then try saying 'yesss!', even 'thank you', and looking forward and up to a hill, a spire, the sky. (To understand why we suggest this, contrast it with looking down and saying 'no'.)

Never lose hope. If it seems to be slipping away, phone a friend but choose one who will support and encourage you – avoid the Eeyores.

Smile. Research has shown it sends feel-good hormones called endorphins rushing through your mind and body. You feel better. So does everyone else. Smiles make friends.

Examine the wobbliness. If you've done something wrong, put it right. Most likely you haven't and it's an old tape replaying in your head and body. Have a few drops of Bach's Rescue Remedy and count up the good healthy positive things in any situation. If the wobbliness persists, repeat again. If it is really troubling you, consider talking therapy of some kind and/or homeopathy.

Reach out to other people. Be nice – it's so much easier. Pay compliments. Listen, really listen.

Notice good things. Even tiny ones: store them up to remember at night and when things are difficult.

Never give up on passion. (We heard novelist Edna O'Brien say that, and she's now in her late seventies.) Yes, we do mean the physical sort of passion! And being passionately interested in people and things of all sorts. Be passionately creative too: paint, sing, play an instrument, garden, take photos – whatever you enjoy, do it!

Cultivate peace. We can't really tell you how – try seeing what makes you feel peaceful and doing more of it. Or it may be a case of 'being' rather than 'doing'.

Make yourself look as *GORGEOUS* as you can. *Wear colours*, put on **make-up**, brush your hair

Hang on to your marbles

Fewer lines and a trim waistline are all fine and dandy – but in the bigger scheme of things, nobody would question that keeping your brain sparky and your memory sharp(-ish) is going to do more for your quality of later life than pretty well anything else in this book

'Not fade away' is a BIG theme of *The Anti-Ageing Beauty Bible* – and it applies just as much to our brains, as well as to hair, complexion, eyebrows and so on.

Memory loss is probably the biggest brain-related anxiety we experience, once we hit a certain age. We're not talking about full-blown dementia, such as Alzheimer's disease – though that prospect can be seriously angst-inducing, especially if there's a family history – but about the Craft (Can't Remember a Flipping Thing) moments that strike everyone, usually kicking in around perimenopause. Naturopathic physician Dr Mosaraf Ali explains, 'Anxiety, depression, physical fatigue and anything which causes less blood flow to the brain weakens the ability to store or recall memories.' So: when you bump into someone unbelievably familiar but you can't remember their name (or how you know them), stress or exhaustion are the most likely explanations.

The good news is that, as experts agree, there are many, many lifestyle steps that we can all take to improve our memories.

Eat oily fish. It's rich in omega-3 essential fatty acids (EFAs), which researchers world-wide agree are vital for brain function; they have been shown to help depression and general mental acuity, as well as helping age-related memory loss and just possibly helping to prevent dementia (research is ongoing). These brain-friendly lipids can't be manufactured by the body, and must come from our diet. And the richest source of omega-3 EFAs is oily fish. So if you're vegetarian, like Jo, take them in the form of supplements (see page 180 for our suggestions). Everyone should also consume lots of dark green vegetables such as spinach, watercress, dried seaweed and spirulina (all of which also contain B group vitamins – see box opposite), walnuts, flax and hemp seeds and their oils, try these over vegetables and we like them stirred into baked beans... Phosphorus may also help the brain, and is needed for the body to absorb those vital B vitamins; it's found in oily fish and also in nuts (including walnuts, Brazil, cashew, peanuts, pecans and pine nuts), eggs, lentils, soya, wholegrains and – yay! – chocolate (the darker the better). You can self-test to see whether you are deficient in omega-3 EFAs with a simple at-home blood test (see DIRECTORY).

Do sudoku or quizzes or crosswords. And/or play a lot of Scrabble. All of these help with memory. The general principle is that exercising your brain with any different routines and new tasks is effective. Learning to play the piano (it's never too late), a new language, even finding your way around a new city – any new skill – gives the memory area of your brain a vital workout.

Train your brain with an App. Every day at 8am, Jo's iPhone reminds her: 'It's time for your brain training.' She spends five minutes doing online games (matching shapes, colours, etc) which improve attention and memory, and speed up thinking time. The App is Brain Trainer by Lumosity (www.lumosity.com) and is available via iTunes. Graphs help you chart your progress – and the alarm is a reminder to do the brain exercises. (Although as your memory improves, the hope is you won't need a prompt.)

Eat ten almonds a day. They contain an incredible array of nutrients and are the richest source of vegetable protein. Soak them in room-temperature water for 24 hours, peel off the skins, crush and eat with a teaspoonful of Manuka honey, to benefit from micro-nutrients essential for brain function. Or add to muesli.

Support your memory with supplements. Ayurvedic practitioner Sebastian Pole prescribes Brahmi Plus, which combines organic herbs including gotu kola and bacopa monnieri, which increase memory and enhance concentration; it also lowers anxiety, clears your mind and revitalises your intellect. (We're sold on it.) We're also considering taking phosphatidylserine (PS), a phospholipid which has been shown to improve memory and mental acuity, due to multiple functions which basically help your brain cells talk to each other. (We're told Memory Lane by Power Health is a good formulation.)

Massage your head, neck and shoulders. This not only helps quell anxiety, but boosts blood flow to the brain. We are particularly keen on scalp massage as stress shortens the muscles in the scalp, making the scalp all but immobile in very frazzled people. Firm pressure with the pads of the fingers is pretty darned miraculous – or better still, book in for an Indian

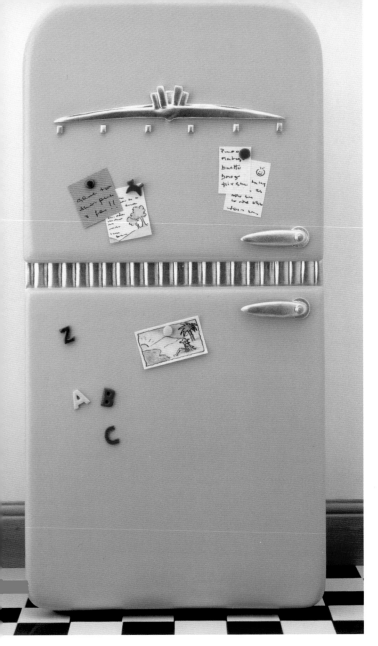

BE ON THE BALL WITH B VITAMINS

Over the past decade, research has increasingly shown that taking high doses of three B vitamins (B6, B12 and folic acid) can help age-related memory loss. These B vitamins help keep homocysteine (an amino acid) at a healthy level. Raised homocysteine may increase the risk of Alzheimer's and heart disease. Taking the vitamins probably won't help if you don't have a mild degree of memory loss but won't harm you and may help other things, eg, stress. If your brain is as sharp as a needle, we think it makes all-round good sense to eat plenty of foods containing these Bs. Find vitamin B12 in meat and fish, with folic acid and B6 in asparagus, lentils, most beans and leafy green vegetables (see our Supergreens Facelift Diet, page 176 – and combine the benefits for face and mind!). For specific supplements of the vitamins, see page 180.

yoga – nature's greatest anti-ageing wonder, in our opinion – see page 204.)

Avoid alcohol, coffee and cola-style drinks. Alcohol in particular is linked with poor memory (and not just in a where-the-hell-did-I-leave-my-keys-after-that-second-bottle-of-champagne way); if you are experiencing regular Craft moments, try cutting down or cutting out alcohol and seeing if that makes a difference, because it does affect the way brain cells communicate. (We're not suggesting that anyone becomes a nun. A special occasion is a special occasion, but for many people a few glasses of wine a day is a habit that's surprisingly easy to give up, once you've made the link with positive improvements.) Caffeine can exacerbate stress – and there's some evidence that, over time, the gradual increase of stress hormone (cortisol) levels in the blood can prevent the brain laying down a new memory, or from accessing existing ones.

Get plenty of sleep. We all know that when we're sleep-deprived, we can hardly remember our own names, let alone phone numbers and the fact we have to pick up our dry-cleaning. Sleep is the brain's way of processing events into memories. For more wisdom on better sleep, see page 208.

Head Massage, which many massage therapists are trained in. Use Google to find someone near you.

Don't multi-task. OK, so for most women this is like telling you to stop breathing. (Men, of course, are another matter…) But studies have shown that memory-related tasks can suffer in the hands of multi-taskers. At the very least, focus on doing – and finishing – one thing at a time. Practise mindfulness (more on page 144). You can sit still to do a waking mindfulness meditation – heck, you can even practise it while washing up. It's all about bringing your consciousness gently back to what you're doing. Whether that's walking, daydreaming – or doing the dishes.

Practise Iyengar yoga. The Cobra pose, which enhances circulation, may be of particular help to your brain. (For more on

And if all else fails, write it down. Whoever said you were meant to remember everything: birthdays, anniversaries, shopping lists, To Do lists, not to mention matching every name in your bulging address book to a face…? Be kind to yourself: the pressure we put our brains under is unprecedented in the history of humanity. Try not to stress out when your memory fails you, or feel it's the start of a slippery slope – it only makes things worse. It happens to us all. Stop, take a deep breath and let your mind rest for a moment. And remember (little joke!) that's what pens, paper, diaries, iPhones and online reminder services were meant for.

Be mindful of life's pleasures

Forget diets. It's time to enjoy your food, eat just the right amount through 'mindful eating' (and lose that middle-age spread effortlessly)

As the years go by, it's ridiculously easy for the pounds to roll on. For most women after the menopause, the evidence is probably lurking around your waistline (we tend to gather fat around our middles due to a shift in the ratio of oestrogen to testosterone). Clothes are tighter. Maybe there's a muffin-top that didn't used to be there. And suddenly, you get as excited over a new pair of Spanx control pants as you once did over frilly, skimpy smalls.

Traditionally, women have turned to extreme diets to combat excess pounds. Trouble is that diets tend not to work long term because they're hard to stick to (and some you shouldn't stick to 'cos they are just plain dangerous).

But there is new thinking that part of the reason we gain weight is that in our busy, stressful world, we're simply not paying attention to what we eat. Think on this. What did you last eat? What did it taste like? Smell of? Did you really enjoy it? Chances are you just don't remember… We're so used to filling our tummies with food like we fill our cars with fuel that we mostly do it on autopilot. Mindlessly. While we do six other things. (Multi-tasking can be a disadvantage sometimes.) The result is that, often, we eat far more than we need because we just don't notice what we're doing. And we pile on the pounds. Because we've eaten too much. Simple!

But it's also quite simple and fun to practise 'mindful eating' – as well as eating well, of course (it won't work if you eat mindfully mashed potato, pasta, cakes and puds for every meal). The bottom line is: it's all about loving your food! 'Mindful eating' is a new (well, old but rediscovered) approach, which is proving very helpful for people who want to lose weight on a permanent basis, not the see-saw of weight loss and gain that's so familiar from so many diets.

So: let's start again…

Go and make yourself something you really enjoy. Needn't be complicated but take enough time to make certain it tastes and looks delicious. Find your favourite place to eat, sitting at a table. Or treat yourself to a coffee or tea and lemon tart at your favourite patisserie.

Now…start by taking a few slow breaths to relax. Look at the food. Notice the colours, texture, smell. Then take the first mouthful. Don't do anything else at all. Just look and taste and smell. Swallow slowly, chewing thoroughly if necessary. Go on to the second mouthful and do the same. Finish your food in the same way, deliberately paying attention to it. That's what mindfulness is – being fully aware of what's happening. With food, it's the sensations and thoughts that occur as we eat. The colours, aromas, textures, flavours, even sounds of the food. And drink – think of the sensation as you taste the chocolate powder on a cappuccino, encounter the cool milky foam, the contrast with the hot, intensely-flavoured coffee.

If your mind wanders, just bring it gently back to what you're consuming. Sometimes it's helpful to say it to yourself, aloud or in your head: 'Now I'm biting into a peach, through the furry skin into the flesh, feeling the juice run down my chin…'

If you like to read or watch TV when you're eating on your own, try to do one thing at a time. So stop reading while you take a mouthful, taste, chew, swallow. Then pick up your book. You will focus on both more completely. (Ideally, ditch the book and switch off the TV.)

If you're eating with friends, it's still possible to be mindful. The key is to do it slowly – and lovingly. So often when you eat out, the food which your host/ess (or the restaurant chef) has cooked and cosseted like a baby is dispatched without anyone really appreciating it. Thinking and talking about each part of the meal is a compliment. So it's win-win!

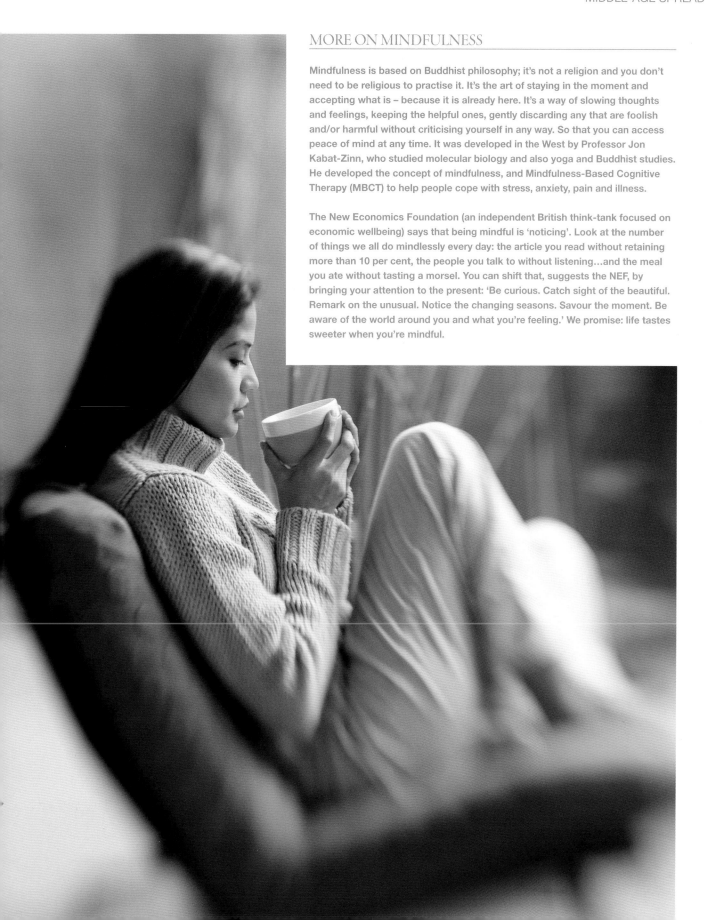

MORE ON MINDFULNESS

Mindfulness is based on Buddhist philosophy; it's not a religion and you don't need to be religious to practise it. It's the art of staying in the moment and accepting what is – because it is already here. It's a way of slowing thoughts and feelings, keeping the helpful ones, gently discarding any that are foolish and/or harmful without criticising yourself in any way. So that you can access peace of mind at any time. It was developed in the West by Professor Jon Kabat-Zinn, who studied molecular biology and also yoga and Buddhist studies. He developed the concept of mindfulness, and Mindfulness-Based Cognitive Therapy (MBCT) to help people cope with stress, anxiety, pain and illness.

The New Economics Foundation (an independent British think-tank focused on economic wellbeing) says that being mindful is 'noticing'. Look at the number of things we all do mindlessly every day: the article you read without retaining more than 10 per cent, the people you talk to without listening…and the meal you ate without tasting a morsel. You can shift that, suggests the NEF, by bringing your attention to the present: 'Be curious. Catch sight of the beautiful. Remark on the unusual. Notice the changing seasons. Savour the moment. Be aware of the world around you and what you're feeling.' We promise: life tastes sweeter when you're mindful.

Minimise those
bad (facial) hair days

Stop yourself turning into a moustachioe-d lady – here's the lowdown on hair removal

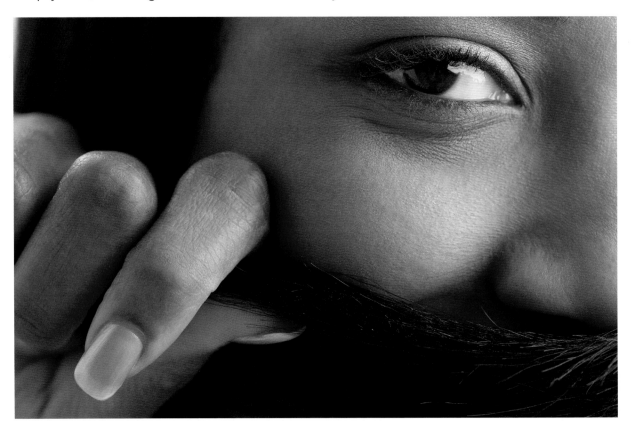

One of the most common questions we're asked is how to get rid of moustaches and, to a lesser extent, other areas of facial hair. We recommend having an appointed 'facial hair buddy' who will tell you when you're sprouting, and you can reciprocate. Mole hairs, in particular, make a break for it after menopause and, as eyesight fades, they can be easily missed.

Now conversely, one of the great blessings of ageing is that elsewhere on the body hair becomes finer and may even disappear altogether (hoorah!). But if you're still fighting excess hair anywhere on the face/body, here's a useful rundown of all the removal techniques you need to know about.

One warning with moustaches: depending on the density of down on the rest of your face (we all have it so don't have conniptions!), completely removing your moustache may leave an obvious hairless patch. In this case, electrolysis is a good option

as the therapist can just take out the coarser, more visible hairs. Alternatively, you could have the whole of your face threaded (but that's quite high-maintenance, so be warned).

Never shave your face. We differ about shaving for legs: Jo does, Sarah doesn't. (If you do, make sure to use a razor dedicated for just this purpose – Jo favours the Gillette Venus range.) But shaving a moustache leads to stubble, and you eventually end up having to do it every day, and fretting over someone feeling a bristly upper lip when they kiss you.

First try bleaching – not so much removal as a disguise. Many of us grew up with crème bleach, and for fine, sparse moustache hairs, it's still an option. However, some testers report that it can sting so much, particularly on your face, that you end up red-skinned, with varying shades of ginger facial hair because you've had to wash it off too soon. Bleach comes in different versions for face and body: get the right one! And please read and follow the instructions to the letter: do a patch test first, every time, don't use with Retin-A, or fruit acids of any kind, and only use on the areas it's listed as safe for.

Experiment with tweezing. Simple, cheap and great for eyebrows, but not recommended for more than the odd stray hair on the rest of your face as it may irritate hair follicles, causing sensitivity and even scarring.

Melt hair clean away with a depilatory cream. These relatively cheap products dissolve hair at the base of the follicle and are useful for legs and underarms (though you'll need to do it often), less so for the face as even dedicated facial versions may irritate sensitive skin, and may not remove all the hairs.

Find a good salon, and try waxing. With waxing, warm/hot wax is applied to skin, then ripped off with a muslin strip bringing the hairs with it. It's usually effective for upper lip and fine hair on the sides of your face, but not suitable for coarser hair on the chin. Never let the therapist use a metal knife for this: it may burn your skin – they should only ever use a wooden implement, and we like salons best which provide a hygienic pack in which every single spatula is used once only, rather than repeatedly dipped.

Get sweet on sugaring. Sugaring uses the same procedure as waxing except that the sugar tends to stick only to the hairs not the skin – so it can be more comfortable. It does need a skilled practitioner to be effective.

Or try threading. (We love threading.) This is an ancient method of hair removal practised in Asian countries. A pure, thin twisted cotton thread is rolled rapidly over untidy areas. As well as shaping brows, skilled practitioners can remove hair anywhere on the face, all over if desired. It's not painful in our experience, but not comfy (it 'pings'). Again it's temporary and needs upkeep.

For permanent hair removal, look at electrolysis. A fine needle conducting an electric current is inserted into the hair follicle, destroying it. You may need several sessions with some maintenance later, but it's an ideal option for a small number of coarse facial hairs, although it is impractical for larger areas, according to consultant dermatologist Dr Nick Lowe of the Cranley Clinic, London.

Laser hair removal is another option. Here, the hair follicle is effectively cauterised with a laser. It's a perfect choice for upper lip hair, says Dr Lowe. Advances in technology mean that any hair with pigment in it can be lasered. (Which usually precludes

treatment of white or grey hair.) There used to be a problem treating coloured skin but new lasers protect tanned, Asian or black skin from losing pigment. These newer modified lasers incorporate cooling technology, says Dr Lowe, who uses the Alexandrite 755 nanometre laser, which cools the skin with a high-flow jet of cold air.

Be aware: laser hair removal won't give you results overnight. (And it's expensive.) It will take between three and six sessions to get the optimum reduction of hair growth, depending on the thickness. And please note: reduction not permanent removal. 'None of the lasers will totally and permanently remove all hair, but this method will achieve up to 70 or 80 per cent in a lot of patients, and patients can come back for maintenance sessions,' advises Dr Lowe. To help extend the time between maintenance (and minimise regrowth), he recommends a prescription cream called Vaniqa, which interferes with some of the proteins that form hair. On the positive side, Dr Lowe says laser hair removal usually works extremely well, and is also useful for ingrowing hair.

> *Appoint a facial hair buddy who will tell you when you're sprouting*

Don't go near lasers if you have pigmentation problems. Laser hair removal is not suitable for anyone with vitiligo (patches of de-pigmented skin) as it may stimulate new areas. Anyone with eczema, psoriasis, hives or urticaria should have a patch test first.

Beware of IPL. Many beauty salons offer treatment with IPL (Intense Pulsed Light), as do some cosmetic surgery clinics. However, Dr Lowe advises caution: 'I've seen so many patients that have had burns and blisters, loss of pigment and scars.' (Dr Lowe uses IPL systems for removal of thread veins, sun spots and for rejuvenating skin.)

And be very careful where you have any laser or IPL treatment. Dr Lowe cautions against booking laser hair removal at beauty salons: you should go to an experienced trained physician at a reputable clinic. We recommend you follow the same guidelines for this as any 'cosmetic tweak' such as Botox, etc, to optimise your chances of the best outcome – see page 46.

A final caution: very occasionally with these high-tech methods of hair removal, hair growth may be stimulated instead of reduced, due to the technology not delivering enough energy to the hair follicle; usually the problem can be overcome by switching to a different laser system. But it's another big argument for going to someone who is trained properly and experienced.

'The only real
ELEGANCE
is in the mind;
if you've got that,
the rest *really*
comes from it'

Diana Vreeland

Nourish your neck (and keep it swan-like)

As our necks start to sag and the texture looks crêpey, our hearts begin to sink. The reality is that the skin is much thinner on the neck than on our faces, and thus more easily damaged. (And we do tend to overlook it.) So, no more neglect – just lavish it with loving care

To misquote Nora Ephron, don't feel bad about your neck.

We love Nora Ephron (screenwriter for *Heartburn*, *Julie & Julia*, etc), and author of the hilarious collection of essays, *I Feel Bad about My Neck*, in which she writes: 'One of my biggest regrets – bigger even than not buying the apartment on East Seventy-fifth Street, bigger even than my worst romantic catastrophe – is that I didn't spend my youth staring lovingly at my neck. It never crossed my mind to be grateful for it... Of course now I am older, I'm wise and sage and mellow. And it's also true that I honestly do understand just what matters in life. But guess what? It's my neck.'

We agree with Nora that necks can be angst-inducing. But we say: any neck – even 'turkey neck' (that unpicturesque term for a sagging neck) – can be improved, with targeted and diligent TLC.

Make like a Frenchwoman and 'double-moisturise'. One of the key issues with the neck is crêpiness, as the skin on the neck has relatively few oil glands and without moisture and lipids, it can start to look papery super-fast. Get into the habit of applying everything you put on your face right down to the bra-line. At the same time, sweep any body lotion up to your chin, so it gets twice the nourishment. Your neck and chest should be part of your 'cleansing zone', but avoid using a scrub on the neck, although a muslin cloth (used with cleanser) is fine.

And consider a targeted neck product. For our testers' favourites, and ours too, see overleaf.

Protect your neck with an SPF15 plus. As dermatologist Dr Nick Lowe tells us, 'The neck is easily damaged by sun exposure as the skin is much thinner than it is on other parts of the face, and its support structure is not as effective.' So the ceaseless battering of UV light breaks down collagen and elastin, leading to sagging. Any SPF you apply to your face – your first line of defence against ageing – should be applied to the neck, the chest and the décolletage, religiously. End... Of... Story. If you tend to 'miss' the sides of the neck because your hair's in the way, scoop it off your face pre-application. If you do have 'age spots' on your neck and chest, see our recommendations for treating these on page 190.

Avoid wearing perfume in the sun. Many a woman's list of neck woes includes pigmented areas either side of the neck. Certain fragrance ingredients – generally citrus-derived – contain psoralens, components which over-stimulate the pigment-producing cells. This produces localised brown patches (medically called Berloque dermatitis), that look like a streak of brown pigment rather like a raindrop running down a window pane. (Plus the alcohol in the scent dries out the skin.) The solution? If you want to enjoy a summer fragrance in the sun, try spritzing it on your clothing rather than your skin. (Check first, of course, that it doesn't discolour the fabric: you can try it on a tissue.) Or wear a ribbon around a wrist or your neck, drenched in scent, à la Marie Antoinette and her mob. Spritz a hankie with scent and tuck it in your bra – or your swimsuit, as long as you're not planning to get wet. And, of course, enjoy liberally after dark. Just be certain to cleanse away the fragrance the next morning with a wet flannel, before you go anywhere near the sun.

Take up yoga. One of the key reasons women develop 'turkey neck', double chins and those 'necklace rings' on the neck is because underlying muscles are weak. So neck firming is yet another reason to add to the list of why embracing yoga is a good idea (more on page 204). It's fantastic, fantastic, fantastic for strengthening the neck and the jaw and – as we've observed in previous books – we know seventy-something yoga devotees who have sharp jaw-lines and smooth, swan-like necks. And we want to be like them. It's not just us. Esteemed dermatologist Dr Karen Burke observes: 'If you do yoga you can postpone facelifts for years. People have those sharp jawlines because they're doing a total stretch.'

Raise the height of your computer screen. Whether you use a laptop or a full-size screen on your desk, you should make sure that it's high enough for you to look straight at it, rather than looking down.

Embrace polo-necks, pashminas, scarves and pearl chokers. If you really still feel Nora Ephron-ish about your neck, short of surgery/lasers (we'll come on to that), camouflage is your best option. These all hide a multitude of sins. Not everyone suits a polo-neck, but if you generally look better with a scoop- or a v-neckline, you can create a flattering optical illuson that draws attention downwards by hanging a necklace or rope of pearls over the top. Wear earrings, too, which distract the eye from your neck. But you have to trust us: nobody looks as unforgivingly on your neck as you do.

As a last resort, there's surgery. And fillers. And Intense Pulsed Light (IPL) treatments. We are going to point you in the direction (not for the first time in this book) of Wendy Lewis, who is the fount of all cosmetic surgery wisdom. In her book *Plastic Makes Perfect* (see ANTI-AGEING BOOKSHELF), she devotes several pages to all the options, which range from 'plastysmaplasty' (to tackle 'turkey wattle') to liposuction and the fillers Restylane and Perlane. But any procedure to do with the neck is A Big Deal (remember: your main artery and all the important nerves go through the neck); botched neck treatments happen. If you can afford any of these procedures, you can afford to talk to Wendy first: she is completely independent and not affiliated with any doctor, but knows better than anyone on the planet who's best at what.

And if you still feel bad about your neck, read Nora Ephron. Because at least there's someone who feels worse about hers than you do.

'I look forward to getting older when looks should become less of an issue, and when who you are is the point' Susan Sarandon

Neck treatments: *our award winners*

Why do so many women buy neck creams, only to leave them languishing on the bathroom shelf? Is it a belief that nothing can make a difference to this notoriously hard-to-treat area? Certainly, the key with any neck treatment is ritualistic use – preferably twice a day (and it does no harm to shield the area with an SPF15 during daylight) – and a high pleasure factor helps to encourage that ritual. If you follow our testers' recommendations and are religious with any of the following creams (the victors from among more than 40 trialled just for this book), you may be as pleased as they were

AT A GLANCE

Clarins Super Restorative Décolleté and Neck Concentrate

Liz Earle Superskin Concentrate

RéVive Fermitif Neck Renewal Cream SPF15

Liz Earle Skin Repair Moisturiser Dry/ Sensitive

This Works Perfect Cleavage for Neck & Chest

Lulu's Time Bomb Trouble Shooter Neck, Jaw & Chest Firming Cream

REVIEWS

Clarins Super Restorative Décolleté and Neck Concentrate

 This fluid treatment is instantly skin-firming, moisturising – and features a combination of plant extracts for its age-defying power (we really don't think you need the complicated, Linnaean list of specific botanicals!). It is also said to lighten pigmentation spots, used over time, through a vitamin C derivative. Clarins recommend a specific one-minute massage technique to enhance the effects (you'll find it slipped inside the box).
Comments: 'Such a treat – can't emphasise how much I loved the silky texture and beautiful smell: you're advised to massage it in so it's a treat that way too: neck and décolletage appreciably smoother and softer, less fragile and with a slight gleam – lovely, lovely, lovely!' • 'fine lines have much improved, some disappeared, and deeper ones less noticeable; texture and sink-in-ability faultless' • 'very definite improvement in neck area especially, much smoother, less crêpey, necklace lines much less visible, looks younger and smoother – am so pleased and impressed!'.

Liz Earle Superskin Concentrate ❀❀

 A high-scorer in previous books, a stellar performer in the facial oil category here, and a favourite of Jo's… Well, Liz Earle sent another ten bottles of this to be trialled as a neck treatment, and they obviously knew what they were doing: the argan- and rosehip-rich oil, turbo-charged by vitamin E, came up trumps here too. (NB: the aromatic essential oils are said to aid restful sleep, as a bonus.)
Comments: 'Very noticeable difference immediately; greatly improved smoothness, which continued with use; skin feels softer and smoother, the biggest difference is to fine lines which are far less noticeable – a fantastic product' • 'neck felt and looked plump and smooth; healthier, fresher skin' • 'skin looks and feels beautiful, and younger because smoother' • 'I love, love, love this product! Smells great, feels great and makes my skin look great! Neck is certainly less craggy, has eliminated all signs of crêpiness and dryness, lines finer and less visible, skin moisturised and supple'.

RéVive Fermitif Neck Renewal Cream SPF15

 We often wonder why more neck creams don't incorporate an SPF, since the neck's so vulnerable to sun damage. Hallelujah: this one does (a chemical sunscreen, note), in a luxurious, softly rose-scented cream with special firming agents from wheat protein and barley extract, plus what RéVive call their 'youth molecule'.
Comments: 'Skin immediately lovely and velvety to touch, supple and plumped up; with regular use, everything is smoothed out and fine lines much

This Works Perfect Cleavage for Neck & Chest

8.28/10 We're personally delighted that this product from our beauty editor friend Kathy Phillips's range did so well here, having previously had so many anecdotal good reports. With larch extract, yellow algae and pomegranate, rose oil, patchouli and tonka bean, it's sensually-scented, the packaging's chic – and Kathy's own smoothly swan-like neck is Perfect Cleavage's own best advertisement. (Though the yoga – which she's practised daily for decades – may help…!) Testers particularly liked its effect on the décolletage.

Comments: 'Nice texture that's easy to spread, sinks in very quickly and smells absolutely lovely; the wrinkles on my neck look much better and I have had less spots since using' • 'less crêpiness with this lovely serum – I have gone and bought a couple more, which says it all' • 'dryness and texture improved, encouraged me to put cream much lower down than just my neck – lives up to its promise of being tightening, nourishing and shimmering!' • 'loved this product, which improved fine lines, crêpiness and made neck look younger and smoother'.

more faded, neck looking much younger' • 'skin on neck and décolletage feels much firmer, softer and looks better – more supple, wouldn't have believed that this product could make such a change' • 'skin looks glossier and firmer – just loved this product and think it does an amazing job'.

Liz Earle Skin Repair Moisturiser Dry/Sensitive

8.41/10 Interesting! This everyday moisturiser from Liz Earle did well in previous books as a neck treatment, even though it's not specifically labelled as such. Once again, they sent us ten pots to be specifically trialled for this book. And guess what? Once again, Skin Repair got a great score from this entirely new bunch of neck-conscious testers. Packed with plant avocado and borage oil, echinacea, pro-vitamin B5, antioxidants – all the botanicals which are the signature of Liz's so-successful range, in fact.

Comments: 'Fantastic: the skin on my neck drank up this product like it had been stranded in the desert, immediately became plumper, smoother and felt more comfy; neck looks much younger and healthier – you absolutely must try it!' • 'gave a kind of "soft focus" effect to lines' • 'skin felt instantly nourished by this rich, light cream, absorbs like magic, have never used a cream that made my skin feel so soft, supple and moisturised – would like to score it 12/10!'.

♡ WE LOVE...

From being too lazy to use anything at all on her neck, full-on neck panic now has Jo veering between two favourites. The serum-like Liz Earle Superskin Bust Treatment is now (at Jo's own suggestion!) going to be rebranded as Neck & Bust Treatment, because it's also fantastic for this purpose. But the incense-y smell of Neal's Yard Remedies Rejuvenating Frankincense Firming Neck Cream also inspires Jo's slavish devotion. Sarah has always slathered moisturiser on her (long) neck and chest and now slops on facial oil too (any, all!), which is very effective.

Lulu's Time Bomb Trouble Shooter Neck, Jaw & Chest Firming Cream

8.25/10 This formula from the ever-youthful singer's age-defying range was created to firm skin and lighten age spots, blending 'chrysanthellum extract' (to target jaw-droop), vitamin E, pea extract, shea and sunflower seed butters, plus white truffle extract. Happily, it smells gorgeously of Lulu's favourite lavender oil, rather than a risotto…!

Comments: 'Loved this thick cream that absorbed like a lotion and felt incredibly hydrating; definite improvement in fine lines and sagging under chin, jaw contour looks more pronounced, neck looked considerably younger and smoother' • 'really liked this product, nice texture, smells lovely, did improve my neck – made it very soft and smooth' • 'neck did feel very smooth and tightened, soft and supple'.

'Lift' your face – without surgery...

(Yes, it's possible.) Maybe you want to look your best for a special occasion. Or perhaps your face would love a boost after a stressful time. But you're not up for surgery, fillers, dermabrasion or lasers – so what's to do...? Here are the (non-surgical) fixes that we know really work

Try CACI. Over the years we've been in the beauty business, we've pretty much tried out all the non-surgical facelift systems. These mostly involve probes carrying low-voltage electric currents which are moved over your face to make the muscles jump around and work harder, giving a temporary lift – sometimes versions of these are used in tandem with facials. Of the many that have been launched over the past two decades, the one that has stood the test of time world-wide is CACI, which stands for Computer Aided Cosmetology Instrument. From the one original option (CACI Classic), there's now an almost bewildering range – which extend to microdermabrasion and ultrasonic peeling, and beyond the face to include CACI for bust enhancement, stretch

marks and cellulite. We honestly don't know how well all that works – but we do know that for a temporary (24 to 48 hours) boost, a CACI treatment can be rejuvenating. (And just lying still for an hour or so is a big bonus for many busy women.) For longer-term results, CACI recommend ten to 15 treatments and then maintenance sessions every four to six weeks. (Worth considering, we'd say, if you enjoy it, like the results and your budget permits.)

Find a great facialist. For our money, a good facial with massage by skilled hands can give some gorgeous instant results. (On page 79 you'll find our favourite facialists, but talk to girlfriends and investigate local talent – you might find a hidden magic-worker just around the corner. (Tell us if you do, at www.beautybible.com!) Some facialists undoubtedly have healing hands; indeed one of our fave raves Emma Hardie (who now has a lovely skincare line with products that regularly feature in our award winners) started out in the early 1990s with her own natural lifting and sculpting facial. Sarah wrote about it for *YOU magazine*, other beauty editors (including Newby Hands, formerly of *Harper's Bazaar*'s) endorsed it – and Emma has become a legend in natural rejuvenation.

Get the needle! We swear by facial acupuncture. And believe us, the needles truly aren't scary. (The only version we did find too much to take was electro-acupuncture, where the needles carry a current which is progressively increased. You need to be made of sterner stuff than we are for that.) Sarah really loves a treatment from Annee de Mamiel, formerly a successful banker who studied acupuncture after recovering from cancer. Annee treats your whole body, explaining: 'Beauty is about being balanced on the inside, in every way – physically and psychologically. If you feel good about yourself, it reflects in the way you look. Dry, wrinkled, saggy skin mirrors what is happening in your body, so I look at the roots of the problems and treat those too.' For instance, the common problem of vertical lines between your eyebrows can relate to liver energy not flowing properly (frowning too much is a factor too!), so as well as needling the lines themselves, Annee treats the liver. As well as acupuncture, she makes up specially blended oils for each client plus a herbal tea to take home. Annee incorporates stimulating Tui Na Chinese massage (to invigorate the skin) and lymph draining massage and acupressure to relax you from top to toe. An increasing number of acupuncturists now offer facial acupuncture; ask friends for recommendations. (Jo sees a fab Hove-based therapist called Steve Mason for this.)

Just say 'ouch'. Much the most painful treatment Sarah has endured is having the muscles inside the mouth at the base of the tongue released by osteopath Vicky Vlachonis in London (who learned it from French obstetrician Michel Odent). As she wrote at the time, 'The results are extraordinary: any downward drift perks up and the contours of your face seem redefined – truly a non-surgical facelift moment.' And the pain is definitely worth the

TIP

If there's one low-tech gizmo we'd recommend for ironing out your face at home it's Sarah Chapman's Facialift, an odd-looking contraption with eight small knobbly cogs on a handle which rotate as you push them up and down your face. Good for massaging in product, or simply for stimulating the skin tissue and encouraging lymph drainage.

> '**BEAUTY** is about being balanced on the inside. If you feel *good* about yourself, it reflects in the way you **LOOK**'

gain, according to Carine Roitfeld, former French *Vogue* editor, who recently revealed that this internal facial massage is her secret for looking younger. 'They put on gloves and massage inside because all your stress is in your jaws. It hurts very much, but is my beauty secret,' she says. NB: if you want to try this do make sure you go to a practitioner who has really learnt this technique: you don't want to be a guinea pig.

Do it yourself. If you haven't got the time, budget or opportunity to have a treatment, you really can achieve wonders by yourself. Start by sipping some still room-temperature water, then spend a moment or two focusing on your breathing, as Annee suggests:

● Do this breathing exercise throughout the day: inhale through your nose to a count of three, exhale through your mouth for five, then pause for a second or two and let your body and mind go still and release tension.

● If possible, apply an instant face reviver (see page 212 for our testers' top-scoring products).

● Massage your face to relax muscles, allowing oxygenated blood to flow freely and toxins to be released, leaving you with a fresher, brighter complexion, less puffiness and fewer wrinkles. (See page 78 for guidelines.)

● Practise some yoga, or lie flat on your back for five minutes (more if you have it), knees bent, eyes closed (with damp teabags over them if possible). In your mind's eye, see blue sky – and as stray thoughts pop into your brain, convert them into clouds and let them float away.

Think nice thoughts. Your skin and face reflect your state of mind. If you're stressed, you run the risk of looking pinched and peaky. Try thinking of a couple of nice things that have happened to you today – remember someone you love and, if you're having an iffy day, that you never know what delicious thing might be around the next corner. Even if life is really tough (and it happens to everyone), there's almost always something positive. Gratitude and hope are great beautifiers.

Night treatments: *our award winners*

Here you'll find the treatments which – according to our testers – really do transform mere slumber into beauty sleep. Because of the body's repairing rhythms, most cellular patching-up happens while we're slumbering, so that many 'miracle' treatments are specifically designed to be used overnight. And because we don't need to slap on make-up over the top, night creams tend to be richer. Here are the night-time products our testers loved – out of over 90! – with some truly spectacular scores, and new/updated entries for this edition. (For day-time miracle treatments, turn to page 16 – also see Korres's entry, right…)

AT A GLANCE

Elemis Pro-Collagen Oxygenating Night Cream

Crème de la Mer Moisturizing Cream

La Prairie Anti-Aging Night Cream

Korres Thyme Honey 24-Hour Moisturising Cream

REN Omega 3 Night Repair Serum

Lancôme Génifique Repair Youth Activating Night Cream

LP Skin Therapy Overnight Replenish Cream

REVIEWS

Elemis Pro-Collagen Oxygenating Night Cream

 9.37 / 10 This outstandingly high-scorer is the night-time 'sister' product to a cream that's excelled in previous Beauty Bible books. Said to increase oxygen levels in the skin by 'up to 41 per cent', it combines an anti-ageing hexapeptide, marine extracts, antioxidants and Padina pavonica, a potent algae to boost firmness and elasticity. Luxuriously priced too.

Comments: 'My skin just drunk it in, skin was plumped up and very soft, helps with wrinkles because it's so hydrating; someone I hadn't seen in a while complimented me on a healthy glow' • 'skin looks much fresher and plumper in the morning, smooth and calm; does enhance radiance, dehydrated areas have improved dramatically and wrinkles greatly reduced' • 'skin looks better in every way, clear, soft and glowing, skintone more even and calmer' • 'this is the best night cream I have ever found, my hormonal skin has never looked better'.

Crème de la Mer Moisturizing Cream

 9.33 / 10 Crème de la Mer resubmitted this legendary rich cream – created by a NASA scientist to deal with severe chemical burns, and based on a 'Miracle Broth' including marine ingredients – for this updated edition, and it rose even further up the charts. New comments for this 'cult' product – which we've observed is suitable for even the most sensitive complexions and requires a special 'massage' technique.

Comments: 'Skin brighter, softer, amazing reduction in crêpiness round eyes and mouth; friends commented on how "well", "fresh", "been on holiday?" I looked' • 'I grew to love the special massage technique which has delivered slow but sure improvements' • 'cheeks more plumped up and less old and saggy' • 'I'm saving up to buy more!' • 'lives up to all the hype' • 'noticeable reduction in fine lines on treated side' • 'really impressed' • 'skin brighter, illuminated' • 'improvement in bigger wrinkles and grooves' • 'I may have to start a Crème de la Mer money box to save up for my next jar!'.

La Prairie Anti-Aging Night Cream

9.08/10

Again, a luxe-priced winner – though not as pricey as some La Prairie supercreams. Rich in peptides, it also features an extract of green micro-algae (again, to help production of collagen and elastin), plus La Prairie's signature Exclusive Cellular Complex.

Comments: 'LOVED it! Inside the silver box is a silver jar with a spatula and when you apply the cream skin feels nourished and has a radiance' • 'my skin is glowing and silken, more toned, lines beside eyes less visible, and two rather large frown lines between my eyebrows have lessened; I'm its biggest fan' • 'my mature fair skin looks younger, definitely addressed fine lines particularly around my mouth – I've had compliments – and my husband has bought me some more of their range' • 'most fine lines reduced, some bigger wrinkles too, and I am told I look younger'.

Korres Thyme Honey 24-Hour Moisturising Cream ❀

9.03/10

An impressive, lusciously honey-scented entry from Korres, a fast-growing Greek natural brand. Thyme honey is rich in antioxidants, as well as helping to maintain skin's ideal moisture level. Oops: our testers were asked to put it through its paces as a night treatment but it's designed to be used in the morning too.

Comments: 'I absolutely love the honey smell, so good you could almost eat it! Left a soft, velvety feel to my skin, hydrates well for 24 hours; people say my skin is glowing' • 'skin felt instantly nourished, smooth and renewed when I used it for the first time; sinks in within a few seconds, my skin is in a lot better condition and plumper, so fine lines not so apparent; my two daughters say my skin certainly looks better' • 'a little goes a long way' • 'skin plumped up the first morning after I applied it, had a pretty immediate effect with less obvious lines and much fresher!'.

REN Omega 3 Night Repair Serum ❀ ❀

8.93/10

Rich and unctuous, this, and certainly not something for applying under make-up. Blended with rosehip seed/gold of pleasure/coconut and wheatgerm oils, it has generous levels of omega-3 fatty acids. We could have categorised this as a facial oil, or a

serum, but went by REN's stated purpose for their product: 'To ensure skin gets its beauty sleep'.

Comments: 'Skin looked more luminous after 48 hours; liked the rich but light texture which was very quickly absorbed into skin, definitely enhanced radiance; very pleasant smell – like honeysuckle' • 'skin softer, more rested-looking, brighter and healthier – I look like I've had more sleep than I have, even my husband said I looked young and fresh-faced – does it come in industrial-sized vats?' • 'it makes a real difference to my skin, more so than many products that claim anti-ageing benefits'.

Lancôme Génifique Repair Youth Activating Night Cream

8.75/10

The boffins in L'Oréal's labs harnessed ten years of research to create this light-textured, neroli-and-citrus-scented cream, which they claim 'revives the activity of the genes responsible for reinforcing the skin's barrier function'! They further promise 'one night's all it takes to obtain a more rested appearance...'

Comments: 'Really like sleep in the jar: I could tell the difference having used this: skin was soft, smooth, clearer, more radiant' • 'smoothed fine lines; skin felt and looked plumper, supple and with a healthy glow' • 'my husband has commented a couple of times on how great my skin is looking'.

LP Skin Therapy Overnight Replenish Cream

8.44/10

Dr. Linda Papadopoulos (LP) is actually a psychologist who believes that planning a 'calming nightly routine' will reduce stress, help you sleep better and look more refreshed'. All the more so, it seems, if you apply this – which features baobab oil, from the so-called 'Tree of Life', in the vitamin-rich formula.

Comments: 'The most noticeable change is my appearance in the morning: caught sight of myself in the bathroom mirror and literally did a double take as my face looked radiant and youthful' • 'love this: skin seemed "happier" next day; couldn't bear to finish the jar and will buy again as often as I can justify' • 'with a velvety texture, definitely plumps skin so it looks younger'.

♡ WE LOVE...

Jo once declared Liz Earle Naturally Active Superskin Moisturiser 'the best moisturiser ever, ever, ever' – and still loves it before bedtime. 'It's rich, nourishing and the "plumping" action is amazing,' she says. When Jo had her facial moisture levels checked at a recent launch for a skin cream not so long ago, she scored the highest percentage for moisturisation of any beauty editor. Sarah is devoted to the high-scoring Temple Spa Skin Truffle you can read about on page 17, with a rejuvenating formula including truffles, diamonds and pure gold (gosh!).

TIP

Many people we know swear by a silk pillowcase to sleep on, insisting that they wake up without the 'sleep creases' that can develop in skin as we slumber. Also a silk pillowcase – unlike cotton – doesn't absorb either your skin's natural moisture or the cream you put on, so you're giving your skin the benefit of any anti-ageing ingredients – not your pillowcase...

Give aches and pains plenty of TLC

We're not talking here about the sort of pain that comes with acute illness or injury. This is the general wear and tear that we're all prey to and which can make us look and feel older – so here's our prescription for kissing it better!

Two out of three people suffer neck and shoulder pain in their lives. Back ache is endemic, affecting eight to ten of us, the majority aged between 35 and 55. Then there are the usual headaches, not to mention sore feet (for more about them, see page 96). And none of them are beautifiers: we furrow our brows, the light goes out of our eyes, we stoop or slouch. (And left untended our joints may suffer irreparable damage.) So it's worth having strategies to deal with aches and pains. First of all, prevention – below you'll find the most useful tips we know for everyday stuff. And if despite your best endeavours you do end up in agony, see overleaf for advice.

Stand up straight. Improving your posture reaps heaps of benefits – preventing aches and pains, making you look slimmer, and even keeping you happier. Ears, shoulders, hips, knees and ankles should be in a straight line; pull your tummy button towards your spine. Breathe slowly. (See the box overleaf for more.)

Make sure you can see clearly. Having the right specs will help prevent that tortoise-poke-forward as you peer at a book, the

screen – or the road ahead (as well as stopping you frowning, which should save a few pounds on face creams). Have your eyes tested at least every two years, annually after the age of forty if you have glaucoma in the family (it can result in blindness, so this is vital). Check your lighting: if you're working at a screen, the main source should come from behind it to avoid reflections on the screen. If you're reading, the light source should preferably come from over your left shoulder; in the darker winter months, you will need stronger light than on a bright summer's day. (We like Serious Readers dedicated lamps.)

Keep moving. Our bodies were not designed to sit still for long periods. Neck, shoulder and back aches often come from sitting in a fixed position at screens (laptops are worst of all, see right) and also driving, lifting, etc. The golden rule is: get up and walk around every 30-40 minutes – more if possible. Sip a glass of water as you amble, and you'll be doing double beauty duty.

Position your head correctly. It's very heavy (about 12 pounds) and needs to sit directly on top of your spine rather than poking forward, straining muscles and causing injury. Aim to have your ears, shoulders and hips in a straight vertical line. Lifting your chest and letting your shoulders roll back and down helps; gently push your shoulder blades together (see exercises below).

Have your knees slightly lower than your pelvis when sitting. This helps put the spine into neutral position. If you don't have a chair with an adjustable seat, try putting a couple of folded towels under your bottom, and sit into the back of the chair.

Your screen should be at eye level. Have your forearms at right angles to your body and in a straight line to your fingertips. An arm rest may help. Your mouse should be easily accessible by swinging your hand round, to say 45 degrees maximum. You shouldn't have to lift your elbow or make a claw. RSI sufferers should choose a big 'elephant's foot' mouse or trackball.

Keep the documents you are working on at eye height to avoid squinnying at the bottom of the screen.

Do simple, gentle exercises to keep your circulation moving. A counter-stretch will reverse the hunched position, particularly after using a laptop; imagine you're 'opening like a flower', says Tim Hutchful of the British Chiropractic Association. Reach your arms out to the side, palms up, then open your fingers and turn your palms down to the floor; look gently up to the ceiling, push your shoulder blades together and hold for ten seconds. Follow with a 'chin tuck': pull your chin into your throat as if you are trying to make a double chin and hold for ten seconds. Also shrug your shoulders up to your ears and circle them back and forwards. (For a quick exercise programme for all ages, visit www.youtube.com and put Straighten Up UK! in Search – fantastic if you're feeling tired and/or looking peaky.)

POSTURE

Bad posture is to blame for all sorts of aches and pains. But here's an interesting thing: good posture can actually help to change your mood. If you feel low, you tend to look down, which keeps you feeling, well, low and down. Matters get worse if you hunch your shoulders and clasp your arms or hands in front. 'You're closing off your chest, which means you don't get as much oxygen in your lungs and your brain,' explains body language expert Robert Phipps. 'If you straighten up, open your chest and shoulders, look ahead and around keeping your eye movements horizontal, you start to feel better. Looking down connects with the emotional part of your brain whereas looking up and to the right engages with your future. You will notice your breathing changes, and your whole body lifts.'

Posture is also a vital component of social signalling: 'If you adopt a confident body posture, you project confidence. Barriers and defensive postures signal fear; uncrossing your arms and lifting your chin signals "I'm not afraid". Our minds and bodies are in a constant feedback loop, conveying information. Animals respond purely to body language; humans put a social veneer on behaviour but we always revert to animal instincts,' says Phipps.

A tip: on a first meeting or at an interview, mirror the person's body language for three or four movements, match their rate of talking and breathing, then sit back in your chair. 'At an interesting moment in the conversation, pause, lean forward and drop your voice slightly so they have to come forward to you. They are then mirroring you – through your confident strategy,' says Phipps.

Of course, posture isn't just about your social life. 'Good posture keeps your bones and joints in alignment so you can use your muscles properly and keep them fairly relaxed to avoid painful tension,' explains chiropractor Tim Hutchful. 'It should also prevent your spine being distorted into an abnormal position, which can lead to

LAPTOP KNOW-HOW

Laptop computers have liberated us in many ways but, according to chiropractor Tim Hutchful, the downside is that they can cause considerable damage to your neck and spine, resulting in lots of aches and pains including headaches. 'Because the laptop keyboard and screen are integrated, you risk compromising your neck, shoulders, arms and/or back when using one, so there's potential for problems in all these areas,' he says.

● Taking a small keyboard with you (pack everything in a rucksack so the weight is even) may seem like trouble but it can really help you avoid it.

● Try to work with your arms supported (on a train or plane table, or even on cushions if you're in the back of a car), to avoid neck pain from the muscles that hold up your arms.

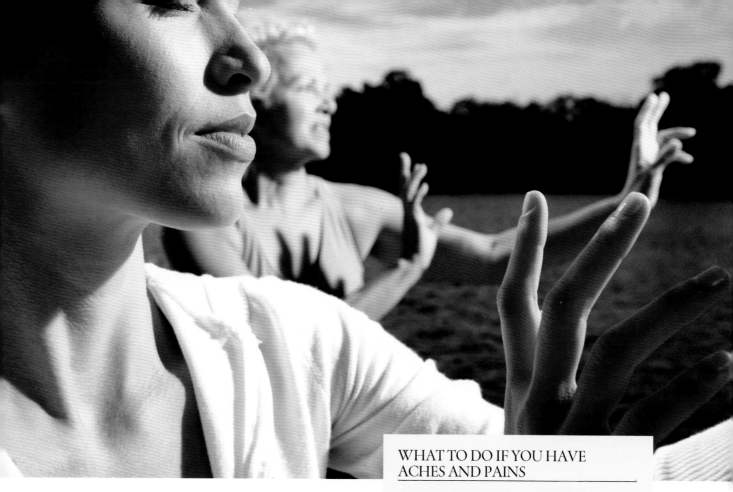

T'ai chi helps many aches and pains, including knee osteoarthritis and fibromyalgia, as well as quality of sleep. It may also benefit bone density, and increase musculoskeletal strength.

pain in different parts of your body. Additionally, if you're evenly balanced, it helps to reduce abnormal wear and tear of joints. Remember that good posture is just as important when you're moving as when you're still,' he adds.

To support your spine, it's vital to strengthen the corset of abdominal muscles between the lower margin of your ribs and your waist, all round. Simply contract those muscles as you sit at your desk or stand at the bus stop. To create a 'cross bracing effect', try the Superman exercise: go down on all fours like a coffee table, arms and upper legs at right angles to your body. Raise your right arm and left leg to the horizontal, hold for five to ten seconds, then swap sides. Repeat five times. (Don't do this if it's uncomfortable.)

WHAT TO DO IF YOU HAVE ACHES AND PAINS

Spray on magnesium oil: it will relax the muscles in that area and should provide quick relief. You can use it several times a day, and before bed. Genius! (Try Magnesium Oil by Better You.)

Take an anti-inflammatory: we don't get on with conventional versions, so took the advice of integrated medicine guru Dr Andrew Weil and keep a stock of Zyflamend by New Chapter, a combination of plants that help reduce pain and inflammation in the joints (can also be used for skin).

Try Bromelain, an enzyme with remarkable painkilling properties, that's been extensively studied for use in digestive disorders (eg, heartburn, reflux and food allergies), also inflammatory conditions (arthritis, sports injuries and skin conditions such as eczema and psoriasis). (Bromelain by LifeTime Vitamins.)

Explore complementary therapies such as acupuncture, chiropractic (try McTimoney chiropractic if you don't like too much clunk-click stuff), Bowen technique, osteopathy and/or cranial osteopathy. Practise (gently) yoga, Pilates or t'ai chi.

'Beautiful YOUNG people are accidents of nature, but beautiful OLD people are *works of art*'

Eleanor Roosevelt

Embrace pearls
(it worked for Grace Kelly)

We love pearls. Ropes and swags of them. As necklaces, chokers, bracelets and don't forget earrings. Real, cultured or plain fake. Sea or freshwater. Vintage or just-strung. Oversized and multi-stranded or neat, demure singles. White, pink, grey or black. With denim or satin, T-shirt, woolly or your most glam glad rags

Forget diamonds – we say: pearls are a girl's best friend. Why?

Because these lustrous baubles are just about the most fabulously flattering accessory for any mature complexion – whether your skin has warm or cool tones. (Michelle Obama looks amazing in pearls. So do Hillary Clinton, Oprah Winfrey and Elizabeth Taylor, which tells you everything you need to know about how they work for every complexion. Think of Coco Chanel, Audrey Hepburn, Jackie Kennedy Onassis, Princess Diana – all draped in them. And not for nothing have English and North American women traditionally been given a pearl necklace and earrings when they came of age.)

Pearls may swing in and out of fashion, but they are always miraculously flattering. Pearls distract the eye. They're lambent like moonlight, creating a sort of 'halo' effect when close to the face – bouncing light on to your skin and making it appear softer and more radiant.

A pearl collar or choker can disguise a less-than-fabulous neck. Dowager duchesses have

LUST FOR THE LUSTRE

Pearlised pigments and, in some cases, real crushed pearl (aka 'nacre') are also being incorporated into skin creams for instant radiance – great in a make-up primer, as it gives skin that 'halo' effect when foundation's applied on top. In make-up, these pearl-esque, light-reflective pigments really can create the illusion of softening fine lines, and minimising under-eye shadows or visible pigmentation.

always known that, but frankly it's a tip that many of us could make use of if neck-angst kicks in. You don't need a title or family jewels for this: Jo, in particular, is constantly on the lookout for great costume jewellery pearls, but also likes real baroque Indian pearls: she first found them in Anjuna Market in Goa, and while a practised eye might be able to tell them apart from much, much pricier versions, we're just not that snooty about our jewels. We just pile 'em on. Timeless. Classic. Minor-miracle-working.

And add a touch of pearl to your skin, too. Pearl is also a word – or rather, a texture – to bear in mind when it comes to creating a finish for your make-up. Applied judiciously – a touch on the browbone, for instance, or even on the eyelid – pearlised eyeshadow helps create a sculpting light-and-shade effect. Fact: too matt isn't good, after forty, because a face looks dry and dusty. You need a little sheen. But use 'the pearl test' when you're buying glimmering shades of any product, ie, does this have more shimmer than a real pearl? In which case it's probably too shimmery, whether you're looking at a lipstick or an eyeshadow.

'There is one piece of jewellery that is equally becoming to everybody, lovely with almost every ensemble, appropriate for almost every occasion and indispensable in every woman's wardrobe... Long live the pearl necklace, from our first date to our last breath!'

Geneviève Antoine Dariaux, *Elégance*

'Not for nothing have women traditionally been given a pearl necklace and earrings when they came of age'

'We can't all look like the *wondrous* Carmen dell'Orefice (STILL a supermodel at 79) but we CAN look pretty damn *good*'

Look good in photos

(And feel better about yourself)

We used to think that a friend of ours – then editor of *Tatler* – was being so grand when she refused to be photographed before lunchtime. Now we absolutely understand what she meant. One of the commonest causes of those 'oh, damn!' moments – when we really feel like we've fast-forwarded a decade or two – is seeing ourselves in a hideous snap. 'Do I really look like that…?' Well, the answer is not really: in real life, people take in all of you (voice, smile, twinkling eyes) – whereas in a snapshot, it's so easy to see only your flaws.

So: we believe in positive reinforcement. It's possible to take a hideous picture of anyone (think of those 'drunken' celebrity shots which caught them mid-blink). But it makes all of us feel better if we can glimpse a photo and go, 'Actually, not looking so bad…'

This may be a cheat, but in the same way that famous people control 'official' images of themselves, we suggest that you only surround yourself with photos of yourself that you really like: from the photos on the mantelpiece to the pix you send to friends. And the photos on your Facebook 'wall', or in your online albums.

There's also a great deal more you can do to look your absolute best in photos than just simply say 'cheese'… We can't all look like the wondrous Carmen dell'Orefice (still a supermodel at 79 as we go to press) but we can look pretty damn good.

Don't be photographed before lunchtime. No, we really mean it: most of the early morning puffiness will have diminished by then – and eyes will appear more awake. (And it also gives time to get to the hairdresser, if required. You think we ever have our official pictures taken without hitting John Frieda first? No. Way.)

Remember: this is no time to go bare-faced. Make-up artist Bobbi Brown recommends a yellow-toned foundation and concealer (rather than anything with a hint of pink), as these look better on film. Use a mattifying foundation, rather than a dewy finish; apply with a sponge sparingly, and use concealer to even out any flaws such as broken veins, under-eye circles. Be aware, though, that pen-style light-reflecting concealers – designed to work on dark circles – can bounce back so much light if used with flash photography, they create a 'reverse-panda' effect. Brush translucent powder over the face and exposed skin on the neckline. Avoid shimmer, as any flash will exaggerate shine.

Use matt eyeshadows. Browns and greys look best in photos, with black or brown eyeliner, close to your lashes on top (and, if you like, bottom) lid. Use black or brown waterproof mascara, as any flash can lead to 'tear-ing', thus smudging your lashes.

Go for an enhanced lip-coloured lipstick. Something mid-rose, or a bit deeper – the colour of your lips only a bit more so. These are the shades we generally recommend anyway, but in pictures bright reds, corals and oranges look super-garish.

Stay out of strong sunlight. This creates major nose shadows and makes you squint. Outdoors, open shade is best – daylight under an awning or a tree. As model Lisa Snowdon says, 'Midday sun is the equivalent of looking at yourself in the mirror under an incredibly harsh spotlight, and is very ageing.'

Try 'the golden hour' instead. As Lisa adds, 'This is the first or last hour of sunlight of the day. This is the optimum time for photographs, when you cannot fail to look your absolute best.'

Pretend the photographer is your best friend. You'll be more yourself and your face will take on a more normal expression.

Relax your mouth. Make-up artist Tricia Sawyer recommends saying A-E-I-O-U to achieve this; to give the face a better shape and diminish a double chin, push your tongue against the back of your top teeth. Try not to crinkle your face into a big grin, as this will exaggerate lines around the eyes, but 'twinkle' with them.

Stand slightly sideways – and follow the beauty queens' advice. Angling the body slightly will make you look slimmer. Then put one foot in front of the other, which miraculously narrows the silhouette of the leg.

Never be photographed from below. This is the fastest-track to double chins and awful photographs. Instead, it helps if the photographer is positioned slightly above you: tilting your face up into the camera is hugely flattering (unless you have a long nose). Shots taken full-on can make a wide face look wider; try tilting your head slightly if the photographer is directly in front of you.

B-r-e-a-t-h-e. Many of us find it stressful having our photo taken, but if you hold your breath you'll look 'frozen'. Breathing out relaxes the face and body; inhaling raises shoulders and can give you a look of panic. So first take a few long, deep breaths.

And if all else fails, retouch. You think Hollywood stars REALLY look the way we see them? Online and on the high street you can get photos retouched. Or change to the more forgiving hues of black and white. Whatever it takes to get a photo you love is fine.

Don't let rosacea give you the blues

It used to be blushing that was embarrassing. Well, nowadays for getting-older women there seems to be an increasing problem with redness and rosacea. If you don't quite love your rosy cheeks (yet), here are some ideas

Although a fiery skin can sometimes affect young women, for others the problem starts as they get older. The causes of redness and rosacea are still pretty mysterious – basically something in the bloodstream triggers the swelling of blood vessels in the skin, causing inflammation (redness and soreness).

The triggers are notoriously individual, including food, alcohol, stress, pollution and perimenopause. There may also be inherited components which predispose people to redness: also it shows up much more on people with thin, fair skins.

However, there are some general guidelines which may help, as we learnt from Marie-Véronique Nadeau, the Californian former chemistry teacher who – after 'struggling' with rosacea from her early thirties – started her own skincare company (Marie Veronique Organics) to help people with problem skins. Here's her advice for dealing with inflammatory skin conditions:

Take turmeric faithfully. This Indian spice is a lifesaver for minimising flare-ups: take a 400mg capsule morning and night. It's hard to get enough by sprinkling it on your food, but do that too!

Use products with zinc oxide. As well as providing sun protection and helping wound-healing, this mineral is anti-inflammatory, so helps with most skin conditions including rosacea and also acne. Apply products which contain it (such as Marie Veronique Organics Moisturizing Face Screen SPF30). Other helpful anti-inflammatory ingredients include emu oil, red raspberry oil and aloe.

Take specific supplements. In addition to a good anti-inflammatory diet (plenty of nuts and seeds, vegetables and fruit, oily fish if you're not vegetarian), Marie-Véronique says it's 'an absolute must' to supplement with vitamin C, vitamin D3 and omega-3 essential fatty acids. (See page 180 for more on supplements.) Rosacea patients may also need more of a specific and powerful antioxidant called SOD (superoxide dismutase), so add that in too. NB: Marie-Véronique advises avoiding iron supplements, particularly if you have severe rosacea, as iron may aggravate it.

Monitor your reaction to 'heating' foods. Caffeine, red wine, curries and so on affect redness-prone people differently (see Maggie Alderson's experience opposite). The only advice is to turn detective and track your own personal response.

Beware the sun (and sunbeds). Ultraviolet light and particularly UVA – the longer-wavelength rays that are linked to skin damage and also now to skin cancers – seem to affect some rosacea sufferers severely. Everyone should take care in the sun – ie, always wear sun protection and never fry your skin. But for anyone with skin sensitivity of any kind, it's wise to avoid sunscreens with a chemical sunblock since they are known to be more likely to cause irritation. Opt instead for sunblocks using minerals, preferably zinc oxide (see left). Additionally, avoid anything with citrus essential oils and any product at all with alcohol.

ROSACEA – WHAT WORKS FOR ME

Novelist Maggie Alderson developed rosacea in 2002, when she was in her early forties. Here, she describes her strategies for making the best of what can be a lifelong condition.

'Tucked away at the top of my bathroom cupboard I keep an insurance policy, in the form of a pack of antibiotics my doctor prescribed for my rosacea. I hate the idea of taking oral antibiotics for anything short of a life-threatening infection, but I keep them there just in case the day comes when I really can't live with the raised and angry red blotches on my face any longer.

'I came close to it last summer after using cheap chemical sunblock on holiday and ending up with cheeks and chin almost as red and sore as the worst sunburn, but I managed to get through it by binning the block in favour of hats and beach umbrellas – and giving up wine with dinner. After eight years with this progressively worsening condition, I have found that what you swallow makes as big a difference – if not more – than what you slap on. Coffee, white wine and spicy food are my worst triggers, but apart from sunblock, the other most aggravating factor is stress. Which is ironic, as having a face like an overcooked pepperoni pizza is pretty stressful itself.

'I have tried legion topical products over the eight years or so I've had the condition, from prescribed antibiotic creams to exotic blue potions from imported beauty companies. Some of them worked for a bit, but none of them will cure rosacea. There isn't a cure but one effective temporary treatment I've found is acupuncture, which can settle down a really bad episode – although I know it will always come back.

'So rather than wasting more time and money searching for the miracle, I've come to accept it and, like someone with a port wine mark, put my energy into concealment. You simply have to wear make-up every day.

'The best conventional base I've found is Giorgio Armani Designer Shaping Cream Foundation SPF20, used with Laura Mercier concealer, but more recently I've been exploring mineral

SUPPLEMENTARY BENEFITS

As well as increasing omega-3 essential fatty acids both in the diet and as a supplement, pharmacist Shabir Daya advises taking a probiotic supplement: 'These beneficial bacteria will help to rid the gut of potential toxins that inflame the skin but more importantly they may ensure that specific "bad" bacteria do not proliferate.' Also try anti-inflammatory herbs such as red clover and echinacea, plus yellow dock and dandelion, which have mild diuretic properties to help eliminate the troublesome toxins. A topical serum with pycnogenol (a powerful antioxidant and anti-inflammatory) may also help, he says: 'It immediately reduces redness and inflammation and also strengthens the collagen matrix and in doing so reduces the capability of these toxins to inflame the skin.'

'I've come to accept it and put my energy into concealment. You simply have to wear make-up every day'

make-up. It takes a bit of getting used to but once you get the hang of layering on the fine dust, the coverage is extraordinary, with a lovely dewy finish which doesn't look – or feel – too make-up-y.

'I'm also seeing signs of improvement to my skin. Bare Minerals claim their products can help rosacea and mine has certainly calmed down significantly since I've been using it. The marks are still there, but they aren't nearly so raised and crusty.

'Most importantly, I know I now have a tool I can rely on to get me out of the house without embarrassment, even if I have the worst flare-up.

'One other tip: as well as the red weals and flaking spots, rosacea makes your facial skin as dry as a crocodile handbag. After sampling every miracle moisturiser on the market, the one that really makes the difference is Superskin Moisturiser by Liz Earle.'

Redness treatments: *our award winners*

We'll be frank: we didn't have incredibly high hopes for these. However, the products here – all of them trialled by panellists who put themselves forward because they have redness or mild rosacea – out-performed our expectations. We are seeing rapid growth in this category of products: redness has suddenly been identified as a 'boom' area by the beauty industry. We trialled plenty of new launches for this update (with two excellent new entries) – but do remember that inflamed conditions are notoriously individual, so what works for some may not work for all

AT A GLANCE

Murad Redness Therapy Recovery Treatment Gel

Avène Anti-Redness Day Protective Moisturising Cream SPF20

Darphin Intral Redness Relief Soothing Serum

Jane Scrivner 'Un' Condition Oil

NB **These products are (mostly) not designed as moisturisers, and many women will need to use them with, not instead of, day and/or night creams.**

REVIEWS

Murad Redness Therapy Recovery Treatment Gel

 8.14/10

Uber-antioxidant goji berry is the key anti-inflammatory agent in this gel (goji has 500 times the vitamin C of oranges, and more beta-carotene than carrots, FYI!). It accelerates the healing of dry, flaky skin, and the light gel also features soothing zinc oxide, azaleic acid, vitamin K and peppermint leaf extract, to reduce sensitivity. Dr Howard Murad helped pioneer the whole category of dermatologist skincare, and this is one of a capsule range within his brand specifically to target redness.

Comments: 'Sank in so quickly and left no residue, and I can't tell you how happy I am with this: my redness has demised, and my acne-enraged nose is a distant memory; my skin looks how it used to before all this started. I had become so self-conscious I hated going out even for the school run; I have spent a lot of money on creams before finding this – it's cleared up a lot of the problem with only the odd blip which is gone really quickly and without stress' • 'nice almost milk-like texture and it worked!' • 'left my face a lot less red than it was before – I now use every morning and will buy more' • 'lovely to use and very good results' • 'rosacea is definitely calmed, the broken veins are the same but I flush much more mildly, less red and less often – the only product I have really seen a difference with'.

Avène Anti-Redness Day Protective Moisturising Cream SPF20

 7.89/10

If you've ever set foot inside a French pharmacy you'll be familiar with this range, which has a particular soothing thermal spa water at the heart of every product and specifically targets 'intolerant' skin (think: sensitivity, hyperkeratosis, rosacea, etc). From the 'anti-redness' collection, this daily moisturiser offers a high concentration of butcher's broom (Ruscus aculeatus) extract, renowned for its constricting action on blood vessels. There's a useful SPF20: redness-sufferers don't always realise that sun protection can play a vital role in easing this worrisome problem.

Comments: 'My skin is now much more even-toned – after a few days skin felt less "angry", more settled and resilient' • 'I hadn't heard of this brand before but now will be trying some of their other products' • 'the pale green colour – to counteract redness – doesn't show up when applied; gave skin a glow and made it soft to the touch' • 'although there's an SPF20, it has none of the grey tint/film I'd associate with that, which is a bonus' • 'skin looks more even and is less greasy, too' • 'fewer spots in the area where my hair touches my face'.

Darphin Intral Redness Relief Soothing Serum

This is part of a recently introduced range from Darphin for sensitive skins, created to help strengthen skin while diminishing the appearance of redness. Calming botanicals include grape extract, antioxidant resveratrol, chamomile, hawthorn and peony extracts, in a gentle baby-pink serum.

Comments: 'After two minutes, my very red sensitive cheeks with thread veins felt soothed, and smoothed; moisturiser glided on; I looked forward to applying this every morning as it cooled my skin and took the extreme redness from my cheeks; skin more even and hydrated and I didn't have to use so much make-up to cover. Colleagues and family have noticed the improvement, which is lovely' • 'finally found something that's gentle and effective, will be investing in the accompanying products. Very, very pleased!' • 'skin looks healthy and not as red' • 'I loved this product, it worked brilliantly – 10/10!' • 'after two weeks my skin was less prone to redness'.

Jane Scrivner 'Un' Condition Oil

Jane Scrivner is kind of a 'poacher-turned-gamekeeper': a health writer and detox expert who we've long respected, and who recently brought out her own acclaimed range. Jane put forward her 100 per cent cold-pressed Moroccan argan oil for this challenging category – and it did creditably well. You might like to know that pump-action 'Un' Condition Oil – which we're told is organic, although the product doesn't carry formal certification – also targets other skin woes, including eczema, psoriasis and extreme dryness; to be honest, testers found it more useful for those skin conditions than straightforward rosacea.

Comments: 'This leaves skin feeling comforted and moisturised' • 'I also enjoyed using this as a treatment for dry areas and the backs of my hands before using hand cream' • 'a good "rescue" treatment for carrying around' • 'the skin around my nose seems a lot less inflamed than usual and slightly less red, so this definitely worked' • 'I had a slight flaky patch on my chin and this oil cleaned it up no problem' • 'my daughter used a few drops of this as a hair treatment and loved it!'.

TIP

A friend with flaming cheeks divulged that her secret soother is a spray of organic Pukka Rosewater which she takes everywhere. (It's in a glass bottle but not too big or heavy for most handbags; at home do keep it in the fridge for maximum effect.)

Serums: our award winners

Serums are hot anti-ageing beauty news. A week never goes by now without several ew serums landing on our desks: there's a real anti-ageing 'beauty buzz' about them. The reason is that it's possible to concentrate higher levels of active ingredients in a serum – so potentially they can deliver impressive results. And you don't have to give up favourite day or night creams because serums are usually designed to be layered with them

AT A GLANCE

Estée Lauder Advanced Night Repair Synchronized Recovery Complex

La Clarée Oliv' Radiance Elixir

Pinks Boutique Anti-Aging Serum

Sarah Chapman London Skinesis Age-Repair Serum

TIP

Allow serum to absorb for a few minutes before applying your moisturiser. Pay attention to areas where skin is thin and easily damaged, such as your neck and décolletage.

So: do the benefits live up to the serum hype? Or are serums just another way to get us to part with more hard-earned cash? They can be very pricey – right up to a heart-stopping £1,500, though these winners were significantly less expensive. Our testers were certainly impressed with the following, and we trialled dozens more for this edition – though there's just one new entry: Estée Lauder's classic rocketed into the top slot with a stupendous score. Just remember, more is not more with these products – like facial oils, you just need a very few drops.

REVIEWS

Estée Lauder Advanced Night Repair Synchronized Recovery Complex

 We dithered over whether to put this legendary serum (it's 30 years since the first version was launched!) into Night Treatments or Serums – 'cos it's a serum used at night...! It was really one of the first anti-ageing treatments to harness mega-antioxidant power to target skin ageing, and this lightweight, easily-absorbed intensive serum is used by millions of women all over the world. (To which you can add many of the Beauty Bible panellists who took part in our ANR trial, from now on...).

Comments: '10/10: my skin felt smoother on the "test" side straight away' • 'after two weeks, fine lines below eye that side not as pronounced and skin felt bouncier, and looked plumper; loved it and will be buying more' • 'applied at night and the next morning, to my surprise, my complexion looked brighter, fresher and more evenly toned: my boyfriend asked if I'd been up early on the exercise bike! Skin looks even better a few weeks on. Amazing!' • 'I had dry flaky patches round my nose and hairline, nothing removed them... But since I started using this I have had no recurrence at all. I've bought more for myself and for my mum'.

La Clarée Oliv' Radiance Elixir

From an organically-certified fave range of Sarah's, the texture of this is more akin to a dry oil than a conventional serum (though 'serums' was the category the brand submitted it for). It's suitable for all skintypes. The key anti-ageing ingredient is an olive leaf extract to fight skin stress and deliver radiance. To be applied morning and evening, massaged into skin with little circular movements. Sarah adores this product – which really does boost

Pinks Boutique Anti-Aging Serum ✿ ✿ ✿

8.57/10 Intended ideally for use under night cream or balm, a Soil Association-certified blend of rosehip, avocado, camellia and jojoba that's packed with antioxidants and sun-damage-repairing botanicals. British-born Pinks Boutique is one of the few organic 'spa' brands around and if you're a wannabe-natural beauty, their website is worth checking out for salon locations.

Comments: 'Skin immediately looked a bit more radiant, with a bit more colour in my cheeks, and after two weeks, crow's feet less noticeable, with overall plumpness and healthy glow. I love, love, love it, definitely improves my complexion and makes it looks less tired; plus my big frown line has magically reduced! I've become slightly obsessed with it…' • 'bottle goes a very long way as you only use a few drops, skin looks brighter and healthier' • 'noticeable difference with the side I applied it to – softer, smoother and plumper – and the other side of my face!' • 'skin looked much more nourished, brighter and younger after just two weeks – woo hoo! Lots of fab comments, thank you!!!'.

Sarah Chapman London Skinesis Age-Repair Serum

 8.5/10 A facial with superfacialist Sarah Chapman is definitely worth the waiting list. More readily available, though, is her skincare line – and this silky serum is one of two winners in this book from her elegant seven-product range. Loads of peptides, vitamin E, aloe vera juice and mushroom extract are delicately and prettily fragranced with jasmine, hyacinth and rose essential oils. Stylish pump-action packaging protects the contents.

Comments: 'Immediate and *big* difference in tone, skin brighter and smoother with no tightness; after two weeks, people mentioned I looked great and younger – fine lines disappeared and skin looked vibrant, really bright and smooth with no dark tones, crêpiness lessened – amazing!' • 'my fine lines have almost gone away!' • 'really a wow product, you only need a small amount for a great difference in the texture of the skin, which really did appear softer, brighter and more rested; definitely reduced marionette lines near nose and mouth, definitely buying – I look as if I've had a good holiday' • 'after two weeks, skin is 80 per cent brighter, andfine lines reduced'.

radiance – and isn't at all surprised that testers feel the same.

Comments: 'My favourite of all the products I tested: smells gorgeous, and while skin was nicer from first use, after two weeks my eye area has definitely improved with fewer fine lines, not so puffy and congested-looking – youthful and firmer; face appears brighter and fine lines are disappearing!' • 'just give me more! I'll bathe in it…' • 'within 24 hours, skin was velvety smooth, after two weeks I am a convert, skin is less crêpey, brighter and the smell is divine: a single drop on my granddaughter's eczema made it less dry and itchy immediately!' • 'my skin beamed at me – dewy, alive – and when I woke the next morning it was plumper, amazingly soft and there were fewer creases, crow's feet softened over time and small crease between my brows definitely softened; stubborn crêpiness improved massively, and skin has a glow about it – I have even been out without foundation on!'.

'Don't hold on to *anger*, or *regrets* – it's AGEING. Kindness is GOOD for the skin'

Marie Helvin

Supergreens Facelift Diet

Give yourself a natural face (and body) lift with this plant-loving diet

We could write a whole book about healthy eating (maybe one day we will). And by now you probably know the basics of what you should and shouldn't be munching for general health maintenance. (And if weight has become an issue, you can read all about a different approach to help you shed pounds in our section on middle-age spread and mindful eating on page 144.)

But here's something wonderful. We truly believe that you have it in your power to slow down the process of ageing (or speed it up, of course, if you do the wrong things). We're not talking about delaying the ravages of time with cosmetic surgery but by what you eat. (As well as other lifestyle steps such as sleep and exercise.)

There are two big processes that cause our skin (and indeed all the cells in our body) to age: dehydration and inflammation. You know the culprits! A poor diet, smoking (you don't, do you?), sun and alcohol, plus late nights, psychological stress, a polluted environment and not enough exercise. But eating plants – mostly fresh greens (mostly raw) – helps to hydrate every cell in your body. And that keeps your skin plump and moist. Add in lifestyle shifts such as more sleep, sun protection and exercise, and your skin will 'bounce-back' – as they call its suppleness capacity – like a Duracell bunny!

Chlorophyll-rich greens are packed with amino acids, which are the building blocks of all protein. Unlike animal protein (where the body has to work to break apart the protein into the separate amino acids), green plants offer you instantly absorbable amino acids to transform into protein.

We learned about this concept by trying a green food supplement called Sun Chlorella from Japan. This superfood settles your gut into a state of delicious calm and efficiency. And when that happens, it helps to 'lift' your face and peachify your skin (Sarah couldn't believe it when she first noticed the transformation after taking Sun Chlorella for a month or so).

The reason? Your skin is the mirror of your digestion and, according to Traditional Chinese Medicine practitioner and nutritionist Nadia Brydon, there are two pairs of energy (Qi) lines called meridians running down your face. If your gut is unhappy, the lines droop and so does your face. Stabilise your digestion and whoosh! The energy is replenished and everything goes upwards.

It's not just your face that sags, says Nadia, because the same meridian runs down through your breasts and stomach. 'When we eat too many foods high in calories and refined carbohydrates and low in micronutrients, we're hastening the sagging in these areas too; eat foods high in micronutrients and low in calories – such as fresh greens – and we help to tone, contract, firm and pull up the droops from the inside.'

The Supergreens Facelift Diet (see overleaf) cleanses the skin from the inside, toning, feeding, hydrating, lifting, moisturising, reducing puffiness and wrinkles – and putting back your glow from top to toe! In fact, the very best face and body lift we can give ourselves is to eat more greens in our diet every day, starting with an anti-ageing supergreen smoothie (see box overleaf). Then do the Supergreens Facelift Diet for two to three days once every three months (minimum).

Try following this diet for two days to start with, preferably over a weekend when you can rest as much as you want to. Do some gentle cardiovascular exercise for at least half an hour a day: walking is fine – dancing if you prefer, or jogging, swimming, hockey. Whatever pleases you.

Do remember this is not meant to be a penance. Make sure you have lovely clean fresh bedlinen, bath towels and nightie; your favourite music and DVDs, a stack of glossy magazines and whatever else you enjoy! Go out if you want to – lead your normal life, just stick to the diet.

It's often fun to do these things with a partner, so ask a girlfriend – or lover/spouse if they're game. But choose someone where there's no tension attached.

'If you starve yourself to the point where your brain cells shrivel, you will never do good work' Cate Blanchett

FRIDAY NIGHT

Prep for your weekend by eating a light evening meal between 6pm and 7.30pm. Always leave at least two hours between eating and going to bed. And do plan for an early night.

SATURDAY/SUNDAY

● First thing, drink a large glass of room-temperature water, with a slice of lemon if liked.

● Follow with half an hour of yoga stretching and meditation, or a walk. Salute to the Sun will start your day beautifully whatever age/fitness you are; for easy-to-follow instructions see www.yogasite.com/sunsalute.htm.

● Apply a hair mask before starting, if you wish.

● Brush teeth and tongue, gargle with slightly salted room-temperature water and splash face with cold water to wake up and contract facial skin cells.

● Before showering, body-brush your whole body with a soft, natural brush or mitten to help stimulate and detox the skin and lymph system. Brush from extremities towards the heart.

● Take a shower, ending with hot and cold hydrotherapy water treatment: alternate hot and cold water for half a minute each, repeat seven times in all. End with hot water before bed, cold water in the morning or before a night out. This contracts and relaxes every cell and moves the circulation, so helping to eliminate toxins.

● Shampoo and condition your hair in the shower.

● Moisturise from top to toe.

● Fill 2 x 1 litre bottles with natural spring (or filtered) water, and sip through the day.

THE DIET

Breakfast
Drink half your Supergreen Smoothie (see recipe right)

Mid-morning snack
● Sip half your remaining Supergreen Smoothie
● 50g soaked almonds and 100g white grapes or raw peas, carrots/cucumber sticks

Lunch
● 100–175g steamed or grilled fresh fish of any sort (just not tinned or frozen)
OR 100–175g fresh tofu
OR half an avocado
● 200–400g mixed salad: make a big salad with some or all of the following: torn leaves of lettuce, rocket (arugula), watercress, basil and spinach; chopped red pepper and cucumber; grated carrot and beetroot, radishes, spring onion; 110g living sprouting seeds, eg, alfalfa, pulses, mung bean shoots; 1 teaspoon pumpkin and sunflower seeds. Dress with 1 tablespoon extra virgin cold pressed olive oil and lemon juice, with salt and freshly ground black pepper to taste
● Pudding: 200g mixed berries
OR 100g papaya
OR 100g apple/pear/grapes
● Sip 350ml natural spring water (more if wished)

Mid-afternoon snack
● Drink remainder of anti-ageing/anti-inflammatory Supergreen Smoothie
● Apple or pear or 100g grapes
● 350ml natural spring water (more if you wish)

Evening meal
● 100–175g fresh organic chicken
OR fresh tofu
OR avocado
OR roasted/steamed vegetable medley seasoned with fresh herbs
● Mixed salad and pudding, as above
● 350ml natural spring water or more if desired

SUPERGREEN SMOOTHIE

Pure rocket fuel! This will help reduce your appetite, rejuvenate your skin and whole body, plus give you endless energy. Drinking it in the morning reduces your appetite for sweet tastes so it helps balance blood-sugar levels. Always store in the fridge in a screw-top jar (or wide-necked vacuum flask) and make fresh daily.

Makes about 1 litre in all. All measurements are approximate, so don't fret about being exact.

Blend together

- 600ml still mineral water
- $1/2$ chopped cucumber with skin and pips
- $1/4$ peeled avocado
- 1 chopped celery stick
- juice of $1/2$ lemon or lime
- $1/4$ teaspoon unrefined salt
- small double handful of mixed green leaves (60–80g) from the following: spinach, chicory, watercress, rocket (arugula), Savoy cabbage, chard, lettuce, kale, bok choy (Chinese cabbage), sprigs of mint, parsley, coriander, basil, etc (you can often buy bags of organic mixed green leaves)
- 5–15 pillules Sun Chlorella A (if not used to greens in diet, use 5 tablets for the first 3 days, then build up to 15 over the week)

Plus, optionally

- 1 clove garlic
- 1-2 slices of fresh ginger (5-10g)
- 1 small chopped spring onion
- $1/2$ apple or $1/2$ pear or 100g papaya, mango or melon to sweeten slightly

If you are constipated

- 1 tablespoon fresh flax oil or ground flax seeds

'Eat food. Not too much. Mainly plants'

Michael Pollan's 'Food Rules'

LOVE THESE FOODS

Organic where possible

- **Fresh vegetables, freshly made veggie soups and juices**
- **Fresh salads**
- **Sprouted seeds and pulses**
- **Fresh fruit**
- **Nuts and seeds (soak nuts for 12 hours at room temperature)**
- **Fresh fish including sushi**
- **Tofu**
- **Lean meat/game**
- **Hot water with slice of lemon**
- **Spring water**
- **Herb teas eg, ginger, fennel, peppermint**

REDUCE THESE FOODS

- **All processed sugar and sweeteners**
- **Processed and tinned foods**
- **Junk foods**
- **Dairy products**
- **Wheat products (especially 'industrialised' bread; if you want to eat bread, look for long-fermented sourdoughs from artisan bakeries)**
- **Red meat**
- **Crisps and peanuts**
- **Pasta and pizza**
- **Any foods with E numbers and additives**
- **Sweets/chocolate**
- **Tap water**
- **Coffee**
- **Fizzy drinks**
- **Alcohol**

Discover the supplements you really need

You could spend a fortune on supplements. Or you could miss them out altogether. Neither are good options for optimal health and beauty, we feel…

Consider investing in these basics. Leading experts worldwide consider these the ones you really should include.

● **Multivitamins and minerals:** research shows that even people eating the best diet possible nowadays are deficient in some essential nutrients. Result: you feel and look under par, you're more likely to get ill and you have less energy all round. Invest in a good product, food state if possible for maximum absorption (and value).
Try: All Natural Perfectly Balanced Multinutrients, which contains vitamins, minerals, antioxidants, green foods (including blue green algae, chlorophyll and spirulina), plus liver-cleansing herbs and probiotics (to keep your gut in great order).

● **Omega-3 essential fatty acid:** our bodies don't make essential fatty acids, of which omega-3 is the most important. We need it for pretty well everything in our bodies, including keeping our skin plump, soft and supple. It fortifies hair and nails too. If not veggie try to eat two portions of omega-3 rich oily fish a week, and consider a supplement. Look for a product with EPA and DHA, either based on fish oil, krill or the plant echium.

Try: Ideal Omega 3 by Ideal Omega, a particularly pure form of fish oil, but for those who don't like fish, or are veggie, try Echiomega from the plant *Echium plantagineum*.

● **Vitamin D:** research suggests that at least 50 per cent of adults are deficient in this 'sunshine' vitamin, particularly as we get older. It's vital for your bones, muscles and the immune system, among other functions. It also helps to ward off low mood and depression. Scientists now suggest taking 1,000-2,000 IU daily.
Try: D Lux 1000 spray by Better You – it tastes of lemon and is absorbed rapidly.

We think it's worth adding in these too: you probably won't need or want to take all of them, so read through and see which seem most relevant to you.

● **Phyto-oestrogens:** we don't take HRT (though we're totally sympathetic to women who've tried everything else and feel it's worth the risks), but we do like plant oestrogens which help to mimic our natural hormones and help with hot flushes, night sweats and vaginal dryness.
Try: Sage Complex by Food Science of Vermont, which contains sage, wild yam, dong quai, red clover and a bunch of other herbs including Siberian ginseng, hops, pomegranate extract, fenugreek seeds and kudzu.

● **Digestive enzymes:** as the years pass, our natural supply of digestive enzymes to process food declines, leading to bloating, wind, bad breath – oh dear!
Try: Extrazyme-13 by LifeTime vitamins – a capsule before a meal should do the trick.

● **Hyaluronic acid:** the latest compound to be dubbed the 'fountain of youth' – and with some justice. A protein that can hold 1,000 times its own weight in water, it plumps up skin cells, so helping to erase fine lines and wrinkles. Levels decline with

> ## 50 per cent of adults are deficient in 'sunshine' vitamin D, particularly as we get older

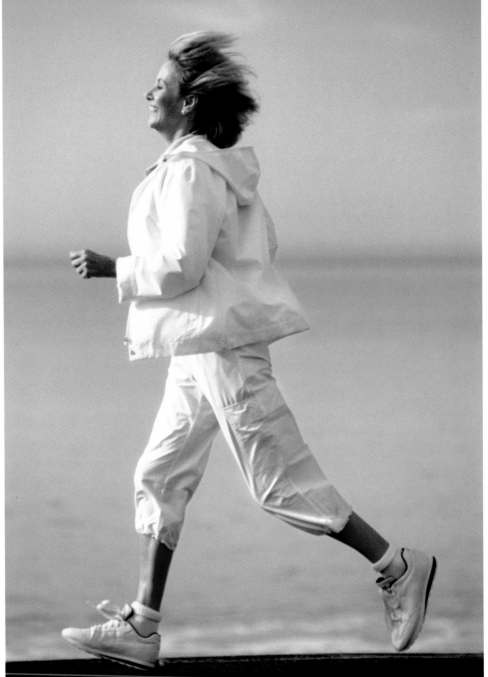

♡WE LOVE...

Jo swears that her bottomless supply of fizz and dash is due not only to her organic diet and daily exercise (yoga and walking) but a supplement called Femergy, which contains the herbs Peruvian maca, Brazilian ginseng plus ginkgo biloba: 'It's a miracle-worker. Two days in a row recently I left the house in a rush and – slapped wrists – forgot my supplements. Result: knackered all day. Today, woke up, took Femergy – and was back to being a little hoppy (not to mention happy) bunny all day long.' Sarah's now a signed-up fan too!

age: as much as 50 per cent by the age of forty. It's also a key factor in keeping joints lubricated and working smoothly. And another thing (or two): it may help dry eye syndrome and also vaginal dryness.

Try: Hyaluronic Acid Capsules High Strength by LifeTime Vitamins, one to two capsules daily.

● **Co-enzyme Q10 (aka Co-Q10):** this vitamin-like compound, which also declines with age, is essential for keeping your muscles (including your heart), gums and immune system in good shape,

and it's vital for anti-ageing in all ways, as well as helping with energy generally. NB: if you take a statin (to lower cholesterol), it's important to take Co-Q10 too as the statin can block production of Co-Q10 and this may create problems in itself.

Try: Super Ubiquinol by Life Extension – ubiquinol is the active form of Co-Q10. Most products are formulated as ubiquinone which is then converted into ubiquinol; taking this supplement as ubiquinol tends to suit people with any sort of digestive problem such as IBS (irritable bowel syndrome) or sluggishness. Take one daily with food.

How to fade your stretch marks

Most women have looked down their body at some point and gasped as they saw the zigzag lines embellishing their skin. We can't really pretend they're gorgeous, so if you can't learn to love them (or at least live with them), we have ways of making them less…

Stretch marks shouldn't be called stretch marks at all – they're really 'hormone' marks. They may happen at puberty (when hormones kick in), pregnancy (ditto) and even sometimes at menopause (which seems especially cruel, if you ask us, considering all the other stuff we have to deal with). It's a bit of a hormonal lottery as to whether you'll get them, but women (and some men) do also get them after weight loss and weight gain (that was Sarah). And the bottom line is that however stretch marks appear on your body, they can cause some distress. So: what to do? Below you will find some general tips – and overleaf, the products our ten women tester panels voted the most effective (and somewhat to our surprise, some really were).

Do as they do in the Mediterranean. Oil yourself. Liberally. Regularly. Olive oil, cocoa butter, shea butter, rosehip oil (which has shown great skin-healing results): all manner of rich and lavish oils will lubricate and nourish the skin. So: anoint your stretch marks at bedtime with oils. When skin is well-nourished, the marks are less obvious. It will also feel smoother and sexier, and more strokeable generally. We're all for that.

Eat foods rich in vitamin K, and plenty of essential fatty acids (EFAs). Vitamin K is a fantastic 'skin-healing' vitamin, found in leafy green vegetables (Brussels sprouts, broccoli, spinach, parsley, okra, mustard greens, peas, artichokes), lentils, kidney beans, plums, liver (if you're not vegetarian) and dairy products. To preserve the vitamin K, all the vegetables should

ideally be consumed raw, or very lightly cooked (save the water for a soup or stock, to reclaim its nutritional value). See page 180 for more about EFAs and their sources.

Live a more holistic lifestyle. This is pretty much the advice that you'll find scattered through this book (because when it comes to looking and feeling fabulous IT WORKS), but eating a good diet, exercising regularly and maintaining a stable weight may have another benefit: it may just help fade your stretch marks. OK, so this is just us speaking (not some doctor with a string of initials after his name), but Sarah used to have shiny stretch marks zigzagging up her hips on either side of her belly. After several years of healthy living – and oiling her body (see left) – she realised the marks had literally vanished. When Jo read this in the answer to a reader's question to www.beautybible.com, she decided to check out her own ancient stretch marks and discovered – to her astonishment – that they had faded too. Not a sign. We can only attribute this to consistent healthy living, and a diet that incorporates plenty of EFAs (plus supplements) and literally mountains of the types of veggies mentioned left.

Try Heal Gel. Anecdotally, Heal Gel has had remarkable results on many different types of scarring (including tough-to-treat keloid scarring). Developed by leading plastic surgeons with a biochemist, this treatment – which also works on sprains, sunburn and bruising – can be worth a shot. You need to apply it two or three times daily, and although you only need a titchy bit, that could prove an expensive option. For other options, trialled by our tester panels, see overleaf.

Buy a tankini. It's tummy stretch marks that really seem to upset the women we know. (Despite the fact that the marks are usually a proud badge of motherhood.) If the one thing standing between you and baring your stomach in public is a network of stretch marks, consider a tankini: the vest top of this style of two-piece swimsuit can be rolled up when nobody's looking, so you get the glorious feeling of air on your skin (and a touch of sun) in the privacy of your back deck/garden, or rolled down in company. Your bikini days may be over, but your tankini days needn't be.

If they really distress you, consider laser or IPL treatment. This works best with pigmented stretch marks; pale or flesh-toned marks don't respond so well to treatment – although there are now re-pigmenting lasers that can help with this. The Lux1540 laser has been approved by the FDA in the US for the treatment of stretch marks, but is only available in a handful of locations. We would certainly suggest only going to a 'master' of laser surgery (local clinics may promise the earth to get your bucks, but as with all high-tech treatments we advise major caution). Be sure you are armed with all the right questions, as per Wendy Lewis's advice on page 46. You may want to consider a pre-treatment consultation with Wendy herself (Wendy works in the US but you can contact her via email and she does consultations on Skype – see

DIRECTORY). Beware: this will be expensive, and at this stage in life it's unrealistic to expect to go back to your smooth-skinned former self.

STRETCH MARKS: THE SCIENCE BIT

Stretch marks – as many of us know – start as fine red or brown lines (sometimes raised) and can deepen to purple on some people. But it's the legacy of stretch marks that causes so much heartache: they fade to a white or silver colour (usually lighter than your natural skintone), but the skin can be much (much) slacker – so it folds and, yes, hangs differently. They're most common on the abdomen, breasts, thighs and buttocks. As well as reproductive hormonal changes, why are stretch marks also linked with gaining and losing weight? According to Dr Eric F Bernstein (Clinical Associate Professor of Dermatology at the University of Pennsylvania School of Medicine, and head of the Scientific Advisory Board of www.stretchmarks.org), 'When people gain weight, our hormones are metabolised by fat cells. Hormones resemble fat and cholesterol, so when we gain and lose weight it affects the hormones in our body – and also the hormones in our skin.' Normal skin is 80 per cent collagen and just 4 per cent elastin, but that elastin is oh-so-important for skin resilience – and stretch marks are basically damaged elastin fibres. According to Dr Bernstein, 'Elastin fibres are the single hardest thing to repair in skin.'

SCAR GAZING

Beat-generation poet Fran Landesman, who's still writing and doing readings in her eighties, wrote a poem called 'Scars' – and it applies just as much to stretch marks (except that wouldn't sound so poetic…). Fran has had grateful fanmail from women who she's helped to come to terms with their scars. You can find the whole thing on www.franlandesman. com – do look. Here's a snippet we love:

Don't be ashamed
Everybody's got scars
From our various wars
On the way to the
  stars
So I'll show you my
  scars
If you show me yours
In the streets and the
  bars
Everybody's got scars
On their way to the
  stars
Everybody's got scars

SKIN TAGS

Skin tags: these tiny little growths, which may be flesh-colour, or sometimes look brown or purple-ish, are not harmful but are often unsightly and can be irritating if they are near or on your eyes, or where clothes rub. An old-fashioned DIY method was to tie a piece of cotton tightly round the base, blocking the blood supply so they eventually dropped off (ligation). However, this carries a risk of infection, so do consult your family doctor or dermatologist who can remove it with a minor surgical procedure. The most common options are cryotherapy (where very cold liquid nitrogen is applied directly to the area), cauterisation (heat is used to burn off the tag, called electrolysis), and excision (the tag is cut off with a scalpel). Your doctor will use local anaesthetic if necessary and provide an antibiotic ointment to prevent infection. If the tag is very close to the eyelid, the procedure may need to be done by an ophthalmologist.

Stretch mark treatments: *our award winners*

Stretch marks are a concern for expectant mothers but as the collagen and elastin in skin break down with ageing, they can be even more anxiety-inducing later in life. (As we say, for some women, stretch marks make an unwelcome appearance at menopause, since they're linked with hormonal upheaval rather than 'stretching'.) This was one of the toughest challenges in the book: can anything lessen or reverse stretch marks? Our testers were rather pleasantly surprised (and so, to be honest, are we!)

AT A GLANCE

Aromatherapy Asssociates Renew Rose Massage & Body Oil

Shiffa Healing Balm

Bio-Oil

This Works Stretch Mark Oil

TIP

One tester trialling the top-scoring cellulite product Thalgo Crème Thalgomince (page 38) noticed that it had a double-whammy effect, not only greatly improving cellulite but also helping to fade her silvery stretch marks. Result!

REVIEWS

Aromatherapy Associates Renew Rose Massage & Body Oil ❀ ❀

 8.75/10

Fascinatingly, Aromatherapy Associates re-submitted this rose, orange blossom and evening primrose-based light oil for the paperback – and in what is an incredibly tough category it came out top once again, scoring an identical mark of 8.75/10! So we've replaced our hardback's remarks with the latest comments. Testers just adored the all-round benefits of this oil.
Comments: 'I have some old stretch marks and new ones especially at my arms where I've lost some weight; the new stretch marks seem to be less angry/visible – but overall it helps perception of them as you feel you're "making a difference"'
• 'marks less prominent and it helped to fade the smaller stretch marks; has a lovely fragrance'
• 'used it on my stomach and marks look softer and skin feels smooth' • 'has a lovely, feminine smell that's almost a substitute for perfume; I also used it on elbows – which have "split" skin – and saw an improvement almost immediately'
• 'reduced redness and also crêpiness on body'
• 'though no effect on long-standing stretch marks, I suffer from arthritis in my back and have trouble sleeping. I used this as a massage oil for my back; it helped me drift into a lovely relaxing sleep and I would purchase this again and again just for that!'.

Shiffa Healing Balm ❀

 8.28/10

A multi-tasking luxury balm created from a blend of organic butters and oils (plus a few synthetic ingredients) by a Dubai-based doctor, this balm was specifically submitted for assessment of its action on stretch marks. To be frank, those results were a bit up-and-down: some testers saw great improvements in stretch marks, others none – but they did generally completely fall in love with the balm's fragrance, texture, and its effect on both mood and dry skin. We say: even if you're unlucky enough not to see an improvement in your stretch marks, you'll enjoy its fall-back position as a face balm/hand cream/foot treat.
Comments: 'I would marry this product if I could; my "white" stretch marks are definitely much better – much less noticeable and I can hardly "feel" them any more' • 'stretch marks are less evident – not totally faded, and although I don't believe there's a product that can magically ease them they are certainly far less noticeable' • 'made stretch marks look better as they were well-moisturised, but all-round my skin was much smoother and healthier after a week – I also used this to treat my son's eczema and it immediately reduced itching and inflammation' • 'my hands were raw and parched from frequent hand-washing – and this really turned the corner for them' • 'a slice of decadence, with multiple uses' • 'once I opened the jar and smelled the balm I was a goner…'

Bio-Oil

8.21/10

Bio-Oil is something of a beauty legend, with many women we know swearing by its effect on scars and stretch marks, as well as an everyday (or rather, everynight) facial oil. We'd never managed to put it through its paces till the trials for this book, and it performed very well in this challenging category. We do need to knock one myth on the head, though: there's a common misconception (echoed in their marketing) that Bio-Oil is 100 per cent botanical, when the key ingredient is mineral oil. (That does happen to be amazing for helping to maintain skin's moisture.)

Comments: 'Lovely fresh smell and after a few weeks, old scars have begun to fade considerably, some gone completely, skin is smoother and less crêpey and in time I think even my older stretch marks will fade: excellent product' • 'also very good on eczema on hands and boobs' • 'absorbs easily and no residue on clothes, skin now looks smoother and improvement in general texture; stretch marks still visible but my C-section scars have nearly vanished!' • 'I've used this as a preventative long term during my pregnancies and through diets and had very few stretch marks, which have faded by now. This is great'.

This Works Stretch Mark Oil ✿ ✿

7.8/10

Our friend, beauty editor and This Works founder Kathy Phillips truly believes in the power of massage to prevent stretch marks (she had a massage every two weeks while expecting her son Oscar). In her range, then, she made sure to include a rich blend designed to counteract the appearance of stretch marks, blending oils of passionfruit seed, gold of pleasure, rosehip seed, alongside coconut and chamomile.

Comments: 'Over one month of use, dark stretch marks faded considerably and some of the new ones had disappeared; skin very hydrated. Wonderful!' • 'just perfect for its job – getting rid of those awful stretch marks; love the fact it's natural too' • 'This Works actually WORKS – what a little miracle' • 'sank in immediately, very attracted to the smell, my skin drank it in and the overall look was improved, as well as helping stretch marks – a marked improvement' • 'a joy to use; divine smell, very nourishing product that leaves skin looking and feeling wonderful, with stretch marks much improved; has definitely made my 17-year-old-marks much less noticeable and I would highly recommend it to any mums-to-be'.

ut sun spots in the shade

Age spots. Liver spots. Whatever you like to call them, they're something we can all live without

Lines we can live with. (Just.) But according to research carried out for Clinique, the problem of uneven pigmentation can be more distressing than wrinkles. The research also identified that from the perspective of a stranger looking at your skin, pigmentation issues ('dark spots', 'sun spots', 'age spots' – or to give them their formal name, 'solar lentigines') can increase your perceived age. Ironically, according to Dr Daniel Yarosh (who's Senior Vice President, Research and Development Basic Science at Estée Lauder), 'Today, these spots are appearing in people decades before their first senior moment. That is a dangerous sign that sun worship is out of control.'

It's fair to say that tackling the problem is one of The Big Beauty Challenges Of All Time (which is one reason we're so tub-thump-y about sun protection everywhere in this book) – but on the upbeat side there are steps you can take if you're troubled by uneven pigmentation.

Never venture out without an SPF30 or over. And please Start Right Now! This is non-negotiable; it should prevent the spots you have from getting any worse, and may actually go some way towards slightly fading them. If you aren't affected by age spots so far? A daily SPF15 (or higher) will go a long way to preventing their future appearance; for a rundown of the daily sun-protective moisturisers which our testers liked best, see page 188. Hand creams with a built-in SPF can be super-useful on the backs of hand/forearms. If you tend to spend a lot of time outdoors, apply regular sunscreen to these vulnerable zones, and remember to repeat after hand-washing (advice which we echo in our HANDS section, page 122).

Wear a hat. If you have sun spots, or seek to avoid their appearance, we also advise: get yourself a fabulous, stylish collection of fairly tightly-woven straw hats, and keep on a peg near your door/s, for easy grabbing when you go out on a summer day (not a baseball cap because the brims aren't big enough, plus they miss your ears which are very vulnerable). Sometimes anti-ageing solutions can be wonderfully low-tech. Wide-armed, large-lensed sunspecs also help.

Try a specific 'age spot' treatment. A vast amount of cosmetic research dollars is currently being channelled into this area of skincare. Dermatologists in some countries can still prescribe hydroquinone for the problem, but in others this skin-lightener has been banned (research showed that it caused mutations in DNA in animal lab tests – though we totally disapprove of those). And even in the US, where its use is popular, treatment with prescription 4 per cent hydroquinone is restricted to a maximum of 12 weeks. We would suggest one of the alternative over-the-counter cosmetic options – and for a shortcut to the most effective, see what really works on page 190.

Apply the product very carefully – don't slap it on before reading the directions. Be aware: most of these treatments take some time to kick in, and there are no overnight miracles here. (You're probably looking at three months minimum, which is longer than most 'miracle' wrinkle treatments take.) Be aware, too, that some are for all-over skin application, and others are literally 'spot-targeted', requiring the use of a cotton bud to apply precisely. Get out your magnifying glasses and read the instructions before throwing out (preferably recycling) the box. Another tip is to apply a thin amount to dark areas at least one

THE SCIENCE BIT

Sun spots, explains Dr Daniel Yarosh, are a direct result of accumulated sun damage, which triggers melanin-producing cells in the skin to lose control and produce too much pigment as a defence mechanism – on the face and chest, in particular, but also the arms and backs of the hands, where they're harder to conceal. Fairer skins are more susceptible – and against a paler background, age spots show up more, too. Jo had one of those 'oh s**t' moments when a dermatologist told her that the dark patches on the side of her face were sun spots, not – as she'd thought/hoped – beauty marks. Which goes to show how easy it is to miss the edges of the face and the outer jaw-line when applying sunscreen. So be sure to smooth your morning SPF into the whole face. Many botanicals have proven pigment-lightening actions, including azaleic acid (from barley and wheat), kojic acid (from fermented mushrooms), retinoic acid and retinols (vitamin A derivatives which are also famously effective against lines), magnesium ascorbyl phosphate (a stabilised form of vitamin C) and liquorice. They all work by inhibiting the melanin-producing enzyme tyrosinase.

KEEP AN EYE ON YOUR MOLES

Most people have ten to forty moles, some many more. Most moles are benign but it's always worth doing a mole check every month or so from top to toe, including your back. If you notice changes in colour (especially if moles are bi-coloured), size, height or shape, or they bleed, ooze, itch, appear scaly, or become tender and/or painful, consult your doctor or dermatologist.

hour before bedtime; this will let it fully absorb into the skin so it won't slide into your eyes when you press your face into the pillow. (Although the products are mild, skin-lightening ingredients can still sting eyes.)

Use make-up to conceal the spot. Once you've got an age spot, what's to do? For a quick fix, turn to make-up. As we explain on page 88, after your primer, dot on a matt, yellow- or peach-based corrector or concealer (deeper peach for women of colour), with a little brush,

then press it in with your finger – don't sweep it on. If needed, top with cream or liquid foundation or brush on a mineral powder base.

Be careful with fragrance. Certain perfume ingredients – particularly some derived from citrus (such as bergamot) – can interact with sunlight to cause permanent pigmentation problems, in the form of 'staining' of the skin, with dark streaks or patches – typically on the neck and chest, where perfume is spritzed or splashed. We counsel: in summer, it's safest to apply perfume to skin for evening only rather than daytime, or put it where the sun won't strike directly. (So long as there's no risk of staining your clothes, fabric is a wonderful 'carrier' for scent, too; more on page 102.)

Zap 'em. The super-high-tech solution is laser treatment, which can disperse these patches of pigmentation, literally 'zapping' the melanin into oblivion. It's painful. It's expensive. If you really decide to go down this route, turn to page 46 and arm yourself with all the advice that you need to shop around to optimise your chances of a safe, effective treatment.

Sun protective day creams: *our award winners*

Repeat after us, please: 'The very best way to stop my face from ageing is to protect it from the sun.' It is never too late to add an SPF day cream into your skincare regime – but it's never too early, either. This goes for all skin colours and types, dermatologists insist, to prevent the signs of ageing. And for anyone already suffering age/sun spots, sun protection is essential to prevent further damage and give any targeted pigmentation treatment the best chance of working. (More about those overleaf)

A good SPF day cream, though, doesn't just offer protection: it sinks in sufficiently well **NOT** to leave skin either greasy or with a white film of sun-protective ingredients on the surface. The following creams – each with an SPF15 or above – fit the bill beautifully, according to our panellists. Optimum protection starts here.

REVIEWS

Clinique Superdefense SPF25

 Another impressively high score for Clinique, who've done very well in this book. Their thinking is that 'stress ages skin, making it dull and lifeless' (we agree!), so alongside the SPF25, there are 'skin de-stressing' ingredients, including a rare red microalgae extract. It's lightweight and – being Clinique – hypoallergenic and fragrance-free.

Comments: '10 out of 10: sank in easily, gave dewy effect and kept skin moisturised all day; good base for make-up and skin doesn't dry out after foundation/powder are applied' • 'skin felt soft and moisturised all day, looks radiant • 'love it! Moisturises very effectively, absorbs very well with no residue, it didn't aggravate my acne and was a very nice base for foundation' • 'you use very little so it lasts a long time' • 'moisturised really well, the best I have tried; sank in well leaving dewy glow and was rich enough for the dry parts of my face'.

Estée Lauder DayWear Advanced Multi-Protection Anti-Oxidant Cream SPF15

 We're long-standing fans of this product, with its cool-as-a-cucumber scent and equally cooling, melts-into-skin texture. Lauder was really the first brand to share research with beauty editors into the important defensive role antioxidants play; in this updated favourite day cream (a new entry in this edition) there's a state-of-the-art blend that neutralises free radical damage, as well as UVA/UVB protection. It is lusciously skin-quenching yet we've always found it a good base for summer make-up. As we've recommended this to readers countless times, we're gratified DayWear makes an appearance here.

Comments: 'Smooth, gorgeous consistency: not watery, not too thick, providing a good level of moisture all day' • 'love it! If you've ever mashed an avocado to use as a face mask and put slices of cucumber over your eyes, the scent of this will be familiar' • 'I have the sort of dry, irritable skin that makes finding a moisturiser problematic – but this ends the search' • 'I've been very happy with how my skin looks while using this effective moisturiser' • 'fewer breakouts since using this' • 'lovely texture – soothing and smoothing'.

♡ WE LOVE...

For day, Jo alternates between two SPF moisturisers (switching when she gets to the end of the product, so there's no risk of the SPF degrading): Dior Hydra Life Pro-Youth Protective Fluid SPF15 is great for summer (it's super-skin-quenching but not greasy), while Sarah Chapman London Skinesis Dynamic Defence Anti-ageing Day Cream SPF15 is more suited for the chillier seasons. Sarah too has several favourites, including all-natural Kimberly Sayer Anti-Oxidant Daily Moisturizing Cream SPF25 (for summer) and our award winner Clinique Superdefense SPF25 (for winter).

Sarah Chapman London Skinesis Dynamic Defence Anti-ageing Day Cream SPF15

8.64/10

Sarah Chapman has become one of our favourite facialists (we're lucky enough to be fast-tracked up her waiting list), offering treatments from a tiny Chelsea clinic for which women fly from around the globe. We're fans of her signature skincare products, including this rich, subtly jasmine/hyacinth/rose-scented daily moisturiser, which is packed with vitamins, antioxidants, omega-rich oils and a broad-spectrum SPF15. A fave of Jo's (see We Love…).

Comments: 'Fantastic! Left skin dewy and well-balanced' • 'easily absorbed rich cream which leaves my very dry skin supple, silky, dewy and clear; I have fallen in love with this product and would buy it again' • 'superb packaging with integral pump, although possibly a bit rich for my shiny skin, which is prone to spots' • 'brilliant product which moisturised well so my skin kept a lovely glow; make-up went on very well after' • very rich cream which felt divine and smelt really nice but subtle' • 'lovely matt finish once it sunk in'.

Crème de la Mer The SPF30 UV Protecting Fluid

8.44/10

Absolutely no question about it: Crème de la Mer has put on a stupendous performance in this book update (see Award-winning Night Treatments, page 156). This is formulated not only to defend skin with an SPF30, but offers 'Hollow Platonic Spheres' (don't you love beauty lingo?) to scatter light and make skin appear more radiant and luminous. Lightweight and transparent enough to work as an excellent make-up primer, while protecting skin against moisture loss.

Comments: 'Usually SPF30 products are really gloopy or hard to blend, but this has a lovely feel and is great under foundation' • 'most products irritate my eyes but this didn't, felt lovely on my skin and protected patches that I'm paranoid about because they're so sun-sensitive' • 'natural effect on skin – slightly dewy and fresh' • 'very smooth, no tightness or greasiness and if you were in a rush you could apply make-up straight away – a real luxury product' • 'nice light, natural fragrance' • 'loved this product!'.

Sun spot treatments: our award winners

In recent years, the beauty industry has declared sun spots (aka brown, liver or age spots) Public Enemy Number One, with lots of launches targeting hyperpigmentation. Bold claims are made – but as we know (somewhat to our surprise) from the first edition of this book, some products really do improve pigmentation

In fact, two new entries here at the top of the 'sun spot' charts put on a very impressive performance. Further down the list scores varied widely, so the averages aren't that high – BUT testers nonetheless loved all these products for their skin-brightening, decongesting, rejuvenating, skintone-evening effects – and would buy them just for that. (Our testers of miracle creams also noted that Melvita Naturalift Anti-Ageing Cream lessened hyperpigmentation, see page 18.)

REVIEWS

Darphin Orange Blossom Aromatic Care ❀ ❀ ❀

8.12 / 10

From a French aromatherapy brand snapped up some years ago by the Lauder empire, this Ecocert-certified facial oil blends seven specifically radiance-enhancing, skin-brightening ingredients including powerfully antioxidant cranberry, lavender, lemon, carrot, bilberry and liquorice (to boost natural radiance) – plus orange blossom, a key ingredient in the aromatic scent that testers loved. Five drops should be applied before your regular moisturiser at night.
Comments: 'Lovely citrussy smell; I like the intense moisturising effect and the fact it's encouraged me to massage my face' • 'I've noticed texture, elasticity and tone of my skin has improved – in one sentence, my skin looks clearer' • 'skin clarity improved and I shall be buying more the minute it runs out – though that'll be a while as it's very long-lasting; my complexion looks much more clear and even after using this as instructed: morning and evenings' • 'after two weeks, age spots (albeit not too significant) were less noticeable' • 'clarity and tone were improved and skin had a fresher, healthier colour; a family member I hadn't seen for months commented on my lovely skin, which was really nice to hear!' • 'I have no sun spots on my face but some small ones on my hands; the treated spots faded so much that after four weeks of using this lovely oil, they were barely visible' • 'luxurious and pampering, quick and easy to use'.

Estée Lauder Idealist Even Skintone Illuminator

8.05 / 10

The shimmery aqua packaging gives a clue to what's inside the dropper-bottle: this high-tech, lightweight oil-free gel-serum is packed with colour-correcting, soft-focus and brightening optics which add glimmer to the skin. This instantly 'blurs' the appearance of age spots while antioxidant rice brand extract and vitamin C, anti-irritant liquorice and gentian, vitamin C and botanical extracts get to work longer term. For some testers, the 'luminosity' washed off at bedtime, while others observed more significant fading of age spots and a significantly more even skintone.
Comments: 'Age spots diminished and less noticeable; my husband, boss and mum said I look better!' • 'glides on easily, like velvet – rich and smooth, but sinks in easily leaving skin soft all day; huge improvement in tone, clarity and age spots are much less obvious – a definite improvement' • 'reduction in discolouration around my nose which I've had for years – redness has all but gone, and helped to fade pigmentation on my cheeks; my skin

looks more even and fresher – a miracle product!' •
'skin looks generally healthier and younger' • 'a light
texture which is velvety on the skin, leaving it fresher
and smoother, clearer and brighter' • 'perks up the
skin immediately; I felt like my hours of sun-
worshipping were less easy to spot, and skin also
looked less haggard and tired' • 'soft-glow effect
"dimmed" the appearance of age spots'.

Dior Capture Totale Radiance Enhancer

This luxurious pale pink serum/cream (at
an accordingly luxe price) is instantly
luminous, so the appearance of
pigmentation and redness are toned down straight
away. (It's as a bit like an all-over light-reflecting
concealer.) Over and above the instant concealing
effect, two testers felt it improved the sun spots on
their faces somewhat, a third said it helped those
on her hands; the rest saw no long-term difference
in pigmentation but voted it a 'miracle' cream for
improving vibrancy, tone and clarity.

Comments: 'Some improvement in sun spots after
two weeks but my skin generally just looked so
much better; fantastic product that made my skin
appear younger and more vibrant' • 'when I finished
the product, age spots weren't as noticeable, skin
more even, with pigmentation faded and so looked
slightly younger' • 'after two weeks sun spots
began to fade slightly and weren't as noticeable; by
the end of the product, they were much less visible
though not completely gone, but I can't see them
after I put on make-up' • 'skin was smoother and
brighter and clearer so I love it and don't want to
stop using it!' • 'no difference to age spots but my
skin is much brighter; I am hooked'.

Origins Brighter By Nature High-potency Brightening Peel with Fruit Acids ✤

This is a brightening solution based on
AHA/fruit acids impregnated into (wet)
pads to swipe over the face, with
high-potency skin-brightening botanicals derived
from coconut and salicylic acid (willow bark),
balanced by soothing cucumber extract, aloe,
Japanese basil leaf and caffeine, plus a
mega-antioxidant complex. In their own clinical
tests, Origins observed results comparable to a
30 per cent glycolic peel.

Comments: 'I have areas of pigmentation on cheek
bones and upper lip; after two weeks using these
slightly abrasive pads there was a slight fading of
age spots, overall skin felt smoother and brighter

immediately, less congested; by the end, the
pigmentation had faded slightly but no dramatic
improvement, however the overall skintone and
clarity has improved' • 'after two weeks, the spots
on my forehead going into my hairline became
micro-sized, and are now unnoticeable, plus my
skin looks a lot younger' • 'no difference in age
spots but the product is definitely peeling away
redness and fellow book clubbers noticed
improved clarity, brightness and more even tone'.

Brush up on tooth wisdom

The thing the majority of people remember most vividly from a first meeting is your smile. (Why do you think Julia Roberts became galactic?) OK, as the years go by, flashing a Californian-babe beam may look out of place but long term, caring for your teeth (and gums) is vital for your appearance, confidence – and your general health

We've become a bit obsessed about our teeth and gums. We're both lucky in that we have quite strong teeth and, partly because we eat well, they aren't discoloured or stained. (Though Sarah had veneers applied in her thirties because of brown stains and shortened teeth due to tetracycline antibiotics as a child.) But we want to keep them that way, and also keep our gums in good shape so that teeth don't get loose. (The thought of putting them in a glass at night is a powerful incentive.) Plus, your whole mouth structure is so important for literally holding up your face – if that gets slack and/or you lose teeth, your cheeks cave in, and that really does age you in a trice. So we're going to spend a bit of time in this section of the book giving you expert advice from London-based holistic dentist Dr David Cook, who has transformed the mouths (and in some cases lives) of several people we know.

So, what ages your smile?
● Stained, discoloured or mismatched teeth.
● Gum disease, which causes gums to recede so teeth look long and horsey; gaps like black triangles often appear at the gum line; loose gums mean teeth may fall out.
● Tooth loss (also grinding, see below) can lead to the lower part of your face looking 'caved in', appearing pinched and shorter with more lines and folds, as well as having gaps (obviously).
● Grinding your teeth at night (bruxism) wears them down, making them shorter and squarer, which distorts the proportions and makes them look less attractive when you're smiling.
● Grinding also causes jaw muscles to bulk up so you get a square-jawed look (not very feminine).

Can the state of your teeth affect your health? In a word, yes...
● Gum disease (aka gingivitis) increases the risk of heart disease, stroke and, in women of child-bearing age, low-birthweight babies. There is also increasing evidence of a link with osteoporosis, type 2 diabetes, Alzheimer's disease and other inflammatory conditions.
● The bacteria that cause gum disease can be passed to others, so partners, children and grandchildren are at increased risk. (Kissing babies is a bad idea if you have gum disease.)
● Poor oral hygiene and gum disease are the primary causes of chronic bad breath (halitosis) and the sufferer is often unaware of the problem.
● Tooth wear and loss can lead to the collapse of your ability to bite down on food – this means your jaw muscles and joints have to work harder, putting strain on them and causing pain and further bite problems.
● Grinding your teeth at night can cause poor sleep patterns, with all its related problems.

WE LOVE...

Dental Miracle, an all-natural green powder with orris root, juniper berry, peppermint, calendula and acacia gum, which leaves your breath fragrant and has a gently abrasive action to leave teeth sparkling clean. It also claims to help 'reinforce' gums, as well as preventing and getting rid of plaque.

'Nothing
makes a
woman
more
beautiful
than the
belief that
she is
beautiful'

Sophia Loren

So what exactly is going on?

Read Dr Cook's advice on common problems and how you can treat them.

Brighten stained and discoloured teeth

As teeth age they tend to get darker, due to stains building up on the surface of the teeth and also penetrating the surface through micro cracks and porosities. Tea, coffee, red wine and tobacco are the main culprits here, and surprisingly herbal and fruit teas are notable culprits too.

A twice-yearly professional clean by a hygienist can work wonders. Once all stain and surface discolouration is polished away you may be surprised at how good your teeth look. After that, using whitening toothpaste with a sonic toothbrush can be very effective at reducing the rate of further stain build-up. (You may need advice from your hygienist on how best to use a sonic toothbrush; also see box page 198.)

Teeth that are badly discoloured or have lost their sparkle and vitality can be rejuvenated with whitening (aka bleaching), using hydrogen peroxide gels which work all the way through the teeth and actually change the colour. Gel concentration and safe application time varies widely, so this should definitely be done under the supervision of a dentist. Provided that tooth whitening/bleaching is done professionally, it is safe, very effective and has few side effects apart from temporary sensitivity. Over-the-counter (or internet) whitening products are usually ineffective and may be damaging due to high acidity, so they should be avoided.

MATCH UP YOUR MOLARS

Misshapen, damaged or worn teeth can be enhanced with porcelain veneers, crowns or onlays to give a beautiful and functional appearance. These techniques can also be used to restore a severely worn or damaged bite, which returns facial balance and gives support to cheeks and lips – (that's why it's sometimes known as the 'dental facelift').

FIX CROOKED TEETH/ BAD BITE

A crooked smile or bad bite can be corrected with braces, and modern techniques are quick, comfortable and can be virtually invisible.

Love your gums

Gum (periodontal) disease is a chronic bacterial infection of the supporting tissue of the tooth (gums and bone). As the body tries to ward off the infection, inflammation develops; over time this leads to bone loss around the teeth. Often this happens with few external signs and little or no discomfort until quite advanced, which is why regular dental visits are so important. If the reversible early stage of gum disease (gingivitis) is allowed to continue into periodontitis, the bacteria and inflammatory cells can leak into the bloodstream and be carried around the whole body contributing to the problems highlighted on page 192.

What you can do:

● Brush your teeth! The first line of defence is hygiene – meticulous, thorough, regular cleaning with a toothbrush and floss will remove bacteria, reducing inflammation and aiding healing. Aim for twice a day at least.

● Regular visits (usually twice-yearly) to your dentist to monitor disease progress, and to the hygienist to clean the mouth thoroughly and advise on effective homecare – every mouth and person is different, so homecare needs to be tailored to individuals.

● Don't smoke – smokers are more prone to gum disease and once established it will progress much faster than in a non-smoker.

● Eat well: a diet low in all forms of sugar with healthy levels of antioxidants is beneficial. There is growing evidence that supplements of vitamin C, coenzyme Q10 and zinc (antioxidants which also act against inflammation) are also helpful. Natural live yoghurt which has both calcium and lactose bacteria appears to help prevent gum problems.

● Take exercise – it can help to reduce inflammation.

● Try to avoid stress as this leads to a higher risk of disease.

● Drink lots of still water (but not fizzy! See page 197).

● Gum disease runs in families, so be extra vigilant if there's a family history. Women are more likely to suffer, which is probably related to reproductive hormones.

● If you have another inflammatory disease, such as diabetes, keep tight control on blood-sugar levels.

● Brush your teeth! Again!

MAKE UP FOR LOST TEETH

Losing teeth at an early age affects your appearance as well as the way they function (or don't…), plus other teeth can drift around the jaw, leading to bite imbalances. Replacing lost teeth as soon as possible helps prevent more complex problems. There are three basic options to replace missing teeth, all of which can work well.

1 **Implant:** screwed into the bone, this is effectively a like-for-like replacement which can last a lifetime and is considered the gold standard.

2 **Bridge:** this uses adjacent teeth to support a replacement unit but can involve damage to the supporting teeth and commonly needs replacing after several years.

3 **Denture:** this is removable and allows easy cleaning, but can be uncomfortable.

Deal with tooth grinding and bite problems

The wear caused by teeth grinding at night and/or from a 'bad bite' (where your teeth are misaligned so they don't meet correctly when you bite) can cause the structure of your teeth to be badly affected. This can lead to problems such as sensitive teeth, receding gums, and broken teeth or fillings.

Grinding your teeth can actually lead to bite problems because of the damage to tooth structure. The whole thing can become a vicious cycle, causing pain in addition to the other problems above.

Additionally, persistent grinding at night prevents the jaw muscles from relaxing and can lead on to muscle spasm, cramps, head and neck pain, even migraines. Night grinding also disturbs sleep patterns, which can lead to tiredness, stress and so more grinding…

What you can do:

● Have your bite, jaw muscles and joints assessed regularly to catch any problems early, before too much damage occurs.

● Many people with a problem will benefit from a night splint – a custom-made appliance worn over the teeth when sleeping to position the jaws so as to allow muscle relaxation and better-quality sleep, and to help prevent further damage.

● If the damage is more advanced or symptoms are severe, your dentist may advise some form of bite reconstruction (potentially surgical); when done correctly this can not only restore appearance but prevent future problems. NB: this needs an expert practitioner.

● Tension in the head and neck due to a bad bite can be relieved by skilful use of complementary therapies such as physiotherapy, osteopathy and chiropractic. Simple exercises and home massage of the jaw can help greatly (as Sarah knows from personal experience).

A colleague who was prescribed a 'bite splint' says:

'From the first night, I slept more deeply than I had in years. I felt better, looked better and people started asking whether I'd had a holiday'

Learn about dental decay – the great enemy for teeth

We all know that sugar is a big problem food in tooth decay. But it's not just eating candy and cake, modern processed foodstuffs often contain hidden sugar, which is tricky to detect. What's more, from a dentist's perspective, natural sugar sources such as fruit and honey are just as problematic. And don't let's even mention fizzy drinks – yet…

To understand what's happening, the all-important link between sugar, acid and tooth decay and what to do about it, we need to know a little bit about the science. (It's riveting, promise!)

Here's Dr Cook's explanation: 'The human mouth is full of bacteria, happily living in the microscopic nooks and crannies and most of them causing no harm – in fact, some give us protection from more dangerous organisms. But certain types love to feast on sugar and the more sugar they eat, the more they multiply. The problem for your teeth is that as the bugs consume sugar, they produce acid (as a waste product) – and that's the agent which attacks and weakens teeth. The acid environment in your mouth also encourages more bacteria, so more acid is produced, and so on…and on…

'The body's defence against each sugar dose is saliva, which neutralises the acid. But this process takes about 45 minutes, during which the acid launches an attack on your teeth, dissolving some of the hard mineral coating of the tooth [demineralisation of the enamel]. Once the saliva has neutralised the acid, the minerals it contains begin to repair some of the acid-damaged enamel [remineralisation]. But if another dose of sugar comes along too soon – continuously sucking sweets, say, through the day, rather than in separate "hits" – effective repair is impossible and the weakened enamel begins to break down and dissolve again. This creates a protected home for more bacteria which can't be completely cleaned off – and a cavity becomes established. The sugar also forms a gungy residue called plaque, which sticks to the tooth.

'But there's an extra threat to your teeth in the shape of acidic foods and drinks, notably carbonated drinks, tea – including fruit teas, coffee, vinegar, alcohol, salad dressing and ketchup.'

What you can do:

● Clean away as much of the bacteria and plaque as possible – brushing and flossing thoroughly, ideally after every meal but at least twice a day.

● If you have snacked on something sugary or acidic (see next point), wait 30 minutes before brushing to allow the acidity in your mouth to become more neutral.

● Remember: the main offenders are sugary foods (including most fruits and fruit juices) and acidic ones (including fizzy drinks, tea, coffee, alcohol, vinegar, ketchup and most salad dressings).

● It is the repeated frequent acid attacks that cause the major damage, so if you want something sugary/acidic, eat it all in one go. Best of all, go for nuts or unsweetened natural yoghurt as a snack.

● Help the naturally protective saliva by chewing sugar-free gum after a meal, preferably one sweetened with xylitol (eg, Trident sugarless gum). This speeds up the neutralisation of acids and the xylitol – a natural sweetener and proven tooth (and bone) strengthener – helps stop the plaque from sticking to teeth.

● Drink plenty of water – this helps flush away acid and keeps saliva flow high.

● End a meal with a little cheese or unsweetened yoghurt: this helps speed up acid neutralisation.

● If you've had a lot of fillings in the past or some of the enamel has been demineralised, you can use a remineralising paste, smeared over the affected areas and left overnight or held in a custom-made tray. This can significantly increase the chance of reversing very early decay (water-based, sugar-free GC Tooth Mousse from your dentist is the most effective).

Know your fillings

Amalgam is a mixture of mercury with silver, copper and tin, which forms a strong, relatively stable material when set. It's been in use as a filling material for over 150 years and continues to be used today, largely because it's inexpensive and requires little skill to place quickly and successfully. So why the fuss? Because mercury is a known poison and extremely toxic. While the majority of the mercury in a dental filling is stable within the amalgam, small amounts are continuously released. If this were anywhere other than inside someone's mouth, it would be classified as an environmentally contaminated zone… Over the past decade, concern about toxicity from mercury in amalgam has increased and many countries restrict the use of mercury-based products.

As a patient, potentially the biggest exposure to mercury is when you are having old amalgam fillings removed. This can be accomplished safely. Check that your dentist understands the risks (you can afford to be blunt). Ensure that a rubber dam will be placed around the tooth to isolate it from the rest of your mouth. Dr Cook normally advises swallowing two activated charcoal tablets before treatment (these mop up any debris that slips past the dam). For more sensitive patients, a clean air supply during the procedure may be advisable, plus specific nutritional supplements afterwards. Once the amalgam is removed, there's a range of options as replacements:

● **Porcelain:** this is very aesthetic, strong and can be used anywhere.

● **Gold:** very noticeable (so unaesthetic), but the strongest and can be used anywhere.

● **Composite resin:** this looks very good and is durable in small- to medium-size cavities, but it is not suitable for back teeth unless they are small.

In Dr Cook's opinion, 'The aesthetics of porcelain outweigh the slightly better strength of gold – particularly "Emax", the latest generation material which is incredibly strong and looks fantastic. But any of the options above can perform very well. However, to get the best out of them requires meticulous technique and is time-consuming, so the procedure will be more expensive than amalgam.'

KEEP YOUR TEETH BEAUTIFULLY CLEAN

The reality is that it's less about what you use and more about how. The basic equipment of a toothbrush with a small to medium head and dental floss is all most people need – if they use it correctly. Having said that, electric brushes, particularly sonic ones, are very effective and there's a wide selection of different brushes specially developed for cleaning between and around teeth and gums.

Every mouth is different, and the correct tools and technique need to be tailored to each individual, so the best advice is to ask your dentist or preferably your hygienist to advise and demonstrate a personalised cleaning routine. Also have it checked after a couple of months to make sure you are managing it correctly. This is probably the best investment of time and money you can make and could save you many times the investment in the future. (For general guidelines, see box left.)

Mainstream toothpastes are all effective (although specific smokers' pastes and powders can be very abrasive and damaging). Fluoride is a naturally occurring element which is incorporated into tooth enamel, making it harder and more resistant to decay. Fluoride toothpaste has been shown to reduce the level of dental decay, so unless your diet and hygiene are perfect, not using a fluoride toothpaste may mean you need more dental work.

The evidence for a protective effect when fluoride is swallowed (in the water supply or as a supplement) is less clear and it can have toxic side effects, so using fluoride like that is controversial. However, if fluoride is applied as a toothpaste in the correct and tiny amount – a pea-size for an adult and half a pea of an appropriate product for a child – and not swallowed, the benefits can be great and the risk is probably negligible. (This is Dr Cook's opinion, which we respect – though we prefer to use natural fluoride-free toothpastes ourselves.)

Another controversial toothpaste additive is sodium lauryl sulphate (SLS): this is a chemical foaming agent common in many household products – shampoo, bubble baths, detergents, etc. It has been shown to cause skin reactions and ulceration. SLS-free toothpastes are available: Dr Cook's favourites are Tom's of Maine Clean & Gentle Care, and Sensodyne Total Care Gel. (We like the Green People and Weleda ranges, which have peppermint-free options suitable for people taking homeopathic remedies.) If you suffer from mouth ulcers, it's worth trying an SLS-free toothpaste.

TEETH-CLEANING TECHNIQUE

Brush your teeth outside and inside for two to three minutes twice daily (at a minimum), after meals, and follow with flossing. If you use a sonic toothbrush, all you need to do is hold the head steady against each tooth where it meets the gum – counting to six on each side. If you're using a manual brush (choose a soft one), hold the brush like a pencil and go round and round gently in little circles on the chewing surfaces of each tooth. The brush should be at a 45 degree angle towards your gum so that the tufts are pressed into it.

TIP

Toothbrush heads harbour bugs, so do change them regularly and particularly after you recover from any infections.

Brightening toothpastes: *our award winners*

A first, for us: we've never trialled toothpastes before. But since a brighter smile can be instantly 'de-ageing', we figured: why not trial brightening, whitening toothpastes alongside all the beauty lotions and potions? With tooth-bleaching procedures more popular than ever, these are the low-tech, daily-use alternative. So: is it possible to brush your way to a brighter smile…? The averages here aren't spectacular but tend to reflect the fact that for some testers they worked really well, while others didn't see much difference. Still, if you're looking for a shortlist of where to head first when looking for a whitening toothpaste, we suggest you start here.

Aquafresh Iso-Active Whitening

 A unique 'foaming-gel' – featuring a special ingredient that activates the gel as you brush – this 'directly targets bacteria to fight a key source of oral malodour'(!), and within the Iso-Active range this is the tooth-brightening option. In a pump-action dispenser (which testers mostly disliked, on the score there was too much packaging and the nozzle didn't work that well).

Comments: 'You apply this just like ordinary toothpaste but thinner, rather like Pearl Drops; teeth feel extra clean and mouth very fresh, better than a normal product, so I would buy though not certain if teeth actually whiter' • 'thick paste that really foamed up when applied, very minty but not so much that it stung, teeth felt really fresh and clean after, my slightly stained teeth look much brighter: did get compliments! I love this and won't be without it from now on, lasts a long time and my mouth feels so much cleaner as well' • 'after ten days of using this, two people in two days asked whether I had had my teeth whitened, so they obviously noticed a difference – though to start with I didn't…' • 'I was very sceptical but I have to say my teeth did look much whiter – I was impressed!'.

Beverly Hills Formula Total Breath Whitening

 Beverly Hills Formula were pioneers in whitening toothpastes, and promise 'whiter teeth in one minute' from what is now a wide range of formulations. This particular toothpaste features an antibacterial formula to help fight plaque (and bad breath) – leaving breath fresher for up to five times longer than a regular toothpaste, so they say.

Comments: 'Nice light toothpaste with minty aftertaste and I definitely saw a difference, my teeth were much whiter and my family noticed; I tried the tip about leaving it on the tongue for a bit before brushing for freshness and this worked well' • 'my teeth do look good and don't feel rough to the touch as they did at first' • 'I have started drinking green tea without milk and noticed how much it stains the cup: I think it would have stained my teeth but this has kept them looking clean and bright' • 'I enjoyed using this and my teeth did look a little bit better'.

AloeDent Triple Action Toothpaste

 AloeDent takes its name from the soothing aloe plant, a key ingredient in this natural toothpaste range, which also combines tea tree oil and green tea extract to fight against bacteria, plus Co-Q10 for healthy gums. The naturally whitening mineral silica is significantly less abrasive, they promise, than conventional stain-removing ingredients.

Comments: 'Really nice taste, no difference in amount of foaming, my teeth felt really clean after' • 'definitely makes my slightly yellow teeth whiter, difference showed up pretty much the first time of use; teeth feel very clean after using too' • 'I thought aloe vera would be horrid but I'm a convert! Teeth feel really clean and mouth fresh' • 'loved the taste – teeth and mouth felt clean and invigorated; though I didn't notice any difference in whiteness, I love this product: it may cost a few pence more but it's really worth it'.

AT A GLANCE

Aquafresh Iso-Active Whitening

Beverly Hills Formula Total Breath Whitening

AloeDent Triple Action Toothpaste

♡ WE LOVE…

Jo uses a natural toothpaste with no specific brightening promises… Sarah particularly likes natural brands with xylitol, a compound that helps prevent bacteria sticking to teeth: these include Xyliwhite Toothpaste, which is fluoride-free, as is Tom's of Maine Tartar Control Plus Whitening Toothpaste, which contains xylitol, zinc citrate and silica (though they appear to contain forms of sodium lauryl sulphate which we don't like so much…).

TIP

Once you've brightened your teeth, keep stain-causing liquids from reversing the improvement by using a straw. (You can do this for hot drinks but it takes a bit of getting used to!)

Tinted moisturisers: *our award winners*

Tinted moisturisers are absolutely brilliant for evening out skintone without making a face look over-made-up. Some, though, are just too moisturising (and so shine-inducing), while others aren't quite dewy enough, so they go on patchily (and need a moisturiser underneath). With a couple of dozen products to trial, we asked our panellists to help us identify which really are 'the business'. Read on for lots of high-scoring new entries in this category, all of which feature an SPF – so no need to 'layer' your summer skincare

AT A GLANCE

Bobbi Brown SPF15 Tinted Moisturizer

Estée Lauder DayWear BB Anti-Oxidant Beauty Benefit Crème SPF35

RéVive Tinted Moisturizer SPF15

Estée Lauder DayWear Sheer Tint Advanced Multi-Protection Anti-Oxidant Release Moisturizer SPF15

REVIEWS

Bobbi Brown SPF15 Tinted Moisturizer

 8.81/10 A heck of a score for this new top-slot tint, which comes in a wider-than-most choice of seven different shades. (Testers put Light Tint through its paces, which is third-from-palest.) A lightweight formula targeted at normal and dry skins, it does feature skin-conditioning jojoba oil and other emollients to leave skin feeling supple; if you're prone to shine, there's also an oil-free version (though we didn't trial this).
Comments: 'Previously I'd always used foundation; though it doesn't cover quite as much, it give me a more natural, youthful-looking product – amazing' • 'impossible to go wrong with this: you can't apply too much (although a little goes a long way) • 'gives complexion a bit of a boost while evening out thread veins, open pores, pigmentation – blends into the face a treat, and doesn't "settle" into fine lines' • 'skin looks healthier, more glowing and I won't leave the house without applying it now' • 'my 18-year-old daughter asked to borrow it as she thinks it looks so natural and makes my complexion radiant' • 'the first tinted moisturiser I've ever liked' • 'glides on creamily, easy-to-blend'.

Estée Lauder DayWear BB Anti-Oxidant Beauty Benefit Crème SPF35

 8.48/10 We're going to let you in on a little industry secret about BB creams, which have been A Big Beauty Buzz lately. In reality, many would previously have been categorised as tinted moisturisers: we've even seen one product hurriedly relabelled with stickers, to reposition it in the hot 'BB' category. Some – as in this case – do contain a higher-than-usual dose of 'light-reflecting pigments', which work to blur imperfections and boost skin's radiance and glow. For those concerned about the sun's ageing effects on the face, this BB also features a higher-than-average SPF35 plus mega-antioxidants, and has the signature cucumber-y scent we personally know and love from the rest of the DayWear range. (Read on for another winner…) In two shades; testers had the 01 Light.
Comments: 'Blends extremely well compared to my usual product, which just sits on my face' • 'velvety product delivering a healthy glow and colour, worn on its own' • 'the perfect holiday product: does the job of a whole shelf-ful – sun protection, foundation, moisturiser, primer' • 'skin looks younger when I'm wearing it – which makes me feel younger'.

RéVive Tinted Moisturizer SPF15

 8.33/10 A sheer, featherlight moisturiser that adds a healthy hint of colour, this is from an advanced skincare range 'infused with Nobel-prize-winning technology' (so RéVive tell us!). A true treatment product, it's packed with antioxidants and vitamins, marine extracts and EGF (Epidermal Growth Factor), to increase cell renewal.

♡ WE LOVE...

Many tinted moisturiser brands simply don't come in a pale enough shade for Jo's very pale skin. (See Mary Greenwell's tip below.) But Dior Hydra Life Pro-Youth Skin Tint SPF20 comes in several shades (Jo's is 01 Natural) and she finds it super-skin-quenching. Sarah is unswervingly devoted to Crème de la Mer's The SPF18 Fluid Tint, in medium, which has a bit of coverage and gives the most fabulous dewy finish. It lasts her through spring, summer and autumn – so justifying a hefty investment.

TIP

Mary Greenwell insists that tinted moisturiser should be viewed more like a lightweight foundation than as something to change the underlying tone of your skin. She prescribes the same colour-matching technique as for foundation: apply to just below your jaw to find the shade that will blend in seamlessly. If you're very pale, you'll need to check out one of the ranges which now offers a selection of shades – many tinted moisturisers are one-shade-fits-all options, and one shade DOESN'T fit all.

Comments: 'I like this; nicely moisturising, with an SPF, covers quite well but not heavy-looking, evens out skintone so it just looks better but not made up' • 'product has slight luminosity which makes skin more alive and full of bounce' • 'maybe not for oily skin but suits my drier skin beautifully' • 'great velvety texture, not too thick or liquid, blended well to look completely even; covered thread veins, small spots and dark marks completely, didn't sit in lines and wrinkles'.

Estée Lauder DayWear Sheer Tint Advanced Multi-Protection Anti-Oxidant Release Moisturizer SPF15

8.3/10

We can't help but be impressed when of dozens of new products submitted for new trials for this book, two contenders

from a single brand make it to the winners' podium. This is an old and oft-recommended favourite of ours, with a touch of magic about it: the light, suits-all-skintypes cream that emerges from the tube is a kind of mauve-y/grey, but then is transformed on contact with skin to a customised shade on every single skintone. Alongside the SPF15 is DayWear's usual cocktail of skin-shielding antioxidants.

Comments: 'Considering I'm 47 this is impressive as it manages to cover all blemishes and fine lines – so light I don't feel I'm wearing any make-up' • 'velvety, smooth texture – so easy to apply' • 'throughout the day skin felt moisturised and looked bright, and I feel it has anti-ageing benefits' • 'did well covering up sun spots'.

Say goodbye to spider veins!

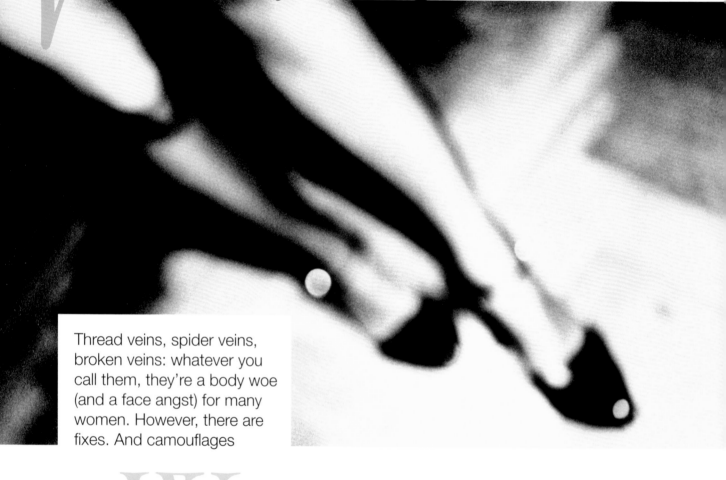

Thread veins, spider veins, broken veins: whatever you call them, they're a body woe (and a face angst) for many women. However, there are fixes. And camouflages

When a truly gorgeous-in-every-way friend in her early fifties was deserted by her (daft) husband, part of her fresh start was to tidy up the 'hated spider veins which creep in at various places up my legs and fan out over my thighs', as she put it. It isn't just legs that can be affected: many women are troubled by the appearance of thread veins on their face (cheeks, forehead, eyelids and around the nostrils), also neck and upper chest. They're particularly noticeable in people with pale thin skin. (And, says Jo, 'certainly the curse of my beauty life – the price for an English rose complexion'.)

The technical name for these clusters of tiny dilated blood vessels (capillaries), which appear just under the surface of the skin, is 'dermal flares'. They're incredibly common and while not serious, they are unsightly. On the legs, they can also lead to heavy aching legs and even pain. 'Little nerves in the veins can be painful if the veins get stretched,' explains consultant vascular surgeon Mr John Scurr of the Lister Hospital in London (our long-time 'veins' expert). They may be worsened by fluctuating levels of hormones, pre- and post-menopause, as well as standing up for long periods. (Men get them too.) Before treating leg veins, Mr Scurr explains that it's vital to have a scan first to check that there are no underlying problems, such as varicose veins (or, at the worst, deep vein thrombosis) – and be aware that varicose veins need to be treated before treating dermal flares. The following two treatment options are Mr Scurr's preferred choices.

For spider veins on legs, consider microsclerotherapy. Getting rid of these 'dermal flares' can be simple – but it's likely to be time-consuming. Mr Scurr recommends a process called microsclerotherapy, where each capillary is injected with a very fine needle containing a 'sclerosant' solution that expels blood from the vein, and leaves the walls of the vein stuck together so the blood can't return.

The sessions last about 20 minutes and are usually carried out by a nurse. Veins may sting a little but shouldn't be painful. A cylinder of tightly rolled cotton wool is stuck on each injection site immediately after to minimise bruising, and legs are wrapped in a light bandage before you leave. Both bandage and cotton wool can be taken off three hours later. Legs may ache slightly for a few days.

If you have a number of flares this process can take several weeks. And while microsclerotherapy is the most effective for legs, it's not appropriate for faces, where laser is the best and safest option.

Electrolysis is another option. In this treatment – suitable for faces as well as legs – an electrical current is passed through a fine needle to cauterise the vein so the blood is absorbed back into the body. (See right for more about facial thread veins.) Electrolysis is available at beauty salons, but you should always have potential 'deep veins' on legs checked out by a doctor first. Make sure you go to an experienced therapist who has the back-up to deal with potential problems, such as infection.

Schedule treatment for the tights season! Microsclerotherapy (and sclerotherapy which can be used for some varicose veins) can leave legs looking a bit battle-scarred so, if possible, time your treatment when you can cover up with black opaques. The process is definitely not a quick fix but, says our friend, it's worth it: 'Wonder of wonders, I now have unblemished thighs and legs. For the first time in years, I can leave the sarong behind when I walk to the pool.'

Remember dermal flares may stage a comeback. Mr Scurr warns that those pesky flares may return and need further treatment. Natural products, either to take internally or rub on, may help. Try Diosmin Complex by LifeTime Vitamins, a combination of natural compounds, or Zinopin Daily, a natural blend developed to prevent DVT for air travellers. Spider Veins Cream by Provenance features glycosaminoglycans (GAGs) that may help repair the damaged capillaries and possibly toughen the outer cell layers, minimising the appearance of spider veins. (Find a source for these in DIRECTORY.)

FACE YOUR THREAD VEINS

Cosmetic dermatologists treat unsightly thread veins on your cheeks and face with state-of-the-art lasers. Individual broken capillaries can be treated with walk-in-and-out lunchtime therapy which doesn't cause any bruising. (But you must, absolutely must, wear a sunblock for at least three months after.) Why not sclerotherapy? Experts including Dr Nick Lowe of the Cranley Clinic, London, and Dr Andrew Markey, say that while sclerotherapy is the gold standard for treating leg veins, they disapprove of using it on the face, because injecting the wrong vein may provoke an emergency and, in the worst-case scenario, lead to loss of vision. (Plus we've heard from a woman who had it done – unwisely – around her nose, that it's agony.) However, if you have developed thread veins during pregnancy, try waiting a few months after the birth because they may disappear on their own. And if you have acne rosacea with inflamed skin that looks like thread veins, you should probably be treated with antibiotics first. (For more on rosacea see page 168.)

In any case, please do make sure you consult a qualified and experienced dermatologist – it is your face after all! We recommend following Wendy Lewis's checklist of questions to ask, even before something which seems as minor as veins treatment (see page 46).

For us, a little bit of concealer (see camouflage suggestions right, and also top concealers on page 91) plus topical treatments minimise the problem very satisfactorily, without recourse to expensive treatments. Also see page 170 for products that have done well for facial redness. And do avoid scrubs or using anything scratchy on your face.

PS Sarah had more veins on her cheeks and round her nose in her twenties than she does now, and can only put that down to taking more care of her skin – with plenty of nourishing moisturiser in cold/windy weather and lots of anti-inflammatory foods and supplements, notably oily fish and omega-3 essential fatty acids (again!) – and leading a calmer life generally. Oh, and not drinking alcohol!

OUR TOP CAMOUFLAGERS

Products we know work include Estée Lauder Maximum Cover Camouflage Make-up for Face and Body and Vichy Dermablend Ultra-Corrective Foundation Cream Stick together with the same brand's Setting Powder. Laura Mercier Secret Camouflage can be very effective for faces, too.

TIP

Visible facial veins often come as a result of sun damage so – once again – please can we remind you to slap on the SPF! And avoid roasting and frying in the hottest parts of the day. And while we're at it, please avoid sunbeds too – they're a short cut to ageing and pose a significant risk of skin cancer. Remember: when it comes to tans, fake it to make it!

Take up yoga.
Just do it, please

For us, this is almost the most important advice in this book. If you do it already, you will know the absolutely miraculous results of an hour or so's practise (sometimes just five minutes is enough to turn you round). Done regularly long-term, yoga can transform your life

We find yoga THE perfect exercise for a more mature body – and for ironing out any wrinkles in our minds. If you've never done it before, it can help enormously with flexibility – and bone strength, too. And there is nothing – repeat nothing – we've found that's better for stress, and for making us feel like we're on top of the mountain of different things we have to juggle. Plus it makes you look fabulous! At the end of a long day – or if you get up in the morning feeling and looking exhausted – the most effective way to go from tired and drab to glowing and gorgeous is to do some yoga. (Just try it.)

Take up yoga for your bones. As yoga teacher Jan Maddern, author of *Yoga Builds Bones*, observes, 'Yoga creates a balanced harmony between the ovaries, adrenal, parathyroid, pituitary and pineal glands, ensuring that the body receives a steady supply of the right hormones for maintaining bone strength and maximum

health and wellbeing. The regular practise of weight-bearing hatha yoga postures offers women everywhere a safe way to build bone strength.' There is even some evidence that yoga can help people who have already developed symptoms of osteoporosis: according to Dr Andrew Weil, the world's leading expert in integrated medicine, two studies have shown that elderly women who took part in regular yoga classes, two to three times a week for between three and six months, saw a slight reduction in curvatures of the upper spine ('dowager's hump'). In one study the control group who didn't practise yoga actually saw an increase in upper spinal curvatures. In another study, older women who did a nine-week yoga programme gained a centimetre in height.

Take up yoga to balance your hormones. Consultant gynaecologist Michael Dooley recommends yoga to all his patients, particularly any going through the hormonal roller-coasters around

menopause. Teachers have always held that certain postures can reduce hot flushes and night sweats as well as promote calm and restful sleep, and this was confirmed by researchers in India. (It also sharpened mental function – yippee!) During the long, slow asanas (postures), certain glands in the body are gently pressurised and depressurised, helping to stimulate and control the hormones produced by those glands. Yoga for menopause should place an emphasis on moving slowly and smoothly.

It is never too late to take up yoga, but

YOU MIGHT LIKE TO READ JO'S YOGA BOOK...

If you'd like to take up yoga for the first time after forty (or at any age, frankly), then you might like to know that Jo has written a whole book about how to do just that. *Yoga for Life* (published by Kyle Books) had been very well-received as a mumbo-jumbo-free, down-to-earth gentle introduction to the whole subject of yoga and meditation, featuring sections on the best sorts of yoga for older bodies, yoga travel and foods that will enhance your practice (as well as your health).

it's also never too early: as Suza Francina, a teacher who writes books about yoga for women (rather than babes) points out, 'If you practise yoga before the menopause, all the poses that are useful for coping with uncomfortable symptoms are familiar, and you can reach for them like an old friend. If you are familiar with restorative poses, then you have the best menopause medicine at your disposal.'

If you Google 'yoga for menopause' you may even be lucky eough to find a specific class in your area, as some teachers are starting to offer this type of yoga specifically (it's a baby-boom thing). Failing that, it's important to explain to your teacher if you have hot flushes, because they can guide you through the more restorative and cooling postures. The use of supportive props such as bolsters, blankets and blocks can help adapt postures so that you avoid gripping or straining, which can cause over-heating. Specific postures that are recommended during menopause include:

● Legs-up-the-wall pose (viparita karani), which is great for grounding.
● Head-to-knee forward bend (janu sirsasana) and seated forward bend (paschimottanasana) for irritability.
● Plough pose (halasana) and Shoulder Stand for hormonal balance.

LESS PAIN, MORE GAIN

Research by the US National Institute of Health revealed that taking regular yoga classes can reduce chronic back pain and enhance flexibility. In a 12-week study, volunteers who took 90-minute yoga classes twice a week showed 42 per cent reduction in pain and therefore reduced their dependency on pain medication. NB: it's vital to find qualified and experienced teachers who specialise in backs, however, as practising the wrong postures can make things worse.

Take up yoga for flexibility. There's a famous concept in yoga philosophy that a person's age is determined by the flexibility of his spine, not the number of years he has lived. (And recent research suggests that stretching the body may help prevent age-related stiffening of the arteries – we'd rather have ours flowing freely.) The improved balance and flexibility that come from regular yoga practise can also help prevent – or reduce the impact – of falls: a stiff body goes down like a ninepin, which is more likely to lead to bone breaks and fractures. And, of course, it's great to hang on to the ability to reach down to your shoelaces or up to a jar on the top shelf, because (even if this seems a long way off) it helps us remain as independent as possible for as long as possible. But we also very much like this quote, frequently repeated by one of Jo's yoga teachers: 'Flexible spine equals flexible mind'. The more we do yoga, the more we find we can roll with life's punches – going with the flow and adapting to change, as well as accepting that change is inevitable.

Take up yoga to tackle your wrinkles. Marie-Véronique Nadeau – who we met when she was visiting from Berkeley, California – is in her sixties, and she's her own best advertisement: almost line-free and with plumped-up, resilient skin. Marie-Véronique (who also has her own skincare line, Marie Veronique Organics) has put together a programme called The Yoga Facelift which we recommend if you feel you can make the commitment to facial exercises. As she says, 'The adage "If you don't use it, you lose it" really applies to the muscles of your face.' Women we know who practise yoga into their later years have sharper jaws and more defined facial contours, as well as glowing skin (it's the improved circulation). We also have a theory that the amount of time you spend 'inverted' helps hair growth, by boosting blood flow to the scalp. (Completely unsubstantiated, but we both have hair that grows like grass.)

Take up yoga for clarity, balance and to quieten 'monkey mind'. In the Yoga Sutras (sacred writings), there's a wonderful phrase: 'Yoga is the ending of disturbances of the mind'. We both find it gives us amazing focus, improves memory – and, when faced with a problem, shows us a clear way to deal with it for a positive outcome. We could cite endless scientific studies to back this up (and explain why), but we can also just tell you: it's true.

So we say, just take up yoga. Don't fret too much about which 'style' of yoga – but we would suggest that Hatha, Iyengar and Scaravelli yoga (which are more gentle) would be most appropriate. We recommend that peri- and menopausal women avoid Bikram (heated) or fast Ashtanga yoga, as these focus on creating heat within the body – and at this phase in life, that's something many of us are trying to avoid. The most important thing is to find a class/classes that fit with your schedule, as you're more likely to go, and the closer to home (or work) the better.

TIP

As well as helping with hot flushes, 'yoga postures and breathing techniques can help reduce general anxiety', comments Michael Dooley. 'If patients are worried about having cervical smears, for instance, I get them to do retention breathing.' (Inhale through your nose to a count of four, hold gently for seven, then exhale slowly through your mouth for eight; repeat five or six times twice daily.)

TIP

Sarah (62 as this book is published) credits years of yoga with enabling her to go on mounting her 16-hand Arab/ thoroughbred horse from the ground – to the amazement of much younger riders who can't do the same – and to calming them both down when he has one of his cadenzas…

Get your Zzzzzs!
How to sleep better

No doubt about it, getting enough good sleep is beautifying. And de-stressing. And energising. All-round wonderful stuff. And every good woman deserves slumber!

Trouble is we don't all get enough sleep. Especially as the years roll by. While some lucky souls can slumber through anything – from thundering traffic and snoring partners, to super-stress – others wake as a feather drops or there's the slightest ripple of anxiety. So, if it's less than restorative, how can you improve your sleep pattern?

As the queens of 'sleep hygiene', doing all the right things to optimise a good night's sleep, we are keen to pass on the stuff we know works. We're both occasionally prone to sleeplessness (and both 'larks' with a tendency to wake up at 4am in summer – or when we're fretting about something, see page 211), so when it comes to sleep aids we've been there, done that, gone to bed in the T-shirt. In other words, we know what works. First of all, get the kit. These are the 'accessories' to good sleep, and the simple steps you can take right now, in your own bedroom, to help get the zzzzzs you need. (See DIRECTORY for sources.)

If you get too hot at night, check out linen. Linen is the most amazingly cooling fabric. On a hot day, you can touch a linen pillowcase on your bed and it will be cool, whereas a cotton pillowcase on the same bed can be room temperature. If you are menopausal or peri-menopausal and you suffer from night sweats or hot flushes, at the very least treat yourself to a couple of linen pillowcases. If you can indulge yourself with linen sheets, even better. A very simple trick to cool down in the night is to flip your pillow over. We thought we were the only people who knew this, but it turns out to be so popular that there is even – we kid you not – a Facebook group called, 'I flip my pillow over to get to the cold side', with nearly one million members when we last looked. (Jo also sleeps in a French linen nightshirt, which has an equally cooling effect.)

And/or buy a Chillow. Again, if you find that you can't sleep because you're too hot at night, the Chillow is an extraordinary innovation that we've heard very good things about. (The Chillow was first brought to our attention by consultant gynaecologist Michael Dooley whose patients were raving about it for hot flushes.) It's made of a patented substance which, when activated by water (you only need to do this once), creates a memory-foam-like layer that you put between you and your pillowcase. (If you don't like the flock-y surface, you can slip it under your pillowcase – ideally linen, see left.) There's a larger version (the Chillow PLUS), originally designed for reducing fevers, which some women prefer because they can wrap it around their pillow and slip a hand underneath while they rest, getting a double cooling whammy. If you're really having a problem with hot flushes, you'll want to know about the Petite Relief Chillow which you keep in the fridge to apply when you're feeling too hot to bear. Another excellent application, for anyone who uses a laptop on their – umm, lap: put the Petite Relief Chillow under your laptop and instead of getting very hot legs, you'll feel cucumber-cool. (And lots of hospitals are now recommending Chillows for hot flushes associated with treatment for breast and prostate cancer.)

'There is no pillow so soft as a clear conscience'
French proverb

And get yourself a Bucky sleep mask. Jo has road-tested just about every sleep mask known to woman, and is convinced that this is the best, the most light-excluding and the most comfortable to wear of any sleep mask out there. It's super-soft and padded, cradling the eyes without pressure. It has soft padding over the nose and cheeks, which avoids even a molecule of light peeking in. The Bucky sleep mask also Velcros around the back (so is infinitely adjustable whatever your head size). There are several designs but the one you want is Eye Shades with Ear Plugs (these are stored in a little pouch on the front). Lots of

SLEEP REGIME

This natural regime is more effective than drugs at re-establishing a sound sleep structure, says psychiatrist Dr David Servan-Schreiber. Go to bed at the same time every night including weekends but get up two hours earlier than usual. Don't nap for more than 20 to 30 minutes during the day. If you wake, get up and read a book or magazine for an hour before going back to bed. Once sleep is continuous again – which may take a few weeks – increase the time you sleep by 15 minutes every three days until you're back to your normal length.

colours, all lined with black – but we think midnight or black are the most alluring.

Have an Aromatherapy Associates Deep Relax bath before bedtime. For many years we have been slavishly devoted to Aromatherapy Associates Deep Relax Shower & Bath Oil. It is knock-out drops for us. (After you've had a few baths with this there's probably a Pavlovian response, so you only have to smell the potent blend of vetiver, chamomile and sandalwood to start to feel sleepy.) Our one caveat: if you do get toasty at night, don't have the water too hot because the effect of heating the body will linger when you slip between the sheets. We love this oil so much we give it to friends for birthdays, then they start giving it to everyone they know, like an aromatherapy chain letter.

Or pour in the magnesium flakes. Magnesium is known as 'nature's tranquilliser' and as well as taking a supplement before bed (which helps with restless legs too), we pour Magnesium Flakes in the bath so this soothing mineral can cherish aches and pains and racing minds. (There's also an oil version.) PS Researcher Dr Paula Baillie-Hamilton tells us that putting magnesium in the bath is a wonderful treatment for over-excited/hyperactive children.

Spritz your pillow. We are both incredibly impressed by the Les Fleurs de Bach range, based on the principles of Bach Flower Remedies. Two products stand out in the quest for better sleep: the Anti-Stress Treating Fragrance is amazingly relaxing (and smells awfully nice, with its blend of sage, lavender, bergamot or eucalyptus). We recommend having two: one for the desk (for moments of stress), one for the night-stand; a few spritzes before bedtime – including on the pillow – help prepare the mind for sleep. (We love the whole Les Fleurs de Bach range, and also recommend the Les Fleurs de Bach Sleep Elixir, from the same range.)

Switch off the standby. There is now evidence that even the little standby light on your TV (if you have one in the bedroom) may affect your sleep pattern – not just preventing you from drifting off but interfering with the depth of your sleep. Only when the bedroom is totally dark will your body start to produce melatonin, which not only regulates sleep but also has an important role in reducing your risk of cancer. So: ditch the digital clock. Switch off any appliance that's on standby, and if you have a multi-gang plug with an orange light that tells you it's working, put gaffer tape over it.

Try a pelmet! Jo recently had a moment of absolute revelation, on a midsummer's morning when light was streaming into her bedroom before 4am: 'Ah – THAT's what a pelmet's for…' With the fashion for curtain poles rather than tracks, pelmets have very much fallen from favour – but perhaps our mothers (and grannies) knew a thing or two about keeping light out of a bedroom. If you really can't bear the look of a pelmet, try installing blackout blinds on the windows underneath, which can cover the top of the window but be half rolled up in the night, allowing air in. Meanwhile, if you have to sleep in a house where someone needs the landing light on, we suggest putting a rolled-up towel or a draught excluder at the bottom of the door, to prevent light seepage there.

Invest in a truly fabulous bed. Never, ever buy a new bed without trying it in a store. Or – better still – in a hotel: by popular request many hotels nowadays are offering for sale the actual beds that guests slumber peacefully in. (Jo is right now building up to buying one of the beds from her favourite London sleeping spot, The Langham hotel, where she gets a night's sleep like no other.) The beds with the best reputations are Hästens (made in Sweden out of bundles of horsehair, cotton, flax and pure new wool), and Hypnos (who make beds for the Queen, upholstered with cashmere, silk and lambswool). We are also impressed with the organic beds by Abaca. Some of these are very far from cheap. However, considering we spend one third of our lives in bed, we feel that investing in a great bed is probably as important as choosing a safe car as both are so essential to life.

Treat yourself to good pillows, too. It's up to you whether you like hard or soft, but make sure you replace them regularly. Do 'the pillow trick': hold out your arm, place the pillow over it – and if it flops down either side, it's definitely overdue for replacement. By reputation, the very best pillows are Hungarian or Siberian goose down, which are both very soft. Personally, we've always been impressed with Ikea pillows (they know a thing or two about sleep in a country with such long winter nights), although annoyingly they aren't quite the same size as standard UK pillows. Close enough to fudge it, though. When you want to treat yourself, try www.thebestbedlineintheworld.com for pillows: Jo's came from Claridge's (a generous gift from Clarins – she didn't nick them!), and are – as she puts it – 'like a blissful firm cloud…'.

WHAT TO DO IF YOU WAKE UP IN THE WEE SMALL HOURS

Many older women get off to sleep fine but then wake between 3am and 5am. Often they can't get back to sleep; if they do, it's usually not restful slumber. Whatever the cause – and some swear it can be the phases of the moon – the result is a loss of energy and focus, and a feeling of having to drag yourself through the day until the next broken night. As well as the general advice on the previous pages, experts suggest the following ways to woo sleep; we've tried their advice and it works.

● Relax in the evening; don't drink coffee, tea or cola after 6pm and avoid fatty or sugary foods and excess alcohol which your body has to process during the night; cool your body by walking barefoot, opening a window, wearing light night clothes and having a warm bath.

● Dim lights through the evening: until electric lighting became commonplace, people naturally downshifted with the onset of dusk. Today, the light assault continues until we go to bed and we still expect to fall asleep immediately. Which is dotty since the sleep hormone melatonin needs darkness to switch it on. Last thing at night, spend a few moments gazing at the vast velvet darkness of the night sky.

● Try this delicious drink to calm the nervous system. Stir together over gentle heat: 250ml organic full-fat cow's milk or almond or rice milk, 2 teaspoons organic ground almonds, 2 cardamom pods, 5 strands saffron and a pinch of nutmeg. Strain and add one teaspoon honey, Manuka if possible.

● Take one to two capsules of Valerian and Ashwagandha Formula by Pukka Herbs before bed. Keep a capsule handy to take if you wake.

● And if you do wake up, refuse to fret about missed sleep: until recently, people took it for granted they'd wake in the long periods of natural darkness and talk, make love, tell stories or let their minds roam. Lie there and think of all the nice things you've done this year.

● Breathe: lie flat on your back, eyes closed, one hand on your chest. Inhale for a count of four, hold for seven, then exhale slowly to eight: visualise waves shimmying up a beach, hovering for a moment, then receding gently… slowly… into the sea.

● Low blood sugar may rouse you, so have a small banana and/or a small pot of organic natural yoghurt (plus teaspoon!) by your bed, also a glass of still water with a few drops of Bach Rescue Remedy in it (dehydration can lead to poor sleep and bad dreams).

● If anxieties beset you, remember that around 4am is the 'dark hour of the soul' when your brain can't process worries – thus the jangling cacophony in your head. Keep a pen and paper by your bed, and write them down.

● If you toss and turn for more than 15 minutes, turn on the radio (we love the BBC World Service), read a trashy novel (nothing stimulating), do the ironing or washing-up (nothing energetic).

Instant face revivers: our award winners

Sometimes, what you really want is to LOOK GOOD RIGHT NOW – the instant confidence-boost of a product that perks up your skin, makes you look radiant, peels back the years – especially after a short or disturbed night, before a Big Night Out, or if you've been poorly. Masks are pretty brilliant – see page 82 – but there are also serums, spritzes, gels and (as of this edition) even gadgets which make you look as if you've had eight hours' peaceful and restorative slumber. We know some of them work (see our favourites in We Love…) and our testers do too now!

REVIEWS

Clarisonic Plus

 8.69/10 We're selfishly delighted this sonic, vibrating, massaging, brush-headed (and pricey) skin gizmo's done so well – because now when we're bombarded with questions as to whether Clarisonic really works, we can say definitively: 'yesssssss!' They sent us the Face & Body kit (with two heads) and the accompanying Refining Skin Polish, but we asked panellists to try it with their regular products. (See also Award-winning Anti-Ageing Eye Creams, pages 52–3.) NB: most testers reported long-term, not just instant, skin improvements.

Comments: 'Unprompted and without knowing I've been using something different, friends have commented on how fresh I look lately even on days when I start at 6 am.' • 'I've absolutely fallen in love with this and am raving about it to everyone I know – the first thing I noticed was how soft and smooth my skin looked, with a definite bloom' • 'skin definitely "de-aged"' • 'complexion definitely more radiant after each use' • 'gave a glow and face felt more radiant after use – and oooh, the extra pleasure of feeling I'm cleansing away all the dirt!'.

Clarins Beauty Flash Balm

 8.56/10 Well, what do you know? Clarins invented this beauty category with the creation of Beauty Flash Balm over 30 years ago, winning countless awards before this one.

According to our testers, it's still a wow, living up to its reputation as 'Cinderella in a tube'. With radiance-boosting ingredients, Beauty Flash Balm 'sets' to a comfy, firming film which makes skin look instantly fresh and gorgeously glowy.

Comments: '10/10! My skin felt lovely instantly, no tautness, make-up went on with no sliding or greasiness, there's nothing to compare to this' • 'skin looked brighter and plumper, fresher and more radiant, and it evened out skintone; fantastic product' • 'slight tingling sensation at first, which felt invigorating; very effective, quite a few people remarked on how bright and radiant my skin was' • 'skin looked dewy, glowy and radiant, lovely!'.

YSL Top Secrets Flash Radiance Skincare Brush

 8.5/10 Somewhat in a class of its own, this: a big fat squeezy tube with a brush at one end to dispense fatigue-erasing light-reflective pigments over the face. It basically harnesses the same sort of line-blurring, complexion-smoothing technology as world-beating Touche Eclat Radiant Touch – with extra energising caffeine and something called 'grains of Paradise' – but in primer format, for the whole *visage*…

Comments: 'Really impressed: skin looks more radiant with or without foundation; also photographs well – perfect for weddings or other special occasions' • 'skintone instantly lighter, brighter and benefits were still apparent throughout the day' • 'gave a silky, dewy look to my skin and

ANTI-AGEING
**AWARD
WINNERS**
BEAUTY BIBLE

♡ WE LOVE...

**In Jo's book, there's
still almost nothing to
rival Guerlain Issima
Midnight Secret,
known to insiders as
'eight hours' sleep in
a bottle' (especially
since these days,
Jo merely dreams
of getting eight
hours' kip…). After
a poor night's
sleep, Sarah adores
Guerlain's Midnight
Star – little vials
of genius with a
radiance-boosting
effect, which smooth,
revivify and rejuvenate
your complexion.
(Wagonloads
please…)**

friends commented I looked less tired' • 'a good
product for emergency use during the party
season or when you've been ill'.

Liz Earle Superskin Concentrate

We'll admit that we hadn't thought of
using this facial oil as an instant face-
saver until the brand put it forward for this
category. But now we have, we're impressed at
how this aromatic blend of vitamin E and plant oils
(avocado, rosehip, argan) does speedily revive the
skin. (The chamomile, neroli and lavender
fragrance is especially lovely.) If you wanted to use
this before going out, we'd suggest applying,
leaving to sink in, then blotting firmly with a tissue
before applying make-up. Most testers loved it so
much they chose to use it every night!

Comments: 'Top marks, made my skin really soft
and plump, face uplifted and spirits too! I've been
recovering from a hysterectomy and this has really
balanced and evened out my skin, people say I
look really well and healthy' • 'I was worried about
using an oil on a spotty area, but it has really
cleared my skin and sorted out the dry areas, it's
done wonders' • 'skin felt gorgeous!' • 'made
skintone perkier and more even, skin felt comfy
but supported – like Spanx for the face…' • 'wore
this just with some concealer and blush' • 'loved
the smell of lavender which really helped to relax
me at bedtime'.

TIP

'To brighten your skin,
fill a basin with warm
water and add several
drops of lavender
essential oil. Dip a
face cloth in the water
then lay over your face
for a few moments.
Repeat five times.'
– Ole Henriksen

Directory

The following includes stockist contacts for the brands featured in these books. But we also suggest that you first visit www.beautybible.com and have a look at the INSIDER DISCOUNTS section (it's one of the buttons along the top), as many of the brands featured in this book are available at very nice discounts from a handful of websites which we consider to be 'Beauty Bible-approved' sites (www.victoriahealth.com, www.lovelula.com, www.HQhair.com, www.beautyexpert.co.uk and www.lizearle.com which often put together special kits just for Beauty Bible) – all offering great, swift service and a terrific selection of ranges. A good place to start. (NB: all the brands in INSIDER DISCOUNTS are listed alphabetically.)

Beauty Bible Beauty Steals is available as an App for your iPhone – go to www.beautybible.com and click on the icon on the pink splash page for more info and to order.

All the supplements mentioned in this book, plus advice and information, are available from Victoria Health, tel: 0800 3898 195, www.victoriahealth.com

A

Abaca, tel: 01269 598491, www.abacaorganic.co.uk

AD Skin Synergy, from Victoria Health, tel: 0800 3898 195, www.victoriahealth.com

Aerosoles, available via www.aerosoles.com and from stores in Paris

Alida, from Victoria Health, tel: 0800 3898 195, www.victoriahealth.com

AloeDent, from Victoria Health, tel: 0800 3898 195, www.victoriahealth.com

Alterna, tel: 01179 270435, www.alternauk.com

Amanda Lacey, www.amandalacey.com

Dr Andrew Markey, the Lister Hospital, tel: 020 7730 1219, www.thelisterhospital.com

Dr Andrew Weil, www.drweil.com

Anastasia Achilleos, at Urban Retreat, tel: 020 7893 8333, www.urbanretreat.co.uk

Andy Wadsworth, My Life Personal Training, tel: 07889 940888, www.mylifept.com

Annee de Mamiel, tel: 07516 099010, www.demamiel.com

Aquafresh, www.aquafresh.co.uk

Aromatherapy Associates, from Victoria Health, tel: 0800 3898 195, www.victoriahealth.com

Aussie http://www.aussiehair.com/uk

Aveda, tel: 0800 054 2979, www.aveda.co.uk

Avene, www.avene.co.uk

B

Balance Me, www.balanceme.co.uk

Barbara Daly, www.barbaradalymake-up.co.uk

Bare Escentuals, tel: 0870 850 6655, www.bareescentuals.co.uk

Barefoot Botanicals, from Victoria Health, tel: 0800 3898 195, www.victoriahealth.com

BareMinerals, see Bare Escentuals above

Bastien Gonzalez, tel: 07766 663271, www.bastiengonzalez.com

Beech Sandals, from Victoria Health, tel: 0800 3898 195, www.victoriahealth.com

Benefit, tel: 0800 496 1084, www.benefitcosmetics.co.uk

Beverly Hills Formula, from Victoria Health, tel: 0800 3898 195, www.victoriahealth.com

Bliss, tel: 0808 100 4151, www.blissworld.co.uk

Blood test (at home): Ideal Omega 3 Test Kit from Victoria Health, tel: 0800 3898 195, www.victoriahealth.com

Bobbi Brown, tel: 0800 054 2988, www.bobbibrown.co.uk

The Body Shop, tel: 0800 092 9090, www.thebodyshop.co.uk

Botanicals, tel: 01664 464005, www.botanicals.co.uk

Bourjois, tel: 0800 269836, www.bourjois.co.uk

Bowen technique, tel: 01373 832340, www.thebowentechnique.com

Bucky, www.amazon.co.uk

Bumble & bumble, tel: 0800 014 7424, www.bumbleandbumble.com

Burt's Bees, tel: 0845 423 8718, www.burtsbees.co.uk

By Terry, www.byterry.com

C

CACI, tel: 020 8731 5678, www.caci-international.co.uk

Caudalie, tel: 00800 4429 2424, www.caudalie.com

CCS, tel: 01276 674000 www.ccsfootcare.co.uk

Cellulite Busting Kit, from Victoria Health, tel: 0800 3898 195, www.victoriahealth.com

Champneys, www.champneys.com

Chanel, tel: 020 7493 3836, www.chanel.com

Chantecaille, tel: 0208 740 2085 www.uk.spacenk.com,

Professor Charles Clark, tel: 020 7935 0640, www.charlesvclark.com

Chie Mihara, tel: 0034 9669 80415 www.chiemihara.com

Chillow, tel: 08700 117174, www.chillow.co.uk

Chinese herbal medicine: Register of Chinese Herbal Medicine, tel: 01603 623994, www.rchm.co.uk

Christophe Robin, tel: 0033 14020 0283, www.christophe-robin.com

Clarins, tel: 0800 036 3558, www.clarins.co.uk

Clarisonic tel: 0800 988 4864 www.clarisonic.co.uk

Clarks, tel: 08444 995544, www.clarks.co.uk

Clinique, tel: 0800 054 2666, www.clinique.co.uk

Cosmetic surgery: helpful organisations (see also Wendy Lewis, under 'W')
● British Academy of Cosmetic

Dentistry, www.bacd.com

● The British Association of Aesthetic Plastic Surgeons, www.baaps.org.uk

● The British Association of Dermatologists (British Cosmetic Dermatology Group), www.bad.org.uk

● British Association of Oral and Maxillofacial Surgeons, www.baoms.org.uk

● The British Association of Otorhinolaryngologists, www.entuk.org

● British Association of Plastic, Reconstructive and Aesthetic Surgeons, www.bapras.org.uk

● British Oculoplastic Surgery Society, www.bopss.org

● The Care Quality Commission, www.cqc.org.uk

● The European Academy of Facial Plastic Surgery, www.eafps.org

● European Association of Plastic Surgeons, www.euraps.org

● European Society for Laser Dermatology, www.esld.org

● European Society of Plastic, Reconstructive and Aesthetic Surgery, www.espras.org

● General Medical Council, www.gmc-uk.org

● International Society of Aesthetic Plastic Surgery, www.isaps.org

● The Royal College of Anaesthetists, www.rcoa.ac.uk

Cosmetics à la Carte, tel: 020 7622 2318, www.cosmeticsalacarte.com

Cowshed, tel: 020 7534 0871, www.cowshedonline.con

Crabtree & Evelyn, tel: 0800 1114 406,

www.crabtree-evelyn.co.uk

Crème de la Mer, tel: 0800 054 2661, www.cremedelamer.co.uk

D

Daniel Galvin, tel: 020 7486 9661, www.danielgalvin.com

Darphin, tel: 0870 034 2318, www.darphin.co.uk

Dr David Cook, London Holistic Dental Centre, tel: 020 7323 1363, www.londonholisticdental.com

Decléor, tel: 020 7313 8787, www.decleor.co.uk

Dental Miracle, from Victoria Health, tel: 0800 3898 195, www.victoriahealth.com

Dermalogica, tel: 0800 591818, www.dermalogica.com/uk

Dermol 500, from Victoria Health, tel: 0800 3898 195, www.victoriahealth.com

Diamancel, tel: 0808 100 4151 www.blissworld.co.uk

Dior, tel: 020 7216 0216, www.dior.com

Dr Brandt, from Space NK, tel: 020 8740 2085, www.spacenk.co.uk

Dr Hauschka, tel: 01386 791022, www.drhauschka.co.uk

Dr Lewinns www.drlewinns.co.uk

E

Ecco, tel: 01590 679254, www.ecco-shoes-uk.co.uk

Electrolysis: British Institute & Association of Electrolysis,

tel: 0844 544 1373, www.electrolysis.co.uk

Elemis, tel: 01278 727830, www.elemis.co.uk

Elizabeth Arden, www.elizabetharden.co.uk

Ellis Faas, www.ellisfaas.com

Emma Hardie, tel: 01923 839505, www.emmahardie.com

Espa, tel: 01252 352231, www.espaonline.com

Essential Care, from Victoria Health, tel: 0800 3898 195, www.victoriahealth.com

Essie, tel: 0844 800 9396, www.nailsbymail.co.uk

Estée Lauder, tel: 0800 054 2444, www.esteelauder.co.uk

Eucerin, from Victoria Health, tel: 0800 3898 195, www.victoriahealth.com

EyeSlices, from Victoria Health, tel: 0800 3898 195, www.victoriahealth.com

F

FitFlops, tel: 0845 359 9884, www.fitflop.com

G

Garnier, tel: 0800 085 4376, www.garnier.co.uk

Gielly Green tel: 0020 7034 3060 www.giellygreen.co.uk

Gillette Venus, www.gillettevenus.co.uk

Giorgio Armani, www.giorgioarmanibeauty.co.uk

Gossypium, tel: 0870 850 9953, www.gossypium.co.uk

Green Hands, from Victoria Health, tel: 0800 3898 195, www.victoriahealth.com

Guerlain, www.guerlain.com

H

Hästens, www.hastens.com

Heal Gel, from Victoria Health, tel: 0800 3898 195, www.victoriahealth.com

Hypnos, tel: 01844 348200, www.hypnosbeds.com

I

Ikea, tel: 0845 358 3363, www.ikea.com

Ila, tel: 01608 677676, www.ila-spa.com

Inika, tel: 020 7494 4571, www.inikacosmetics.co.uk

Institut Esthederm, from Space NK, tel: 020 8740 2085, www.spacenk.co.uk

J

Jane Scrivner, tel: 07899 906957, www.janescrivner.com

Jason, from Victoria Health, tel: 0800 3898 195, www.victoriahealth.com

Jemma Kidd, tel: 0844 800 2636, www.jemmakidd.com

Jenny Jordan Eyebrow and Make-up Clinic, tel: 020 7483 2222, www.jennyjordan.co.uk

Jessica Vartoughian, www.jessica-nails.co.uk

JetRest eye masks, from Victoria Health, tel: 0800 389 8195, www.victoriahealth.com

John Frieda, tel: 020 7491 0840, www.johnfrieda.com

John Scurr, tel: 020 7730 9563, www.thelisterhospital.com

Joico, available from salons nationwide, www.joico.com

Professor Jon Kabat-Zinn, Mindfulness-Based Cognitive Therapy, www.mbct.co.uk

Jurlique, tel: 020 3205 3845, www.jurlique.co.uk

K

Dr Karen Burke, tel: 00 1 212 754 1100, www.empowereddoctor.com

Kate Logan www.kateloganbeauty.com

Kérastase, www.kerastase.co.uk

Keromask, tel: 01276 674050 www.keromask.com

Kevin Murphy, tel: 01179 270434, www.kevinmurphystore.com

Kiehl's, tel: 020 7240 2411, www.kiehls.co.uk

Kimberly Sayer, from Love Lula, tel: 0870 242 6995, www.lovelula.com

Korres, from www.lookfantastic.com

L

La Clarée, tel: 0800 027 1102, www.laclaree.co.uk

Lancôme, www.lancome.co.uk

Lanolips, from Victoria Health, tel: 0800 3898 195, www.victoriahealth.com

La Prairie, www.laprairie.com

Laura Mercier, from Space NK, tel: 020 8740 2085, www.spacenk.co.uk

Lavera, tel: 01557 870266, www.lavera.co.uk

Lee Stafford, www.leestafford.com

Liz Earle Naturally Active Skincare, tel: 01983 813913, www.lizearle.com

L'Occitane, tel: 020 7907 0301, www.loccitane.com

L'Oréal, tel: 0800 030 4032, www.loreal-paris.co.uk

Lotus Journeys, www.lotusjourneys.com

Louise Galvin, tel: 0800 334 5933, www.louisegalvin.com

LP Skin Therapy, tel: 0800 0287321, www.lpskintherapy.com

Lulu, tel: 0844 800 1694, www.lulusplace.co.uk

Lumosity, www.lumosity.com

M

MAC, www.maccosmetics.co.uk

Margaret Dabbs, tel: 020 7487 5510, www.margaretdabbs.co.uk

Marks & Spencer, tel: 0845 609 0200, www.marksandspencer.com

Mary Kay, tel: 0800 318 288 www.marykay.co.uk

Mason Pearson, tel: 020 7491 2613, www.masonpearson.com

Matrix, tel: 0845 601 0122, www.matrixhaircare.co.uk

McTimoney Chiropractic, tel: 01491 829211, www.mctimoneychiropractic.org

Melvita, tel: 0800 138 7045, www.melvita.com

Michael Dooley, The Poundbury Clinic, tel: 01305 262626, www.thepoundburyclinic.co.uk

Monu, tel: 0870 220 9094, www.monushop.co.uk

Moroccanoil, tel: 0800 310 1133, www.moroccanoil.co.uk,

Dr Mosaraf Ali, The Integrated Medical Centre, tel: 020 7224 5111, www.integratedmed.co.uk

Murad, from Victoria Health, tel: 0800 3898 195, www.victoriahealth.com

MV Organic Skincare,

tel: 020 3075 1006, www.mvskincare.co.uk

MyFace Cosmetics, tel: 0844 335 6492, www.myfacecosmetics.co.uk

N

Nadia Brydon, practitioner of Western and Chinese herbal medicine, acupuncture and homeopathy, email: nadia@chanters.fsnet.co.uk

Nails Inc, tel: 020 7529 2340, www.nailsinc.com

Natio, from Debenhams, tel: 08445 616161, www.debenhams.com

Neal's Yard Remedies, from Victoria Health, tel: 0800 3898 195, www.victoriahealth.com

New CID Cosmetics, www.newcidcosmetics.com

Dr Nick Lowe, The Cranley Clinic, tel: 020 7499 3223, www.drnicklowe.com

Nivea, www.nivea.co.uk

No7, www.boots.com

Nude, tel: 0800 634 4366, www.nudeskincare.com

Nuxe, www.nuxe.com

O

Ojon, tel: 0870 034 2454, www.ojon.co.uk

Ole Henriksen, www.olehenriksen.com

OPI, tel: 01923 240 010 www.lenawhite.co.uk

Origins, tel: 0800 054 2888, www.origins.co.uk

The Organic Pharmacy tel: 0207 351 2232 www.theorganicpharmacy.com

Orly, tel: 01827 280080, www.orlybeauty.co.uk

Oskia, tel: 01600 710710, www.oskiaskincare.com

P

Paul & Joe, www.paul-joe-beaute.com/en

Paul Mitchell, tel: 0845 659 0012, www.paul-mitchell.co.uk

Percy & Reed www.percyandreed.com

Per-fékt, www.perfektbeauty.com

Pevonia tel: 01449 727000 www.pevonia.co.uk

Philip B, www.philipb.com

Phylia de M, from Victoria Health, tel: 0800 3898 195, www.victoriahealth.com

Pilates:
● **The Pilates Foundation**, tel: 020 7033 0078, www.pilatesfoundation.com

● **Body Control Pilates Association**, tel: 020 7636 8900, www.bodycontrol.co.uk

Pinks Boutique, tel: 01332 204804, www.pinksboutique.com

prAna Yoga Mats, from www.yogastudio.co.uk

Provenance, from Victoria Health, tel: 0800 3898 195, www.victoriahealth.com

Prtty Peaushun, www.prttypeaushun.com

Pure Lochside tel: 0800 0214245 www.purelochside.com

Pureology, tel: 0800 783 3026, www.pureology-uk.com

R

REN, tel: 020 7724 2900, www.renskincare.com

Repêchage, www.repechageuk.com

RéVive, www.reviveskincare.com

Revlon, tel: 0800 085 2716, www.revlon.com

Rigby & Peller, tel: 0845 076 5545, www.rigbyandpeller.com

Rimmel, www.rimmellondon.com

Rodial, tel: 020 7351 1720, www.rodial.co.uk

Roja Dove, www.rojadove.com

S

Sarah Chapman, tel: 020 7589 9585, www.skinesis.com

Sebastian Professional, www.sebastianprofessional.co.uk

Sensodyne, www.sensodyne.co.uk

Serious Readers lamps, tel: 0800 028 1890, www.seriousreaders.com

Seven Wonders, from Victoria Health, tel: 0800 3898 195, www.victoriahealth.com

Shavata Eyebrow Shapers stencil kit, 0208-993 8333, www.shavata.co.uk

Shiffa, tel: 01606 596929 www.zuneta.com

Shoe Therapy, www.shoetherapy.com

Shower water filters:
● Ethical Superstore, tel: 0845 009 9016, www.ethicalsuperstore.com
● Pure Showers, tel: 0800 612 7174, www.pureshowers.co.uk

Shu Uemura, tel: 020 7240 7635, www.shuuemura.co.uk

Sisley, tel: 020 7591 6380, www.sisley-cosmetics.co.uk

Soap & Glory, www.soapandglory.com

Space NK, tel: 020 8740 2085, www.spacenk.co.uk

St Tropez, tel: 0115 983 6363, www.st-tropez.com

Steve Mason, tel: 01273 771441, www.brightonacupunctureand-massage.co.uk

Su-Man Hsu, tel: 07779-151347, email: su-man@blueyonder.co.uk

Sue Devitt, from Harvey Nichols, tel: 020 7235 5000, www.harveynichols.com

Suqqu, www.suqqu.com

Susan Posnick, www.susanposnick.com

Suzie Mitchell, tel: 01424 430389, www.spaghetti-tree.com

T

T'ai chi:
The UK T'ai Chi Association, tel: 020 7407 4775, www.taichiuk.co.uk

Taryn Rose, from Footwise, tel: 01483 455586, www.footwiseuk.com

Temple Spa, from Victoria Health, tel: 0800 3898 195, www.victoriahealth.com

Terra Plana, tel: 01458 449081, www.terraplana.com

Thalgo, www.thalgo.com

This Works, tel: 020 8543 3544, www.thisworks.com

TIGI, www.tigihaircare.com

Tim Hutchful, The British Chiropractic Association, tel: 0118 950 5950, www.chiropractic-uk.co.uk

Tom Ford, www.tomford.com

Tom's of Maine, www.tomsofmaine.co.uk

Trilogy, from Victoria Health, tel: 0800 3898 195, www.victoriahealth.com

Trish McEvoy, www.trishmcevoy.com

Tweezerman, www.tweezerman.co.uk

U

Ugg, tel: 01475 746000, www.uggaustralia.com/gb

Upper Canada Soap, tel: 01277 220842, www.uppercanadasoap.com

V

Vaishaly Patel, tel: 020 7486 7705 (products); tel: 020 7224 6088 (clinic), www.vaishaly.com

Vaseline Intensive Care, www.vaseline.co.uk

Vichy, tel: 0800 169 6193, www.vichyconsult.co.uk

Viscotears, widely available at chemists

W

Weleda, from Victoria Health, tel: 0800 3898 195, www.victoriahealth.com

Wendy Lewis, tel: 00 1 212 861 6148, www.wlbeauty.com email: wl@wlbeauty.com Wendy Lewis Beauty Forum: www.beautyinthebag.com facebook.com/beautyinthebag twitter.com/beautyinthebag

Wild Organics, tel: 01955 609064, www.wildorganicsbeauty.com

X

Xyliwhite, from Victoria Health, tel: 0800 3898 195, www.victoriahealth.com

Y

Yes to Carrots, from Victoria Health, tel: 0800 3898 195, www.victoriahealth.com

Yes to Tomatoes, from Victoria Health, tel: 0800 389 8195, www.victoriahealth.com

Yoga:
British Wheel of Yoga, tel: 01529 306851, www.bwy.org.uk

Youngblood, tel: 0845 246 4666, www.ybskin.co.uk

YSL, www.ysl.com

ANTI-AGEING BOOKSHELF

Food Rules by Michael Pollan (Penguin)

Healing Without Freud or Prozac by Dr David Servan-Schreiber (Rodale International)

I Feel Bad about My Neck by Nora Ephron (Black Swan)

The Lowdown on Facelifts and Other Wrinkle Remedies by Wendy Lewis (Quadrille)

Plastic Makes Perfect by Wendy Lewis (Orion)

The New Yoga for People Over 50 by Suza Francina (Health Communications)

Yoga and the Wisdom of Menopause by Suza Francina (Health Communications)

Yoga Builds Bones by Jan Maddern (Element)

The Yoga Facelift by Marie-Véronique Nadeau (Conari Press)

The Ultimate Natural Beauty Book by Josephine Fairley (Kyle Cathie)

DVD:
Yoga for Beginners by Patricia Walden (from www.yogastudio.co.uk)

Index

Acknowledgements

This book is the result of decades of research. We would like to thank all the friends, colleagues and experts worldwide who have helped us so generously over the years. Also our doughty and dedicated teams of testers, without whose commitment to trialling products and writing up their findings, Beauty Bible wouldn't be here.

A vast vote of thanks to our illustrator David Downton (who's also included in the dedication), who has surpassed himself – and made us laugh a lot too: our Beauty Bible publications would not be so stylish and beautiful without his support and super-talented input.

Particular thanks to:

Maggie Alderson
Bobbi Brown
Nadia Brydon
Dr Karen Burke
Sarah Chapman
Professor Charles Clark
Dr David Cook
Margaret Dabbs
Barbara Daly OBE
Shabir Daya

Carmen dell'Orefice
Michael Dooley
Roja Dove
Liz Earle MBE
Mary Greenwell
Terry de Gunzburg
Newby Hands
Tim Hutchful
Eve Lom
Dr Nick Lowe
Lulu
Trish McEvoy
Lorna McKnight

Annee de Mamiel
Dr Andrew Markey
Laura Mercier
Suzie Mitchell
Marie-Véronique Nadeau
Tim Petersen
Philip B
Kathy Phillips
John Scurr
Gill Sinclair
Dr Andrew Weil
Andreas Wild

Photo acknowledgements

We would also like to thank a raft of beauty PRs who supported us so efficiently with our project but would need an extra book to include them all. But special thanks go to Emma Dawson and her team at L'Oréal; Sarah Griffiths and her team at Estée Lauder Companies; Julietta Longcroft and Tom Konig Oppenheimer at TCS (who went so far as to appoint a special 'Beauty Bible Liaison Officer', Ellie Howden, who we also thank); Nancy Brady and all at NBPR; Jenny Halpern and her crew at Halpern PR; Jo Fox Tutchener and Michelle Boon at Beautyseen; Rick Havemann at www.avea.co.uk; Fiona Dowal, Owen Walker, Max Flower and the team at Modus Dowal Walker; Phily Keeling at Chanel; Lesley Chilvers at Bourjois; Kate Hudson and Helen Mitchell at Guerlain; Jazz Kaur at Benefit (who helped us with this book wearing her former Guerlain chapeau); Aude Chatelin at Dior; Carri Kilpatrick and the Kilpatrick PR team; Kelly Marks and all at Pure PR – plus everyone at Liz Earle (especially Kim Buckland, who set up Liz Earle Naturally Active Skincare with Liz herself).

Thanks to our publisher Kyle Cathie, as ever, and to our colleagues at YOU magazine, Sue Peart, Catherine Fenton and Rosalind Lowe.

And, of course, to our wonderful Beauty Bible team (see dedication).

Title page Plainpicture/beyond

p7 Adrian Peacock, Charlotte Murphy

p9 Icon Photo/C.Watts

p10-11 Kellie Hindmarch

p14-15 Photolibrary/D&L Jacobs

p20 www.urbanlip.com

p22 Photolibrary

p26 Rex Features/T.Logan

p32 Getty/E.Estabrook

p35 Camera Press London/Brigitte

p36 Plainpicture/Ableimages

p39 www.urbanlip.com

p40 www.urbanlip.com

p45 Camera Press London/B.Coster

p46-47 www.urbanlip.com

p50-51 Photolibrary/Photoalto

p52-53 Photolibrary/B.Lark

p54 Photolibrary/Superstock Inc

p57 www.urbanlip.com

p58 Corbis/S.Prezant

p61 Trunk Archive.com/A.Bettles

p63 Getty/Superstudio

p65 Photolibrary/Imagesource

p66 Getty/J.Tisne

p67 Getty/B.Yee

p69 Photolibrary/M.Constantini

p71 Photolibrary/Photoalto

p75 Photolibrary/S.Zulawinski

p79 www.urbanlip.com

p81 Photolibrary/J.Feingersh

p83 Photolibrary/B.Vogel;

p86 Camera Press London/*Journal für die Frau*

p92 Getty/P.de Villiers

p94 Photolibrary/C.Sharp

p97 Photolibrary/T.Kruesselmann

p98 Plainpicture/applypictures

p106 Trunk Archive.com/H.Salinas

p106 Camera Press London/J.Veysey

p106 Corbis

p106 Photolibrary/Z.Smith

p106 Getty/A.Mo

p107 Rex Features/Col Pics/Everett

p107 Camera Press London/J.Veysey

p107 Camera Press London/C.Djanogly

p108 Getty/Tedfoo

p115 Trunk Archive.com/Pamela Hanson/ Hair: Julien d'Ys/Make-up: Stephane Marais

p122 Photolibrary/It Stock RF

p125 Photolibrary/F.Wirth

p129 Photolibrary/B.Erlinger

p132 Photolibrary/A.Oliel

p133 www.urbanlip.com

p139 Photolibrary/Photoalto

p140 Photolibrary/B.Lark

p143 Getty/Dorling Kindersley

p144 Photolibrary/R. Kaufma/L. Hirshowitz

p146 Photolibrary/Radius Images

p151 www.urbanlip.com

p153 Photolibrary/M.Burkhart/Corbis

p154 Photolibrary/Stockbrokerxtra images

p158-159 Photolibrary/Fancy

p161 Photolibrary/Fotosearch

p165 Getty/B.Fraker

p166 Tim Petersen

p168-169 Photolibrary/Pixtal Images

p171 Photolibrary/Corbis

p173 Photolibrary/F.Cirou

p177 Camera Press London/Titti Fabi

p178 www.urbanlip.com

p179 Photolibrary/J.Klee

p181 Getty/A.Rohmer

p182-183 Photolibrary/Tetra Images

p185 Photolibrary/C.Chiossone/Photex

p186 Magnum Photos/Robert Capa/International Centre of Photography

p189 Getty/T.Barwick

p191 www.urbanlip.com

p193 Photolibrary RF

p194 Photolibrary/Uppercut Images

p196 Photolibrary/M.Anderson

p201 Photolibrary/Emotive Image

p202 Photolibrary/P.Leonard;

p204-205 Photolibrary/Innerhofer Photodesign

p207 Getty/LaCoppola-Meier

p208-209 Magnum Photos/Eve Arnold

p210-211 Arcangel/R.Musyhiar

p213 www.urbanlip.com

Acknowledgements page www.urbanlip.com

We would like to dedicate this book to the Beauty Bible 'team' who worked so hard to help us make it happen: Sally Cole, David Downton, Amy Eason, David Edmunds, Jessie Lawrence, Ben Lovegrove, Liz Murray, Jenny Semple, and also to our divine agent Kay McCauley, who we want to be like – and look as good as – when we grow up...

This edition first published in Great Britain in 2012 by
Kyle Books
an imprint of Kyle Cathie Ltd
23 Howland Street
London W1T 4AY

email: general.enquiries@kylebooks.com
www.kylebooks.com

First published in hardback in 2011 by Kyle Cathie Limited

ISBN: 978 0 85783 168 2

Josephine Fairley and Sarah Stacey are hereby identified as the authors of this work in accordance with Section 77 of the Copyright, Designs and Patents Act 1988

A Cataloguing in Publication record for this title is available from the British Library

Text © Josephine Fairley and Sarah Stacey 2012
Illustrations © David Downton 2011
Design © Kyle Cathie Limited 2011

Design: Jenny Semple
Illustrations: David Downton
Copy editor: Liz Murray
Picture researcher: Sally Cole, Perseverance Works Ltd
Production: Gemma John, Sheila Smith and Nic Jones

Colour reproduction by Scanhouse in Malaysia
Printed and bound in China by C&C Offset